T0214776

Concept Analysis in Nursing

Concept analysis is an established genre of inquiry in nursing, introduced in the 1970s. Currently, over 100 concept studies are published annually, yet the methods used within this field have rarely been questioned. In *Concept Analysis in Nursing: A New Approach*, Paley provides a critical analysis of the philosophical assumptions that underpin nursing's concept analysis methods. He argues, provocatively, that there are no such things as concepts, as traditionally conceived.

Drawing on Wittgenstein and Construction Grammar, the book first makes a case for dispensing with the traditional concept of a 'concept', and then provides two examples of a new approach, examining the use of 'hope' and 'moral distress'. Casting doubt on the assumption that 'hope' always stands for an 'inner' state of the person, the book shows that the word's function varies with the grammatical construction it appears in. Similarly, it argues that 'moral distress' is not the name of a mental state, but a normative classification used to bolster a narrative concerning nursing's identity.

Concept Analysis in Nursing is a fresh and challenging book written by a philosopher interested in nursing. It will appeal to researchers and postgraduate students in the areas of nursing, health, philosophy and linguistics. It will also interest those familiar with the author's previous book, *Phenomenology as Qualitative Research*.

John Paley was formerly a senior lecturer at the University of Stirling, and is now a visiting fellow at the University of Worcester, UK. He writes on topics related to philosophy and health care, including research methods, evidence, complexity, spirituality, the post-Francis debate about compassion and nursing ethics.

Routledge Advances in Research Methods

Freedom of Information and Social Science Research Design
Edited by Kevin Walby and Alex Luscombe

Defending Qualitative Research
Design, Analysis and Textualization
Mario Cardano

Researching Ageing
Methodological Challenges and their Empirical Background
Edited by Maria Łuszczyńska

Diagramming the Social
Relational Method in Research
Russell Dudley-Smith and Natasha Whiteman

Participatory Case Study Work
Approaches, Authenticity and Application in Ageing Studies
Edited by Sion Williams and John Keady

Social Causation and Biographical Research
Philosophical, Theoretical and Methodological Arguments
Georgios Tsiolis and Michalis Christodoulou

Beyond Disciplinarity
Historical Evolutions of Research Epistemology
Catherine Hayes, John Fulton and Andrew Livingstone with Claire Todd, Stephen Capper and Peter Smith

Concept Analysis in Nursing
A New Approach
John Paley

For more information about this series, please visit: www.routledge.com/Routledge-Advances-in-Research-Methods/book-series/RARM

Concept Analysis in Nursing
A New Approach

John Paley

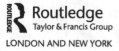
Routledge
Taylor & Francis Group

LONDON AND NEW YORK

First published 2021
by Routledge
2 Park Square, Milton Park, Abingdon, Oxon OX14 4RN

and by Routledge
52 Vanderbilt Avenue, New York, NY 10017

Routledge is an imprint of the Taylor & Francis Group, an informa business

British Library Cataloguing-in-Publication Data
A catalogue record for this book is available from the British Library

Library of Congress Cataloging-in-Publication Data
A catalog record has been requested for this book

ISBN: 978-0-367-14968-0 (hbk)
ISBN: 978-0-429-05414-3 (ebk)

Typeset in Times
by Deanta Global Publishing Services, Chennai, India

Contents

vi *Contents*

Figures

Preface and acknowledgements

I first came across Hans-Jörg Schmid's book on 'shell nouns' in 2016. It got me wondering about the relation between two questions: 'What are concepts?' and 'What functions does the word "concept" have?' Ironically, shell nouns don't play a major role in the final version of this book – they appear briefly at the beginning of Chapter 9 – but they pushed open a door, and a lot of other stuff poured in.

Another irony. Some readers have suggested that I have not been as critical of the nursing literature on concept analysis as I could/should have been. However, I've come to recognise that, although Walker and Avant misunderstood the methods that philosophers use – the methods they used in the 1950s and 1960s, anyway – they and their successors share many of the assumptions made about concepts by philosophers and psychologists. This is true irrespective of whether those assumptions are right or wrong. In any case, this is not primarily a criticising-other-writers book. It's more about exploring a different line of thought, and experimenting with its practical implications.

I hope it's clear that the book is intended primarily for a nursing audience (given that 'concept analysis', as opposed to 'conceptual analysis', is a term found almost exclusively in the nursing literature). There is some discussion of technicalities in philosophy and psychology, but it's confined mainly to parts of Chapters 6, 7 and 11, plus the notes. Inevitably, there is rather more on certain aspects of linguistics; but none of it is desperately difficult even if some of it is unfamiliar.

A lot of people have helped me with this, more than I can remember. I would particularly like to thank Elisabeth Bergdahl, Martin Lipscomb, Trevor Hussey, Juan Diego González Sanz, Nancy Sharts-Hopko, Peter Allmark, Beverly Whelton and Cecilia Malabusini. Elisabeth, Martin and Trevor made extensive comments on the first draft. Elisabeth and Cecilia explained some of the ways in which English differs from, respectively, Swedish and Italian (which led to further reflection on the Anglo-centric nature of the discussion).

I did a workshop on ideas related to this book at the University of Worcester in February 2020. I'd like to thank all those who attended for their questions and comments, many of which confirmed that I hadn't yet worked out how to explain what I thought I was up to.

I'm grateful to Dr Kaye Herth for permission to quote several items from the Herth Hope Scale. Thanks also to Jabeen, who provided the artwork and figures.

The examples are peppered with the names of friends, colleagues and family members, purely because it amused me to think of Linden acquiring the concept of money, Frank climbing Everest, Martin chopping carrots, Rosie drinking Prosecco, Derek digging his way out of prison, Steph and Lewis shifting furniture around. Random names would have done just as well, but they wouldn't have been as entertaining.

Lynda has provided the laughs, the warmth, the help with the crossword, and all the comforts of home – figuratively and, during the lockdown, literally. This time round, she also provided hours of animated discussion, given that she finds the unexpected quirks of language more interesting (and considerably more intelligible) than phenomenology. My gratitude to her exceeds anything that I could conveniently express in a short paragraph.

None of these people are responsible for the mistakes, poor arguments and errors of judgement that occur in the following pages. I'm confident there are some, even if I'm not sure which ones they are.

Finally, the COVID-19 pandemic began during the writing of this book. As a result, I was unable to check the page numbers of some quoted extracts. This is a very minor inconvenience, compared to what large numbers of people have had to endure. However, I need to point out that, in such cases, I have cited the chapter number instead (books), or left the reference incomplete (articles). There aren't many of either.

Glossary

Anaphoric reference

The use of words to refer back to something previously mentioned, without having to mention it again. Pronouns are frequently used in this way 'Kath studied the article. It was, she thought, poorly written'. In the second sentence, both 'it' and 'she' are anaphoric, referring back, respectively, to the article and Kath. Contrast **Cataphoric reference**.

Attributive adjective

An adjective placed immediately before a noun. 'Leo was wearing brown shoes'. Contrast **Predicative adjective**.

Cartesian theatre

A picture of the mind (derived from Descartes) which compares it to an 'inner' theatre, where thoughts, emotions, sensations and perceptions are 'displayed' or 'enacted'.

Cataphoric reference

The use of words to refer ahead to something which has not yet been mentioned, but which is about to be. Pronouns are frequently used in this way. 'They've done it! Chelsea have won the cup!' In the first sentence, both 'they' and 'it' are cataphoric. Contrast **Anaphoric reference**.

COCA

The Corpus of Contemporary American English, a database of English sampled from American sources since 1990. COCA is freely available online, hosted at Brigham Young University, and can be analysed statistically. As of 2020, it contains one billion words. See **Corpus**.

Collocate

A term used in **corpus**-based linguistics. Collocates of a 'target' word are those which appear close to it in sampled texts. In searching the corpus, the degree of closeness can be specified. Collocates (4,2) of a target word would be those which are among the four words immediately preceding the target, and the two words immediately following it.

Compositionality

The idea that the meaning of a sentence is derived from the meaning of its individual constituents, and can *only* be so derived. 'The cat sat on the mat'. Contrast **Construction Grammar**.

Construction

In linguistics, a syntactic pattern which can be used with different permutations of words. 'He hit it out of the park'. 'They threw him into the river'. 'She drank him under the table'. These are all examples of the CAUSED MOTION construction.

Construction Grammar (CxG)

An approach to linguistics according to which the grammatical construction in which a word appears can 'coerce' the sense it has. Contrast **Compositionality**.

Corpus

The name given to large databases consisting of passages sampled from 'real world' text or speech. A corpus can be used to study groups of words occurring together regularly. **COCA** is one example.

Count noun

A noun used to refer to discrete items. 'Book', 'piano', 'day', 'proposal'. Count nouns have plurals, and can be preceded by numbers, 'Two books', 'three days'. They cannot be used to start a sentence, unless preceded by a **Determiner**. 'Cup was overflowing'...? Contrast **Mass noun**.

Derivative

A word derived from another by (usually in English) the addition of a prefix or a suffix, often changing the part of speech category the word belongs to. The adjectives 'hopeful' and 'hopeless' are derivatives of the noun 'hope'. Contrast **Inflection**, and see **Morphology**.

Determiner

A term used to refer to related classes of words: articles ('the', 'a'), demonstratives ('this', 'those'), cardinal numbers ('one', 'ten'), quantifiers ('all', 'most'), possessives ('your', 'its') and a few more. They are used to specify the reference of the noun that follows them, whereas adjectives are used purely to describe.

Dual-life noun

A noun that can be both a **count noun** and a **mass noun**. 'Would you like a coffee?' 'There's an awful lot of coffee in Brazil'.

Ellipsis

The omission from a statement of something that, in the context, is understood. 'As darkness fell, hope faded'. In a news story about a disaster, 'hope' would presumably refer to 'hope of finding survivors'. In context, however, this is understood and does not need to be made explicit.

Exophoric reference

The use of a word, often a pronoun or demonstrative, to refer to something not otherwise mentioned in the text. 'They're late again!' (where the people referred to by 'they' are never explicitly identified). Understanding this kind of reference requires relevant knowledge of the context. Compare **Anaphoric reference** and **Cataphoric reference**.

Grammaticalised

In some expressions, a word loses its normal lexical meaning, and comes to serve a purely grammatical function. 'He's going to finish it'. Here, the verb 'go' loses its sense of movement, and is used to construct a future tense. It is said to have been 'grammaticalised'.

Head noun

The noun which, in a **noun phrase**, is qualified by the other elements in the phrase. 'Water' in 'boiling water', or 'consultant' in 'the very tall management consultant'. 'Concept' in 'the concept of justice'.

Inflection

The use of (usually in English) a suffix to create a modified form of a root word, without changing its part of speech category. The verbal forms 'hopes', 'hoped' and 'hoping' are all inflections of the verb 'hope'. Contrast **Derivative**, and see **Morphology**.

Intensifier

A word, often an adverb, used to 'intensify' an adjective. 'She's really cool'. 'That's very odd'. 'He's enormously rich'.

Mass noun

A noun used to refer to non-discrete items, substances or aggregates. 'Mud', 'information', 'furniture', 'cutlery'. They don't have plurals, and can't be preceded by numbers: 'two muds', 'four furnitures'? They can be used, without a determiner, to start a sentence. Contrast **Count noun**.

Metonymy

A figure of speech in which an expression is used to refer to something associated with it. 'Buckingham Palace said that the Queen would no longer wear fur'. Here, 'Buckingham Palace' does not refer to the building, but to people staffing it.

Modal verbs

Verbs like 'can', 'could', 'may', 'might', 'will', 'would', 'must' and 'should'. They indicate likelihood, ability, permission or obligation. They are unusual in that they don't add 's' or 'es' for the third-person singular: 'I work, you work, she works', but not 'I can, you can, she cans'.

Morphology

The branch of linguistics which studies the structure of words, and how they are related by inflection and derivation. See **Derivative** and **Inflection**.

Natural language

A naturally occurring language, recognisable as such. Hopi, Swahili, English. Examples of languages which are not natural include computer languages, Esperanto and Klingon.

Nominal

In linguistics, a term used to refer to expressions which have the function of a noun. It includes **Noun phrases**, gerunds ('Walking is healthy'), and nouns themselves. They may involve other nouns ('A cup of tea'), or words which are usually adjectives ('The good').

Nominalism

The philosophical view that only particular objects exist, or 'really exist'. This rules out numbers, properties, relations, sets, meanings and other non-spatiotemporal 'entities'. Contrast **Platonism**.

Noun phrase

Any phrase which, as a unit, has the same function as a noun (i.e., it can be used as a subject or object of a verb). 'The tall management consultant with the spectacles wants to talk to you'. See **Head noun**.

Platonism

The philosophical view that there exist (and 'really exist') such things as abstract, non-spatiotemporal objects. This might include numbers and other mathematical objects, propositions, properties, possible worlds. Contrast **Nominalism**.

Polysemous

A polysemous word is one which means, or can be used to mean, different things. 'Get' can mean 'go' ('Get out'), 'acquire' ('She got the tickets'), 'become' ('Get real') or 'understand' ('He doesn't get it').

Predicative adjective

An adjective which is part of a predicate and does not precede a noun. 'The shoes Leo was wearing were brown'. Contrast **Attribute adjective**.

Propositional attitude

Verbs like 'believe', 'doubt' and 'hope' can all be followed by 'that', followed by a clause. 'I believe that Elvis is alive'. 'I doubt that Elvis is alive'. 'I hope that Elvis is alive'. Philosophers call the 'Elvis is alive' part a 'proposition', and the 'believe'/'doubt'/'hope' part a 'propositional attitude' (because these verbs signify different cognitive attitudes towards the proposition).

Reductio ad absurdum

A form of argument which begins with a certain premise, performs a series of logically valid steps, and ends with an absurd conclusion. When this happens, it is taken as a proof that there is something wrong with the premise.

Representation

A term used to refer to something that represents something else. In the philosophy of mind, a mental representation is a hypothetical inner state (or a process) which, in some symbolic sense, represents an aspect of reality.

Semantics

The branch of linguistics concerned with meaning.

Syntax

The branch of linguistics concerned with how individual words are combined to form sentences; or a term used to refer to the system of 'rules' underlying the way in which this combining is done.

1 Aims, methods, conventions

What sort of thing is a concept? What are people referring to when they use the word 'concept'? What does it mean to say that Jones doesn't understand the concept of risk, or that Andrew Jameton introduced the concept of moral distress, or that Ford's Model T was a revolutionary concept in automobiles, or that children acquire the concept of false belief by the time they are four to five years old, or that in the 1940s early ambulation was a whole new concept in postpartum care? If we acquire, or have, or possess a concept, what sort of having is that, and what exactly is it that comes into our possession? Is a concept a mental item, an ability, or an abstract entity of some kind?

I think the first of these questions takes us down a cul-de-sac. Ask what sort of thing a concept *is*, and you are already committed (a) to the assumption that it is *something*, and (b) to the project of trying to determine its nature. The important question – 'Is there, in fact, any such thing?' – has been answered by default. I would rather ask: 'How do we use the word "concept"? What does using the word permit us to do that is useful?'

1.1 Two aims

My *first aim* is to make the following claim more plausible than it will seem now:

> The word 'concept' is extremely useful, to the point of being indispensable. Nevertheless, the word doesn't *name* anything. In soundbite terms, 'there are no such things as concepts'.

Humour me. Suppose, just for a minute, that this claim is true. In that case, there can be no such thing as concept analysis, since there is nothing to analyse. However, there might be an alternative that scratches the same itch. This alternative would not be an analysis of 'concepts'. Instead, it would be an investigation of interesting words and expressions. In nursing, rather than 'analysing the concept of hope', we could explore different uses of the word 'hope' – as a noun, as a verb – and the different functions it can have in a range of grammatical constructions: positive statements, negative statements, first-person uses, third-person uses, with or without ellipsis and so on. (This is not at all the same thing as doing concept analysis, as will become clear.)

My *second aim* is to illustrate this alternative with two case studies.

1.2 Two expressions

The expressions chosen for the case studies are of interest for different reasons. 'Hope' is a common-or-garden term which has come to have clinical significance. There is now a sizeable literature on hope in health care. 'Moral distress', in contrast, is an invented phrase, coined in 1984. The 'concept' of moral distress has been the subject of intensive academic discussion in nursing and, more recently, other health care disciplines.

In summary: Part I makes a case for saying that there are no such things as concepts; but there *are* such things as words, used in a variety of ways. Part II explores the uses of 'hope' and 'moral distress', as an example of a different approach.

1.3 Summary of the argument in Part I

The claim that 'there are no such things as concepts' seems massively implausible, so throughout the first half of the book, I'll have to beg the reader's indulgence, particularly as the discussion draws on material which, for some people, will be unfamiliar. I don't think this material is intrinsically difficult, but its unfamiliarity may require a bit of patience.

Here is a single-paragraph summary of the argument in Part I:

> Concepts are usually treated as if they were objects of some kind, whether abstract entities or mental items. They are said to have structures, boundaries, components and attributes. They are, supposedly, the constituents of thoughts and the building blocks of theory. Part I argues that, although 'concept' is an indispensable word, there are no such things as concepts *in this familiar sense*. Concepts are neither abstract objects nor mental states. The word 'concept' is invaluable, for reasons I explain, but it doesn't name anything.

And now a brief chapter-by-chapter summary:

[2] We generally think of 'the concept of hope' (for example) as a singular something which underlies the various uses of the word 'hope'. 'Hope' *expresses* the same concept whenever it is used, irrespective of the grammatical construction it appears in. This is a familiar picture of the relation between words and concepts. In this chapter, I outline an alternative picture. The function of the word 'hope' varies with the constructions it occurs in; and the expression 'the concept of hope' is just a way of referring (vaguely) to the overall pattern of usage.

[3] We assume that nouns are naming words, and the assumption is more deeply entrenched than we realise. 'Concept' is a noun, so it must name something. However, this chapter shows that many nouns don't name anything at all, even if they are extremely useful; and some nouns don't always name things, even if they sometimes do. The non-naming functions of nouns – or any other type of word – vary with the linguistic context in which they appear.

[4] One important non-naming function of nouns is this: to refer to something without naming it, or (more often) to refer to a domain of things without naming, identifying or describing any of the items in that domain. This function is most visible in words such as 'things' and 'stuff'; but other nouns also perform this function in certain linguistic contexts. These contexts include anaphoric reference and some types of metonymy. (Terms such as these are explained in the Glossary, and more fully when we get to the relevant chapters.)

[5] The expression 'the concept of X' has this referring-without-naming function. It enables us to refer to a large, ill-defined, diverse domain of things – how X is understood, thought about, discussed; how the word 'X' is used, and with what purpose; how Xs are identified; and so on – without identifying, or needing to identify, any of those things. Concept possession is explained in a similar way, with a further observation: if someone 'has the concept of X', it does not follow that there *is* 'something that she *has*'. Many idiomatic uses of the verb 'to have' are such that, if someone 'has an X', there is no 'X' that she possesses.

[6] We generally assume that there *must* be concepts. In this chapter, I consider two 'indispensability arguments': there must be concepts because, if there were not: (a) we could not categorise things, could not have beliefs and could not make judgments; (b) there would be nothing to serve as the constituents of thoughts or propositions. I show why, given the preceding discussion, these arguments do not have any traction.

[7] 'The concept of X' is not a singular something which explains the various uses of 'X'. It is rather an expression which permits us to refer, in vague terms, to the pattern of usage associated with 'X'. So 'concept analysis' – if it is supposed to lead to a 'definition', or a list of the concept's structure and attributes – is a non-starter. The alternative is to explore the uses of 'X', bearing in mind that the same word can have many different uses, and that its function varies with the grammatical constructions in which it occurs. This approach combines Wittgenstein's methods with something called Construction Grammar. (I introduce the latter in Section 2.4; see also the Glossary.)

There will be several things here that seem, in varying degrees, unclear, too vague or obviously wrong. That's the price of an ultra-short summary. However, I hope this overview gives a general indication of the direction of travel.

1.4 The hypothetical reader

One way in which I try to make the reading, especially in Part I, more user-friendly is to have occasional conversations with someone called *Reader*. This figure is obviously hypothetical, though what she says is based on conversations I've had with friends and colleagues. They occur where I have a suspicion about what the (real) reader might be thinking. The conversations are also an opportunity for a change of style. They are as informal as I can make them, and sometimes report what was in fact said by someone eager to explain to me why I was wrong.

For example, I've suggested that: 'there are no such things as concepts'. A familiar reaction to this claim is something like:

Reader: No, that's ridiculous. We talk about concepts all the time. How can there not be any?

Me: If we want to prove the existence of something, is it enough to point out that we use the corresponding word all the time? For example, we use the word 'if' all the time. Does that prove that 'ifs' exist?

Reader: 'If' isn't a noun. Obviously 'ifs' don't exist. 'If' isn't that kind of word. Stick to nouns. 'Concept' is a noun.

Me: 'Unicorn', then. That's a noun. But the fact that we use it, and understand it, doesn't prove unicorns exist.

Reader: Oh, come on! Everyone knows that unicorns are mythical. But you can't say everyone knows concepts are mythical.

Me: No, I can't. But we're discussing a particular argument: 'We use the word "X", therefore Xs must exist'. All I'm saying is: this argument, *on its own*, doesn't work.

1.5 Style of argument

There's a remark of Wittgenstein's that I really like: 'Philosophy is like try-ing to open a safe with a combination lock: each little adjustment of the dials seems to achieve nothing, only when everything is in place does the door open' (Wittgenstein 1981: Ch. 6). I originally found this cited in Millikan (2017: 10), and it struck me as a neat summary of my experience in writing the book. I sus-pect that it will also reflect the experience of reading it (Part I, anyway). One-paragraph summaries may be useful, but there is a fair amount of detail in every chapter because I try to cover the bases. I think the reader will need a degree of patience as each dial is turned, perhaps too slowly, into position.

I don't regard any of the arguments as conclusive, and I never claim that such-and-such a view is wrong. Well, hardly ever. Nor do I suggest that a par-ticular view (call it V) *must* be right. The world is not that simple. Language is not that simple. I am usually more inclined to suggest that V is a good fit for some circumstances, and that W is a good fit for other circumstances. There isn't necessarily a single theory that covers every case. Here is an indication of what this often involves. Instead of saying 'You ought to believe V', I will say: 'Just try V on for size. Don't dismiss it out of hand. Think about how it links to other stuff, and look at how it deals with some otherwise puzzling questions. There isn't a knock-down argument that proves V is right, and I'm not going to pretend that there is.'

Much of Part I is more like trying to get someone to see two faces instead of a vase (in the image below) than it is a logical argument. 'See that as the nose, see those as the lips. See that as the chin … and now see the mirror image of this face on the opposite side of the vase'. Each of these suggestions is one of the dials on Wittgenstein's combination lock, and it may take a while before you get the 'Aha!' moment.[1]

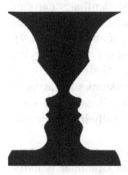

So Part I involves the philosophical equivalent of saying: 'There's a different way of seeing this'. This is one reason why I try to have a conversation between writer and reader, insofar as that's possible. There's no single argument that gets you from the vase to the faces, and which works for everybody. A change in the 'way of seeing' requires a dialogue. Of course, the philosophical equivalent will be nowhere near as straightforward as the vase and two faces. But that's the general idea.

1.6 Speaking of Wittgenstein…

There's no getting away from the fact that there is a fair amount of Wittgenstein in this book. For some readers, Wittgenstein will have a reputation for being enigmatic, difficult, even scary (though Husserl and Heidegger have him beaten all ends up). In fact, he uses very simple language, lots of examples, and consistently avoids jargon (unlike H&H). The problem is: he's trying to dislodge an entrenched picture of language, so some of the things he says are extremely counter-intuitive. What I would suggest is that, if you do have doubts on this score, you can read this chapter and the next, then skip to Section 7.7. From there, you can proceed directly to the chapters on 'hope'. You can come back to Part I later (given that some aspects of Part II won't make sense otherwise).

1.7 Concept conventions

Two chapters in Part I use a typographical convention, adapted from philosophy and psychology, which helps to distinguish between things, concepts and words. Things are referred to using normal font (dog). Inverted commas are placed around words ('dog'). Concepts are referred to using small capitals in bold (DOG). These entities have different attributes. Dogs bark, and are often kept as pets.

Concepts, however, don't bark; and no one keeps the concept DOG as a pet. Words can be put in italics ('*dog*'). The animals, dogs, can't be put in italics. Neither can the concept DOG.[2]

1.8 Linguistics

A lot of Part I draws on linguistics. Some terms will be familiar: 'parts of speech', 'noun', 'verb' and so on. Others go slightly beyond this basic level: for example, the difference between a 'count noun' and a 'mass noun' (Section 1.9). A third group is the kind of thing you might have come across when studying the grammar of your own, or another, language: 'syntax', 'inflection', 'morphology'. Beyond that, it gets more specialised, with expressions such as 'anaphoric reference', 'polysemous' and 'grammaticalised'. The Glossary has short explanations of terms like these; but they're explained more fully in the relevant chapters.

There are two even more specialised fields that I draw on throughout the book: Construction Grammar and corpus linguistics. Construction Grammar is introduced in Chapter 2. Corpus linguistics is the study of the distribution of words in real-life English (or in other natural languages). It involves the analysis of very large databases, called corpora, made up of texts sampled from academic, newspaper, magazine, fiction and spoken-language sources.[3] I make occasional reference to one of these databases: the *Corpus of Contemporary American English* (COCA). This corpus is freely available online, hosted at Brigham Young University. It has one billion words and counting.

I have used COCA to check the range of grammatical constructions in which various words appear; to determine which words occur most frequently in the vicinity of a target word ('concept', 'hope'); and as a source of text examples. Exactly why will become clear as we proceed.

1.9 Count noun, mass noun

A traditional grammatical distinction I refer to frequently, especially in Part II, is that between 'count noun' and 'mass noun'. Count nouns are words like 'biscuit', 'piano', 'prize' and 'father'. They refer to enumerable things, have plural forms ('biscuits', 'prizes'), and take numerical modifiers ('two pianos'). Mass nouns are words like 'spaghetti', 'cutlery', 'equipment' and 'mud'. They refer to aggregates or kinds of 'stuff', and do not have plural forms ('muds', 'two equipments'?).

Most discussions of the difference between mass and count nouns concentrate on words which refer to physical objects and/or substances ('biscuit', 'mud'). However, it is possible to make broadly the same distinction for abstract nouns. For example, abstract count nouns would include 'jump', 'proposal' and 'problem', all of which have plurals and take numeral modifiers: 'The athletes get six jumps'; 'We have two proposals to consider'. Abstract mass nouns might be 'trust', 'information' and 'knowledge'. These don't have plurals, and can't take numeral modifiers ('I have two informations to impart'?).[4]

1.10 The construction convention

As noted in Section 1.7, I sometimes use small caps in bold to refer to concepts. At some slight risk of confusion, I also use small caps, *not in bold*, to refer to some grammatical constructions, a convention adopted in Construction Grammar. Consider the following set of sentences: 'Derek dug his way out of prison'. 'Devala elbowed her way across the room'. 'Lynne blagged her way into the meeting'. 'Alex coughed his way through the interview'. These are all examples of the WAY construction (Hilpert 2014), so called for reasons that should be clear enough. In the same way, the following sentences illustrate the CAUSED MOTION construction: 'Keith kicked the ball out of the garden'. 'Martin chopped the carrots into the salad'. 'The audience booed the comedian off the stage'. 'Howard sneezed the froth off his coffee'.

In summary: *small caps in bold* are used to refer to concepts (DOG); *small caps not in bold* are used to refer to constructions (CAUSED MOTION construction). Generally, the context should make it clear which convention is being used. However, if on any occasion there is ambiguity, I will state explicitly which of the two is in play at that point.

1.11 Other sceptics

In case anybody imagines that the '*no such things as concepts*' claim is completely idiosyncratic, let me mention a few philosophers and cognitive scientists who seem to take a similar sort of view (but for very different reasons). They include Saporiti (2010), Gauker (2011), Harnad (2009), Hacker (2013), Marconi (2015), Turner (2014), Millikan (2017); arguably Wilson (2006), Baz (2017); possibly Machery (2009); going further back, Austin (1961). These writers don't all have the same view, and their arguments differ greatly. But they all think we should 'resist the impulse to consider "concepts" as well-defined entities' (Wilson 2006: 134–5). The author whose position I think I'm closest to is Saporiti. I say more about her paper in Chapter 6.

1.12 Anglo-centrism

This book is, I must confess, Anglo-centric. The examples of usage (found in most chapters) are all in English, some of them being so idiomatic as to almost defy translation. Moreover, *some* of the things I say about these examples could not be said about other-language equivalents, at least not in the same way. This implies that (as an example) what is referred to in English as 'the concept of hope' is not the same as what is referred to in French as 'le concept de l'espoir'. This would be a problem if 'the concept of hope' were a singular something underlying the use of both 'hope' and 'espoir'. However, I don't think it is. 'The concept of hope' refers to the pattern of usage of 'hope', while 'le concept de l'espoir' refers to the pattern of usage of 'espoir' and 'espérer'. There are many similarities, no doubt, between these two patterns; but they are not (I assume) identical. Hence the Anglo-centrism. It would be very interesting to know how far the book's main arguments can be expressed plausibly in other languages.

1.13 A note on the nursing literature

The first draft of this chapter included a history of concept analysis in nursing.[5] But it was too long and – if I'm honest – rather boring, and it didn't fit the 'let's just get on with it' feel I was hoping for. Change of plan, then. I'll assume that anyone interested in reading this book already has a reasonably good idea of what concept analysis in nursing looks like, and confine the potted history to a single paragraph.

So here, in a nutshell, is all you need to know about my take on the story so far.

Concept analysis was introduced to the nursing literature in the 1970s, but the landmark work appeared in the early 1980s (Walker & Avant 1983). This account was based on a single source (Wilson 1963), a book written by a high school teacher for his students. Wilson described analytic philosophy as it was (more or less) in the 1950s. Walker and Avant modified the procedure Wilson described in a number of ways. The most important modification was this: in analysing a concept (let's say X), the analyst must study what is said about X in the literature, and make a note of what comes up over and over again. The descriptions of X that occur most frequently are the defining attributes of X; and defining attributes are what the analyst seeks to identify. In the years since 1983, several more amendments to the procedure have been proposed. However, these discussions have not taken account of the relevant developments in philosophy since the 1970s, and the amendments are all (I would argue) inconsequential. In particular, none of the authors concerned has abandoned the idea that the defining attributes of a concept can be derived, somehow, from the literature (a view which has no counterpart in philosophy). Consequently, Draper (2014) suggested that concept analyses are 'low-grade literature reviews'. Although he got his wrist slapped by Morse (2014) and Knafl and Deatrick (2014), he was right. His essay appeared as an editorial in the *Journal of Advanced Nursing*; and *JAN* subsequently announced that it would no longer publish concept analysis studies.[6] They are still published by other journals.

I'll make no attempt to defend this account.[7] Nor will I spend much time criticising the methods adopted in the concept analysis literature. Instead, I would like to present an alternative way of looking at things, and offer the reader something different to do. My belief is that this 'something different' is more useful and, actually, more interesting than the kind of concept analysis currently found in nursing journals.

Notes

1 According to McGinn (2013: 25/23), Wittgenstein 'does not see himself as out to refute doctrines'. Instead, he wants to 'change the way we see philosophical questions and the sort of investigation they call for'. The image is Rubin's Vase, first published by Edgar John Rubin, a Danish psychologist and philosopher, in 1915.

2 *Reader*: Why do you need a typographical convention to talk about concepts if there are no such things? *Me*: I think you're assuming that we can't talk about things which don't exist. But we can. Phlogiston, the average person, Sherlock Holmes.

3 For an accessible account of corpus linguistics and its potential relation to linguistic philosophy, see Bluhm (2013). Incidentally, don't be put off by the title of the book this chapter appears in. Bluhm's essay is in English and is available online.

4 In recent years the plural 'knowledges' has been introduced in some disciplines, even though it sounds wrong to some people (including me). However, recent work on the distinction between mass and count, which I mention in Chapters 3 and 8, suggests that it is a legitimate usage.

5 'Concept analysis' is a term that is found, almost exclusively, in the nursing literature. Philosophers generally call what they do (or what some of them do) 'concept*ual* analysis'. So the 'new approach' referred to in the book's title is new to nursing, not new to philosophy.

6 The Editor-in-Chief has informed me that the reason for the decision, taken by the *JAN* Editorial Board, was lack of impact. Concept analysis papers were not getting cited. 'We assumed – no citations, probably no reads, no use to anyone, no genuine contribution to any scholarship or debate' (Professor Roger Watson, personal communication, 28th February 2019).

7 I have, however, defended it in Paley (2019).

References

Austin, J. L. (1961). *Philosophical Papers*. Oxford: Clarendon Press.

Baz, A. (2017). *The Crisis of Method in Contemporary Analytic Philosophy*. Oxford: Oxford University Press.

Bluhm, R. (2013). Don't ask, look! Linguistic corpora as a tool for conceptual analysis. In M. Hoeltje, T. Spitzley, & W. Spohn (Eds.), *Was Dürfen Wir Glauben? Was Sollen Wir Tun? Sektionsbeiträge des Achten Internationalen Kongresses der Gesellschaft für Analytische Philosophie* (pp. 7–15). Duisburg-Essen: University of Duesburg-Essen. https://philarchive.org/archive/BLUAPFv1.

Draper, P. (2014). A critique of concept analysis. *Journal of Advanced Nursing, 70*, 1207–1208.

Gauker, C. (2011). *Words and Images: An Essay on the Origin of Ideas*. Oxford: Oxford University Press.

Hacker, P. M. S. (2013). *The Intellectual Powers: A Study of Human Nature*. Chichester, UK: John Wiley & Sons Ltd.

Harnad, S. (2009). *Concepts: the very idea. Review of Machery (2009)*. Department of Electronics and Computer Science, University of Southampton. https://eprints.soton.ac.uk/268029/1/MacheryCommSH.pdf.

Hilpert, M. (2014). *Construction Grammar and Its Application to English*. Edinburgh: Edinburgh University Press.

Knafl, K. A., & Deatrick, J. A. (2014). Commentary on: Draper P. (2014) editorial: A critique of concept analysis. *Journal of Advanced Nursing, 70*(12), 2968.

Machery, E. (2009). *Doing Without Concepts*. Oxford: Oxford University Press.

Marconi, D. (2015). Concepts: Too heavy a burden. In A. Coliva, V. Munz, & D. Moyal-Sharrock (Eds.), *Mind, Language and Action: Proceedings of the 36th International Wittgenstein Symposium* (pp. 497–522). Berlin: De Gruyter.

McGinn, M. (2013). *The Routledge Guide to Wittgenstein's Philosophical Investigations*. Abingdon: Routledge.

Millikan, R. G. (2017). *Beyond Concepts: Unicepts, Language, and Natural Information.* New York: Oxford University Press.

Morse, J. M. (2014). The baby and the bathwater. *Journal of Advanced Nursing, 70*(12), 2969.

Paley, J. (2019). Concept analysis in nursing: Why Draper had a point. *Nursing Philosophy, 20*(4), e12252.

Saporiti, K. (2010). In search of concepts. *Grazer Philosophische Studien, 81*, 153–172.

Turner, S. P. (2014). *Understanding the Tacit.* New York: Routledge.

Walker, L. O., & Avant, K. C. (1983). *Strategies for Theory Construction in Nursing.* Norwalk, CT: Appleton-Century-Crofts.

Wilson, J. (1963). *Thinking with Concepts.* Cambridge, UK: Cambridge University Press.

Wilson, M. (2006). *Wandering Significance: An Essay on Conceptual Behavior.* New York: Oxford University Press.

Wittgenstein, L. (1981). *Personal Recollections* (edited by Rush Rhees). Lanham, MD: Rowman & Littlefield.

Part I
Concepts

2 Concepts, words and pictures

This chapter introduces four themes which recur throughout the book: (a) the importance of pictures in philosophical discussion, and in particular the significance of the (fuzzy) picture we have of concepts; (b) the relation between concepts and words, and two different pictures we might have of that relation; (c) the assumption that the grammar of a sentence has no effect on the meaning of the individual words in the sentence; (d) the claim that 'there are no such things as concepts', and whether that really means what it appears to mean.

2.1 A picture of concepts

According to Wittgenstein, many philosophical problems are the result of over-extending a particular picture. For example, we have a picture of language which misleads us if we apply it across the board, beyond the narrow range of cases to which it applies (Wittgenstein 1963: §1). This picture suggests that individual words are the names of objects, and that sentences are combinations of these names. 'Cat' is the name of a certain type of animal. 'Mat' is the name of a type of material that can be used as a floor covering. 'Sit' is the name of a certain activity or posture in which part of the weight normally borne by the legs is transferred to the buttocks. If we combine these words into a sentence – 'The cat sat on the mat' – we can depict a certain state of affairs, and/or convey information to another person.

Wittgenstein accepts that this picture applies to a particular class of words – for the most part, words which refer to physical objects and visible activities – but suggests that it doesn't work for other kinds of words. Moreover, he suggests, if we try to *make* it apply to other types of words (abstract nouns, for example, or 'mental state' verbs), we are likely to misunderstand how those nouns and verbs actually work.

I will say more about Wittgenstein's picture of language in Section 2.3. Here, I make some preliminary remarks about a certain picture we have of concepts. The picture is simply that concepts are 'sort-of' objects, or perhaps 'quasi objects'. They are things that can be taken apart and analysed, just as physical objects can be. Of course, nobody thinks that concepts *are* physical objects; but the way in which they are talked about does imply that a picture of concept-as-object is lurking somewhere in the background. As Turner (2014: 43) observes, the idea is that concepts are 'shared, object-like things: possessions that one acquires', and that they can be 'subject to a special kind of inquiry', concept analysis.

A brief example. According to Walker and Avant (2005), a concept has an 'internal structure' and can be broken 'into its simpler elements' (64). They further suggest that the analyst is able 'to "get inside" the concept and see how it works' (63). This does imply that they are using physical objects as a point of reference or an analogy. 'Getting inside the concept to see how it works' sounds a little bit like 'getting inside a clock to see how it works'. If you read the passage 'breaking a concept into its simpler elements to determine its internal structure' at the normal pace – that is, without thinking about it too hard – you will almost certainly have this picture, vaguely, at the back of your mind. However, it is not clear how 'breaking into simpler elements' can be done with a mental object, and it is even less clear how it can be done with an abstraction.[1] So this way of talking depends, to a great extent, on not inspecting the picture of 'concept' as the name for something-analogous-to-a-physical-object too closely.

In the nursing literature, this quasi-object picture of concepts has not changed very much over the years. Almost all writers seem to have it in mind, including those who have proposed alternative concept analysis methods (including Rodgers 2000, Norris 1982, Morse et al. 1996, Morse 2000, and Schwartz-Barcott & Kim 2000). All of these authors would agree that concept analysis is 'an inquiry designed to clarify or define a concept by identifying its constituent components and related elements' (Rodgers et al. 2018: 2), and would probably sign up to all or most of the following claims:

- A concept is a type of object: an abstract entity or a mental image.
- It is a singular item and has boundaries distinguishing it from other concepts.
- It is a relatively stable object and has a structure.
- Concepts have components and attributes which can be specified.
- Concepts are the building blocks of theory.
- They are constituents of thoughts and/or propositions.

On the face of it, and in the absence of further clarification, anything which has a structure, components and boundaries, and which can be a constituent or a building block, is something very *like* an object. At any rate, as I have suggested, this way of talking about concepts is ubiquitous; so, even if the authors concerned are only speaking metaphorically, I will refer to it as the 'standard framework'.

Some of the cited authors would argue that they do not accept all of these assumptions. Morse (2017), for example, says that 'concepts are not actual entities', and that they 'do not exist in empirical reality'. In other passages, however, she claims that 'a concept is a mental image', or a 'collection of behaviors', or a 'representation', or a 'word included in the lexicon', or an 'explanatory theory' or a 'name for an idea' (all of which 'exist in empirical reality'); and she insists that concepts have attributes, structures, components and boundaries. Concepts are also said to 'occur', and to have antecedents and outcomes, implying that they are events of a certain kind. Like other nurse authors, Morse does occasionally say something that appears to be at odds with the ways of talking listed above. For the most part, however, she talks in 'standard framework' terms.

In itself, the standard framework may be a perfectly innocuous metaphor. However, in the next section, I'll suggest that it leads theorists in a particular methodological direction, without them realising it, and makes it almost inevitable that they will overlook a different way of doing things. It takes them into a philosophical cul-de-sac, something of which they're not aware because they do not see that they are presupposing a certain picture of what 'concepts' are. The argument, I should emphasise, is not that this picture is wrong, but that (a) it gets over-extended, and (b) there are alternative pictures which open up other lines of enquiry. Focus too much on the vase, and you may not notice the faces.

2.2 Concepts *vs.* words

In Chapter 1, I suggested that there are no such things as concepts, in which case the project of concept analysis would appear to be a non-starter (we have a long way to go before this looks plausible). But I also suggested that there might be an alternative to concept analysis: that is, a purposeful exploration of the *pattern of use* of interesting words and expressions. This section is an initial, and highly schematic, unpacking of this idea. It will briefly sketch the difference between 'analysing a concept' and 'studying a pattern of usage', and indicate why I think this difference is significant.

Nurses (and others) analyse *the* concept of X, Y or Z. For example, there's a growing literature devoted to '*the* concept of hope'. Writers such as Benzein et al. (2001), Cutcliffe and Herth (2002), Miller (2007) and Wiles et al. (2008) use this expression – 'the concept of hope' – unhesitatingly, not pausing to ask whether it actually refers to anything, and not questioning the assumption that the project of analysing *the* concept is a feasible one.

Notice, particularly, the implication of *singularity*. What is analysed is *the* concept of hope; and when a description is offered, or a definition is formulated, it consists of a predicate attached to 'Hope' in the subject position of a sentence: 'Hope is … such-and-such'. 'Hope is a theological virtue, along with faith and charity'. 'Hope is central to life and specifically is an essential dimension for successfully dealing with illness'. 'Hope is a multidimensional dynamic life force characterized by a confident yet uncertain expectation of achieving a future good'. There is only one thing being described, and the predicate which does the describing applies to that one thing in its entirety. This singularity, as I suggested in the previous section, is part of the standard framework.[2]

The assumption is that *the* concept of hope is something – something singular – which is activated (so to speak) every time the word 'hope' is used. Whenever someone says that she's hoping that *x*, *y* or *z*; whenever she talks about there being no hope, or about hope fading; whenever she refers to a hopeless situation, or her feelings of hopelessness; whenever she says 'this is the only thing we can hope for', or suggests that 'there's hope for the future'… in all these situations, *the* concept of hope is being applied. Get the analysis of that singular concept right, and all these expressions will be explained.

Contrast this picture with another one. Suspend, for the time being, the assumption that every use of the word 'hope', with its various inflections and derivatives, can be explained by the analysis of a singular concept of hope. Instead, examine those uses closely. There is quite a rich variety. Here are just a few examples:

(1)   I'm hoping to climb Ben Nevis.
(2)   She's my only hope.
(3)   New Orleans is a city without hope.
(4)   As darkness fell, hope faded.
(5)   There's not a hope in hell that he'll be quiet.
(6)   He has some hopes of raising the money.
(7)   There is no hope of building a perpetual motion machine.
(8)   The review could not hope to be exhaustive.
(9)   Legally, he's in a hopeless position.
(10)   We're the first to admit the hopelessness of the task.
(11)   Hopelessness threatened to overwhelm him.
(12)   There is hope in the industry that the restrictions will be lifted.
(13)   Is there any hope?
(14)   November is the earliest he can hope for.

In Chapters 8–10, I will consider sentences like these, and many more; and I'll suggest that they do not all have the same kind of function. The job that 'hope' does varies in a number of ways, depending on several linguistic factors: whether a positive or negative assertion is being made; whether the mood of the verb is indicative or interrogative; whether the verb is used in the first person or the third person; whether an auxiliary modal verb is used; whether the simple present or the continuous present is used; whether 'hope' is followed by 'that', or 'to'; whether a personal or impersonal ('there is…') statement is being made; whether 'hope' is used as a verb, count noun or mass noun; whether the noun is used in the singular or plural. And that's not counting the adjectives, the adverbs and 'hopelessness'.

So the alternative picture is this: a variegated pattern of usage for the word 'hope'. These uses do not all have the same function, even if some of the word's functions are related. So when I suggest that there is an alternative to concept analysis, the idea is that we should start *here*, and not with the assumption that every occurrence of the word 'hope' *must* express one-and-the-same concept.

To summarise (Figure 2.1):

First Picture: there is a (singular) concept of hope, such that all occurrences of the word 'hope' express (or apply) that concept. Concept analysis should seek to understand and/or define that concept.

Second Picture: there is a rich variety in uses of the word 'hope', and we shouldn't assume that they all have the same function, or that they're all governed by the same singular concept. Concept analysis – or something which occupies

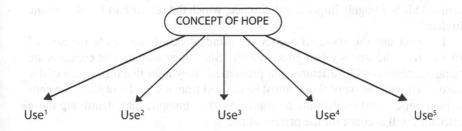

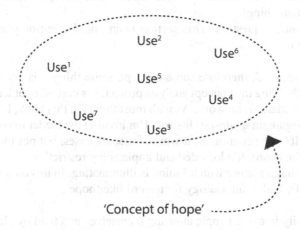

First Picture
Solid arrows to be read as 'explains'
CONCEPT OF HOPE *is the name of a singular object or quasi - object*

Second Picture

Dashed arrow to be read as 'vaguely refers to'
'Concept of hope' is a linguistic expression

Figure 2.1 Use and 'concept': two pictures.

the same slot – should seek to track and understand this variegated pattern of usage.

The *First Picture* takes the singular concept as primary, and use as derivative. The *Second Picture* takes use as primary, and dispenses with the singular concept altogether. In the First Picture, the 'concept of hope' is the name of something which explains the pattern of usage. In the Second Picture, by contrast, the 'concept of hope' is merely a way of *referring to* this pattern, and doing so only in very broad terms. This is a hugely important difference, which the rest of Part I will examine in detail.

I suspect that the standard framework blinds concept analysts to the Second Picture (and the strategy that goes with it).[3] Since they assume that concepts are 'singular objects with structures and properties', they infer that the pattern of use associated with the word 'hope' must be derived from a singular object – the concept of hope – and its defining attributes. So they imagine that identifying those attributes will account for the pattern of use.

2.3 Wittgenstein's field

Reader: Well, okay, so there's a rich variety in uses of the word 'hope'. But why should we *not* assume that they all express the same concept? After all, it's the same word. Why would we use that word if it didn't mean the same on each occasion? Why would we use it if it didn't always refer to the same phenomenon, namely hope? Surely, if we use the same word, we *must* be talking about the same thing!

Me: It's a reasonable question. This section is an initial – but only an initial – response to it.

This idea – same word, therefore same concept, same thing – is another of the assumptions underlying the concept analysis project. It's part of, or at least closely related to, the standard framework. As with most things in this book, I don't have a knock-down argument against it. Instead, I'm inviting the reader to consider the possibility that it over-generalises: it works for some cases, but not for others. If applied across the board, it's lopsided and implausibly restrictive.

Wittgenstein has a picture which I think is illuminating. In this thought experiment, think of the ball as an analogy for a word like 'hope'.

> We can easily imagine people amusing themselves in a field by playing with a ball so as to start various existing games, but playing many without finishing them and in between throwing the ball aimlessly into the air, chasing one another with the ball and bombarding one another for a joke and so on.
>
> (Wittgenstein 1963, §83)

Reader asked: 'Why would we use that word if it didn't mean the same on each occasion of its use? Why would we use it if it didn't always apply to the same phenomenon?' The corresponding question in the 'field' analogy is roughly this: 'Why would we use the ball at all if we weren't doing the same thing with it on every occasion? Why would we use it unless it always had the same function?'

But the people in Wittgenstein's field are not using the ball in the same way on every occasion. The ball *doesn't* always have the same function. And it would be odd to insist: 'It *must* always have the same function, because it is, after all, the same thing, namely a ball'. Analogically, then, I can suggest that it is equally odd to say: The word 'hope' *must* always have the same function, because it is, after all, the same word, namely 'hope'.[4]

Again, there is no conclusive argument here. 'See the use of a word like "hope" as akin to the use of the ball in the field'. This is rather like saying: 'See this part of the image, not as the neck of a vase, but as the space between two noses'. It's about trying to prompt a change in how we see things.

Wittgenstein doesn't generalise. Misleading pictures, like *same-word-so-same-thing*, mislead because they can't be applied across the board. They might fit some words, but not necessarily all. However, what Wittgenstein calls our 'craving for generality' encourages us to think: 'Well, this picture fits *that* type of word, so it must fit all of them'. Typically, the pictures we favour are those which fit physical objects. So a word like 'window' is a reasonable match for the *same-word* principle. Whenever it occurs, it refers to the same kind of physical object.[5] But the same principle may not apply to words for non-physical things such as 'hope'. So the picture of language based on physical objects 'is correct for a certain narrow region of language use but should not be stretched too far' (Kuusela 2008: 43).

There is another assumption that encourages us to treat physical object words and abstract words in the same way. This is the 'analogous grammar' assumption. Wittgenstein (1964: 7) puts the matter like this: 'When words in our ordinary language have prima facie analogous grammars we are inclined to try to interpret them analogously; i.e. we try to make the analogy hold throughout'. The kind of thing he has in mind is the grammar of sentences such as:

(15) She's my only friend.
(16) She's my only hope.
(17) Is there any wine?
(18) Is there any hope?

The grammar of (15) and (16) appears to be identical. Ditto for (17) and (18). Wittgenstein's point is that these 'analogous grammars' encourage us to think that the nouns 'friend', 'wine' and 'hope' function in the same way. In (16) 'hope' seems to play the same role as 'friend' in (15). In (18) it seems to play the same role as 'wine' in (17). So we infer that 'hope', even though it is an abstract noun (unlike 'friend' and 'wine'), can be treated in the same way. Because *they* are names – 'friend' is the name of an object, 'wine' is the name of a substance – 'hope' must be the name of something (a substance, a state, a force, a process) as well. This is not necessarily a conscious inference; it is usually just one we slide into.

Wittgenstein's field suggests that language is messy, inconsistent and fluctuating. It chops and changes moment by moment, not only because the 'meaning' of any particular word can vary, but also because the *same* word is used to perform *different* tasks. Just as the ball's function varies from one minute to the next, so the function of a word like 'hope' varies from one minute to the next. The word's 'meaning' is not a 'halo' (so to speak) which always accompanies the word, and which determines its use in every situation. It is more like a vague gesture towards the wide range of tasks the word is asked to perform.[6]

2.4 Construction Grammar

I have suggested that one implication of the First Picture is that every occurrence of a particular word expresses 'the same concept'. For example, every occurrence of the word 'hope' expresses one-and-the-same concept of hope. This is true irrespective of the grammatical construction that the word 'hope' appears in. Underlying this idea is the assumption that *individual words are the basic units-of-meaning*. If this is true, it is not unreasonable to suggest that the word 'hope' in examples (1) to (14) above must play the same role in each of them. The different grammatical constructions do not affect the meaning 'hope' has, or the concept it expresses.

But suppose it isn't true. Suppose, instead, that the basic unit-of-meaning is a *grammatical construction*. The implication of this would be that, instead of 'hope' playing the same role in (1) to (14), we would have to distinguish between different constructions such as 'hoping that', 'one's only hope', 'could not hope to', 'there is no hope', 'without a hope', 'hopeless situation' and so on. Each of these would have a subtly different function, learned independently; and to talk about the 'meaning' of the word 'hope' – considered on its own – would be a broad, indirect way of referring to those functions.

There is in fact a perspective in linguistics called Construction Grammar (usually abbreviated as CxG), which appears to imply that the meaning of at least some individual words is a function of their role in grammatical constructions. A simple example is 'behalf'. This noun does not exist outside expressions such as 'on behalf of…' and 'on her own behalf'. The word 'behalf', by itself, does not have a meaning which is independent of, and prior to, these expressions.[7] The suggestion is that something similar *might* apply to a word like 'hope': the constructions in which it occurs are primary; and the word, considered by itself, does not have a meaning independent of those constructions. In terms of Wittgenstein's 'field' analogy, it is not the ball which accounts for the various activities in the field. It is the activities which create different roles for the ball. (Much more about the meaning of 'hope' in Part II.)

According to CxG, a *construction* is a unit of knowledge which 'pairs a linguistic form with a meaning' (Hilpert 2014: 10/2).[8] The key idea (for the purposes of this discussion) is that 'meaning' is a property, not solely of the individual word, but of the grammatical construction in which it appears.[9]

This is significant for concept analysis because the 'concept' being analysed is almost always identified with a single mass noun, or a noun phrase. We analyse the concept of *hope*, the concept of *comfort*, the concept of *resilience* and so on. No-one stops to wonder whether conceptual meaning might actually be a property of different constructions rather than nouns and nominal expressions in isolation. If someone says 'there is no hope of that happening', and if someone else says 'I'm hoping to get a promotion', are they both applying the same concept? The reflex answer is 'Yes, of course they are!' However, CxG casts doubt on this natural reaction.

The 'Yes, of course they are!' reaction reflects an idea that 'is widely shared, both among laypeople and among professional linguists' (Hilpert 2014: 2–3). It is sometimes called the 'dictionary plus grammar book model' (Taylor 2012: 8). This model suggests that individual words are the basic units of meaning, and that sentences have meaning because we combine words in a syntactically correct way. If we add to this model the assumption that words have meanings in virtue of the fact that they are names-of-objects, then we arrive at the view that sentences are syntactically correct combinations of names.

For a sentence such as 'the cat sat on the mat', the dictionary-and-grammar model is plausible. 'Cat', 'mat' and 'sat' have individual meanings, in virtue of the fact that they name objects or activities. The full sentence acquires its meaning from the syntactically correct combination of individual meanings, plus the appropriate use of determiner ('the') and preposition ('on'). However, for a sentence such as 'The old buffer has tied up the loose ends, by and large', the model is much less plausible. Knowing the 'individual meanings' of 'buffer', 'old', 'end', 'loose', 'tie', 'large', 'up' and 'by' would be of little help in working out what the sentence as a whole meant.

The dictionary-and-grammar model marginalises idiom, which it regards as a sort of slightly tedious bolt-on to regular, combinatory English. In contrast, one way of thinking about CxG is that it takes exactly the opposite view: *most* of language, both spoken and written, is idiom. The dictionary-and-grammar model works, if it works at all, for a limited range of cases.

The upshot is that, for some words, the constructions they appear in are primary, and their 'individual meaning' is derivative. 'The meaning of a lexical item may vary systematically with the constructional contexts in which it is found' (Hilpert 2014: 17). Indeed, constructions 'may override word meanings'. This is, of course the opposite of the 'building block' metaphor from the standard framework. The 'building block' metaphor portrays a sentence as being assembled out of its component parts. CxG puts that idea into reverse.

As an example, consider two types of construction associated with the noun 'chance'.

(19)   She had a chance to score.
(20)   We met by chance in Paris.

Sentences like (19) embody the construction: CHANCE TO + infinitive verb.
Sentences like (20) embody the construction: finite verb + BY CHANCE.

In (19) 'chance' is a count noun, and is a rough synonym of 'opportunity' ('she had an opportunity to score'). By contrast, in (20) it is a mass noun, and is part of a prepositional phrase. In this construction, it is *not* synonymous with 'opportunity' ('We met by opportunity in Paris'?). The phrase 'by chance' conveys a sense of unpredictability, coincidence, even randomness. To meet 'by chance' is to meet in a way that wasn't planned, intended or foreseen. But it is difficult to find a single word or short phrase that can be slotted into the construction without subtly changing the meaning. 'We met unintentionally in Paris'? 'We met coincidentally in Paris'? 'We met at random in Paris'?

One way of thinking about the difference between (19) and (20) is to say that 'chance' has two distinct senses, and that (19) employs one of these senses while (20) employs the other. The reader, coming to either sentence for the first time, 'selects' the sense which fits the context (perhaps by eliminating the senses which don't fit). This is the dictionary-and-grammar model. Not surprisingly, it raises various questions about how the 'selection' process works, questions which are of interest to psychologists.[10]

An alternative way to think about the difference between (19) and (20) is to say that, in each case, the *construction itself* is responsible for the meaning. The CHANCE TO construction confers the 'opportunity' meaning on 'chance'; while the BY CHANCE construction confers the 'unplanned, unforeseen' sense on it.[11] This is the CxG model. To use the CxG technical term, the construction *coerces* the meaning of the individual word. 'The meaning of the lexical item conforms to the meaning of the structure in which it is embedded' (Michaelis 2004: 25).

So we have a choice. If we adopt the dictionary-and-grammar model, individual words have individual senses, and the meaning of a sentence can be 'computed' by combining the meanings of its constituent words, using the appropriate grammatical rules. On this view, 'chance' has meaning in its own right, independently of the constructions it occurs in. It's just that this 'meaning' resolves into two (or more) senses, which the reader selects from. On the CxG view, however, the meaning of 'chance' is a function of the constructions in which it appears. You don't learn the word's meaning as an independent unit, and later compute the meaning of any construction you find it in. Rather, you learn *the construction itself*.

As I suggested earlier, concept analysis identifies the 'concept' of interest with a noun or a noun phrase, independently of any construction in which the noun or noun phrase appears. So CxG can be regarded as part of the alternative to the standard framework I have been sketching. It is a way of thinking about the plurality inherent in the pattern of usage for any word, in contrast to the singularity of the idea of a 'concept'. It implies that individual words are like the ball in Wittgenstein's field, and that constructions are the equivalent of the activities – diverse as they are – in which the ball is used, and in the context of which it has its different roles. In this sense, CxG is a sort of adjunct to Wittgenstein.[12]

So far, I have sketched two different pictures of language, and two correspondingly different ways to think about the relation between 'concepts' and words. I have not argued that either is right or wrong, although I have suggested that the 'standard framework' applies to only a narrow range of cases. Before closing the chapter, I will return to the claim made in Chapter 1: 'There are no such things as concepts'. Will I really be arguing that, or am I just being provocative?

2.5 No such things?

In an article entitled 'A nice derangement of epitaphs', Donald Davidson (1986: 446) argued:

> There is no such thing as a language ... There is therefore no such thing to be learned, mastered, or born with. We must give up the idea of a clearly defined shared structure which language-users acquire and then apply to cases.

This appears unambiguous, radical and patently ridiculous. However, in the '...' part of the passage, Davidson qualifies the claim he has just made: 'not if a language is anything like what many philosophers and linguists have supposed'.

I can qualify my claim in much the same way: 'there are no such things as concepts, not if concepts are anything like what philosophers, psychologists and nurses have supposed'. And I would add a similar corollary: 'There are no such things to be understood, possessed, or analysed. We must give up the idea of a clearly defined shared structure which concept-users acquire and apply to cases'. We must also give up the idea that this 'shared structure' can be elucidated through 'concept analysis'.

So I'm serious about 'no such things', but the qualification is important. If you think that concepts are 'abstract objects' or 'mental images'; if you think they have components, boundaries, structures and attributes; if you think they are the constituents of thoughts and/or propositions, and that they can be the 'building blocks' of theory ... if *that's* what concepts are supposed to be, then there are no such things.

Defending this view will mean exploring an alternative to the standard framework, along the lines I've begun to sketch, drawing on Wittgenstein's philosophy of language and CxG. It will mean reversing the usual polarity. Instead of taking the 'singular concept' as primary and the pattern of usage as derivative, I will consider the implications of taking the pattern of usage as primary, and suggest that talk about 'the concept of' is no more than a way of referring, in the vaguest terms, to this pattern.

On the alternative view, then, 'concept' talk involves indirect reference to usage. This is why 'concept' is such a handy, indeed indispensable, term. Very roughly, 'the concept of X' is a convenient way of referring to patterns of usage associated with the word 'X'. It is a kind of shorthand. It permits reference to a complex network of uses, without any obligation to identify or describe them (Second Picture).

However, it has one unfortunate drawback. 'The concept of X' is a noun phrase; so we assume that it is the name of something. Ironically, the phrase itself – useful as it is – encourages the belief that there is a singular object, which lies *behind* the pattern of usage, and which explains it (whereas, on my view, it is merely a way of referring to this pattern, or alluding to some of its features). It implies an underlying 'singularity' in a way that 'patterns of usage' does not; and this reinforces the assumption that it has a 'structure' which can be analysed.

An initial stab at a more precise version of the view I want to present is this: 'the concept of X' is a referring but non-naming expression. There is no object, whether abstract or mental, of which it is the *name*; nevertheless, it *refers*. This does not sound quite as dramatic as 'there are no such things as concepts', but it says roughly the same thing. It gives rise to some obvious questions. What is a non-naming word? What is a naming word? What is a referring but non-naming expression? These are the questions that will take us into the next chapter.

Notes

1 Breaking something into simpler elements presupposes the part/whole relation. This relation applies, in the first instance, to objects in space and time. So can it also apply to abstract entities – which, by definition, are neither spatial nor temporal? This is a prominent theme in Wittgenstein: the transfer of ways of thinking about physical space, and physical objects, to 'things' that are not *in* physical space (such as abstract entities and mental states). See Hymers (2017) for a useful discussion.
2 The nursing literature's assumptions about the nature of hope will be discussed at greater length in Section 11.3.
3 Azzouni (2013: 244) suggests that focusing on concepts makes us 'blind to the richness and shiftiness of words as they are utilized in different expressions'. I particularly like the word 'shiftiness' here.
4 I've placed the 'must' in italics to dramatise the conviction that views like this tend to have. The word 'must' in this kind of statement often marks an implicit metaphysical doctrine, giving indirect expression to an unacknowledged picture of how things are ('and how they *must* be!'). In thrall to one picture, as Wittgenstein puts it, we cannot see that there are alternatives. 'Our investigation tried to remove this bias which forces us to think that the facts *must* conform to certain pictures' (Wittgenstein 1964: 43).
5 Or a metaphorical equivalent. 'The eyes are the window to the soul'.
6 Baz (2017: 133) suggests that 'what makes a word suitable for certain uses but not others – call it "its meaning" – is its history, or in other words "former acts of expression"'. The jobs that a word has been asked to do in the past are the starting point for the jobs it can be asked to do in the future.
7 I will return to the 'behalf' example in Section 3.6.
8 My account of Construction Grammar necessarily simplifies. For one thing, there are several different versions of it. Hilpert (2014) is an excellent introductory text.
9 The same idea turns up in lexicography: 'If meanings … are associated with words in context – that is, with phraseological patterns – rather than with words in isolation, some well-known linguistic problems are largely solved' (Hanks 2013: 17).
10 For a review of the relevant literature, see Rodd (2020).
11 There are several other constructions involving the word 'chance'. I discuss some of them in Section 3.4.
12 'Adjunct' in the sense that they are natural allies, even though they focus on different aspects of what Wittgenstein calls 'use' and 'grammar'. Construction Grammar analyses the distribution of words in constructions. Wittgenstein widens the angle, and looks at how they are used in relation to 'language games', which include patterns of behaviour and 'forms of life'.

References

Azzouni, J. (2013). *Semantic Perception: How the Illusion of a Common Language Arises and Persists*. New York: Oxford University Press.
Baz, A. (2017). *The Crisis of Method in Contemporary Analytic Philosophy*. Oxford: Oxford University Press.

Benzein, E., Norberg, A., & Saveman, B.-I. (2001). The meaning of the lived experience of hope in patients with cancer in palliative home care. *Palliative Medicine, 15*(2), 117–126.

Cutcliffe, J. R., & Herth, K. (2002). The concept of hope in nursing 1: Its origins, background and nature. *British Journal of Nursing, 11*(12), 832–840.

Davidson, D. (1986). A nice derangement of epitaphs. In E. Lepore (Ed.), *Truth and Interpretation* (pp. 433–446). Oxford: Basil Blackwell.

Hanks, P. (2013). *Lexical Analysis: Norms and Exploitations*. Cambridge, MA: The MIT Press.

Hilpert, M. (2014). *Construction Grammar and Its Application to English*. Edinburgh: Edinburgh University Press.

Hymers, M. (2017). *Wittgenstein on Sensation and Perception*. New York: Routledge.

Kuusela, O. (2008). *The Struggle against Dogmatism: Wittgenstein and the Concept of Philosophy*. Cambridge, MA: Harvard University Press.

Michaelis, L. A. (2004). Type shifting in construction grammar: An integrated approach to aspectual coercion. *Cognitive Linguistics, 15*(1), 1–67.

Miller, J. F. (2007). Hope: A construct central to nursing. *Nursing Forum, 42*(1), 12–19.

Morse, J. M. (2000). Exploring pragmatic utility: Concept analysis by critically appraising the literature. In B. L. Rodgers & K. A. Knafl (Eds.), *Concept Development in Nursing: Foundations, Techniques, and Applications* (pp. 333–352). Philadelphia, PA: Saunders.

Morse, J. M. (2017). *Analyzing and Conceptualizing the Theoretical Foundations of Nursing*. New York: Springer.

Morse, J. M., Mitcham, C., Hupcey, J. E., & Tason, M. C. (1996). Criteria for concept evaluation. *Journal of Advanced Nursing, 24*, 385–390.

Norris, C. M. (1982). *Concept Clarification*. Rockville, MD: Aspen Systems Co.

Rodd, J. M. (2020). Settling into semantic space: An ambiguity-focused account of word-meaning access. *Perspectives on Psychological Science, 15*(2), 411–427.

Rodgers, B. L. (2000). Philosophical foundations of concept development. In B. L. Rodgers & K. A. Knafl (Eds.), *Concept Development in Nursing: Foundations, Techniques, and Applications* (pp. 7–37). Philadelphia, PA: Saunders.

Rodgers, B. L., Jacelon, C. S., & Knafl, K. A. (2018). Concept analysis and the advance of nursing knowledge: state of the science. *Journal of Nursing Scholarship, 50*, 451–459.

Schwartz-Barcott, D., & Kim, H. S. (2000). An expansion and elaboration of the hybrid model of concept development. In B. L. Rodgers & K. A. Knafl (Eds.), *Concept Development in Nursing: Foundations, Techniques, and Applications*. 2nd ed. Philadelphia, PA: W B Saunders.

Taylor, J. R. (2012). *The Mental Corpus: How Language is Represented in the Mind*. Oxford: Oxford University Press.

Turner, S. P. (2014). *Understanding the Tacit*. New York: Routledge.

Walker, L. O., & Avant, K. C. (2005). *Strategies for Theory Construction in Nursing*: 4th edition. Upper Saddle River, NJ: Prentice Hall.

Wiles, R., Cott, C., & Gibson, B. E. (2008). Hope, expectations and recovery from illness: A narrative synthesis of qualitative research. *Journal of Advanced Nursing, 64*(6), 564–573.

Wittgenstein, L. (1963). *Philosophical Investigations*. Oxford: Basil Blackwell.

Wittgenstein, L. (1964). *Preliminary Studies for the "Philosophical Investigations". Generally Known as the Blue and Brown Books*. Oxford: Basil Blackwell.

3 'A noun is a naming word.' Discuss.

'Concept' is a noun, and nouns are naming words. That's what it says in the dictionary. So 'concept' must be the name of something, or a class of things. Obviously, they are not *physical* things, but they must be objects of some kind: abstract entities, or mental items. They must be objects in the sense that they are identifiable, they can be distinguished from each other, and they are capable of being studied and analysed.

This is the starting position of most of the people I've discussed these matters with. What characterises it is that the metaphysics are 'read off', so to speak, from the syntax (Matthews 2007).[1] We infer what the nature of something is from the logical form of the expressions used to refer to it. In this case, 'concept' is a noun (syntax), so it must name a class of objects (metaphysics). I'll adopt Matthews' terminology, and refer to the way in which we are inclined to 'read the metaphysics off from the syntax'.

The main aim of the chapter is a modest one: to plant a few seeds of doubt concerning the claim that all nouns are 'naming words': that they are 'labels' for things and/or classes of things. I provide a number of reasons for wondering whether this is true in every case. First, while conceding that it is plausible in the case of concrete nouns, we can ask how far it applies to abstract nouns. Second, many words can be used as nouns, adjectives, verbs and adverbs; in which case, the idea that 'nouns' are naming words is problematic from the outset. Third, I suggest that there are many nouns which are difficult to construe as names because they appear in constructions from which they cannot be 'detached'.

3.1 Nouns and names

Most English speakers I have discussed this question with are convinced that nouns *are* naming words.[2] They are 'labels for objects'. It's an idea that gets locked in early. At least it was for my generation. I have a memory of sitting in a classroom, aged 10 or 11, chanting: 'A noun is a naming word, an adjective is a describing word, a verb is a doing word...'. The idea is that every word belongs to *a part of speech*, and each part of speech has a *unique function*. It is a simple and compelling picture.

Dictionaries tend to reinforce the nouns-as-naming-words picture. *Chambers*, for example, defines 'noun' like this:

noun / *(grammar) n* a word used as the name of a person, animal, thing, place or quality, or a collection of these.

Other dictionaries take basically the same line. However, the function of nouns is not always described as 'used as the name of'. 'Refer to' and 'identify' are the most popular alternatives. Merriam-Webster, for example, says that a noun can '*refer to* an entity, quality, state, action, or concept'. The Oxford Dictionary of English says that a noun 'is used to *identify* any of a class of people, places, or things'. Other verbs used to characterise what nouns do include 'represent', 'denote' and 'designate'.

The impression created is that these verbs – '*name*', '*refer to*', '*identify*' – are all used by dictionaries to denote the same relation: that is, the 'label' relation between a noun and the object, or class of objects, it corresponds to. This is illustrated in Figure 3.1. I will call this figure, and several variants, the 'naming diagram'; and I'll refer to what it illustrates as the *noun-name-object* picture.[3]

In applied linguistics and English grammar books, we find statements such as: 'The word class of *nouns* includes words that denote concrete objects in the world around us, for example *bicycle, cat, house, door, planet, vase, pencil, screen*'. This is from *Oxford Modern English Grammar* (Aarts 2011: 42). Like cats, bicycles, houses and planets – in fact, all these examples – are physical objects which can be drawn or photographed. But the obvious question is whether the naming diagram can be extended to other types of noun: abstract

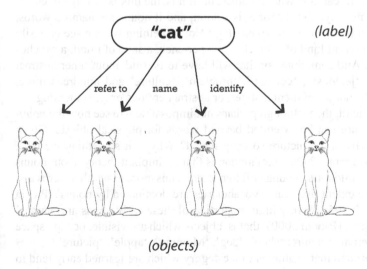

Figure 3.1 Nouns as naming words.

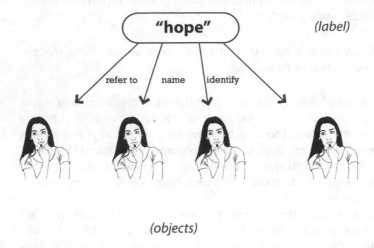

(objects)

Figure 3.2 'Hope' as a naming word.

nouns, or nouns referring to psychological states. For example, does it fit a word like 'hope'? What does the equivalent figure look like? See Figure 3.2.

Clearly, it is not possible to picture *hopes* in the way that *cats* were pictured in Figure 3.1. The best one can do, perhaps, is to have pictures of people hoping. 'These are people who are hoping; what they have are hopes'. But a picture of someone-with-hope is obviously not the same thing as a picture of the hope itself. Hope is not the sort of thing that can be pictured.

So the link between 'hope' and what it names is not, on the face of it, the same as the link between 'cat' and what it names; or, if it is, the link is clearly not established in the same way. Yet if 'hope' is a noun, and if nouns are naming words, then 'hope' must be the name of *something*.[4] Not something we can see or easily portray, but a different kind of 'object': an experience, a state of mind, a psychological process. And something similar will have to be said about other abstract nouns: 'belief', 'jealousy', 'concept', 'problem', 'culture' and hundreds more. They must be the names of mental states, or abstract entities or … something.

It is quite difficult, then – though perhaps not impossible – to see how the *noun-name-object* picture can be extended beyond words for physical objects. Given this difficulty, why is the picture so deep-seated? Why is it something we take, more or less, for granted? One explanation is that an implicit theory about nouns develops during childhood. Young children learn nouns more easily than verbs and adjectives, to the extent that 'early vocabularies are dominated by nouns' (Piccin & Waxman 2007: 295). A very high proportion of these early nouns are 'names' for physical objects (Bloom 2000); that is, objects which are visible, occupy space and have an internal structure: 'shoe', 'dog', 'Mommy', 'apple', 'picture'.[5]

It has been argued that examples of a category which are learned early tend to become the template for the category as a whole (Rosch & Mervis 1975). If this is right, and if learned-early nouns generally refer to physical objects, it would not be surprising if nouns come to be regarded, routinely, as names for objects of *some* kind. Even if the thing named by a particular noun is not a physical/ manipulable object, it is still conceptualised by analogy with objects that are. 'Manipulable object categories come to bias people's expectations about noun meanings more generally ... As a result, when someone uses a noun ... the properties of manipulable object categories become active implicitly and automatically' (Barsalou et al. 2010: 339–340). We saw an example of this in Chapter 2, with Walker and Avant (2005) talking about the 'internal structure' of concepts, 'getting inside' them and 'breaking them into simpler elements'.

It would appear, then, that the *noun-name-object* connection may be a default assumption, appearing at an early stage of language acquisition, and activated subconsciously whenever we encounter a noun. If that's all it is – an assumption – then the idea that nouns are necessarily naming words is worth probing a bit. Perhaps some nouns are not names for objects or object-like entities, whether mental or abstract.[6]

3.2 Parts of speech?

As noted briefly in Section 2.4, the *noun-name-object* picture and the dictionary-and-grammar model go together. The basic units of language, syntactically and semantically, are individual words which can be combined into sentences using grammatical rules. These rules operate on 'parts of speech'.

Take a 'naming' word	*'dog'*
Put an article and a 'describing' word in front of it	*'the small'*
Put a 'doing' word after it	*'was barking'*

'The small dog was barking'. Obviously, the rules are much more complex than this, and sentences are usually much longer and more intricate. But that's the basic idea. Syntactic rules are applied to words-qua-parts-of-speech, and each part of speech has a naming, describing or doing function. It is a widely accepted, often taken-for-granted, linguistic truth.

However, these taken-for-granted linguistic truths are not taken for granted as much as they were. In the first place, the compellingly simple idea that every word belongs to a particular part of speech, and that every part of speech has a distinct function, does not survive an inspection of words we use on a regular basis. 'Some words seem to resist part-of-speech categorization' (Taylor 2012: 68). But 'some' may understate the position. For example, there are hundreds of words that double as both nouns and verbs. Here is just a selection: nurse, study, book, drive, nest, focus, fork, hedge, branch, light, phone, handle, wipe, picture, plate, pen, wonder, dog, trouble, knot, progress, pain, fear, envy, hope. Virtually every page of the dictionary has one; and their noun forms can be concrete or abstract, count or mass.

Similarly, there are numerous words that are both nouns and adjectives: liquid, key, abstract, brief, base, antique, chief, cold, complex, cooler, evil, deep, few, firm, expert, good, first, hollow, half, high, phony, ideal, last, limp, suspect, novel, oval, rash, prize, rank, safe, second, terminal and many more. Quite a few of them are verbs as well. Other words which are both verbs and adjectives include: mellow, faint, moderate, ready, complete, clear, smooth, quiet, narrow, blunt, round, fit, clean, shy, approximate.

There is even a substantial list of words which can be nouns *and* adjectives *and* verbs *and* adverbs: for example, back, better, clean, clear, close, counter, crisscross, damn, double, down, express, fair, fast, fine, flush, forward, free, full, home, jolly, last, light, low, out, pat, plumb, prompt, quiet, right, rough, round, second, short, solo, square, tiptoe, still, upstage, true, worst, well, wholesale, wrong.

Quite where this leaves the idea that 'a noun is a naming word, a verb is a doing word, an adjective is a describing word…' is not immediately obvious.[7] It's not as if the examples listed above can plausibly be dismissed as the 'exceptions that prove the rule'. One possibility is to adjust the basic idea. Instead of saying that 'parts of speech' are *types of word*, we can suggest that they represent *types of grammatical function* a word can have. So that, for instance, the word 'jolly' can have:

A noun function	'They were out on a jolly'.
An adjective function	'He's a jolly sort of guy'.
A verb function	'You can jolly them along'.
An adverb function	'It was a jolly good show'.

This is a reasonable suggestion, and might be regarded as a simplified version of the line adopted by Croft (2001).[8] The implication is that a word like 'jolly' signifies different kinds of thing on different occasions (where 'signify' is a non-committal word referring to the appropriate relation):

Noun function	Signifying *things (not necessarily physical objects)*
Adjective function	Signifying *characteristics*
Verb function	Signifying *actions and activities*
Adverb function	Signifying *ways and methods*

At this point, the question arises as to whether a word like 'jolly' – which can be a noun, an adjective, a verb or an adverb – has the same meaning when it exercises all these functions. Alternatively, we can ask whether it expresses the same concept. The natural temptation is to think that of course it must do. It is the same word, after all, so surely it means the same, and expresses the same concept, whichever of its functions it is performing. (This is the *same-word* principle, referred to in Section 2.3.) However, there are reasons why this reaction might be more difficult to defend than we imagine. Consider, for example, the *Chambers* entry for 'jolly':

adj merry; expressing, providing or provoking fun and gaiety; entertaining, festive, jovial; healthy, plump; splendid, very agreeable.

Vt to make fun of; (*esp* with *along*) to put or keep in good humour, amuse; encourage.

Adv very.

n a party or celebration; an outing, a trip, *esp* at someone else's expense.

The adverb here is the outlier, and could be taken as a different word, given its role as an intensifier. So put that to one side. The other functions are clearly all connected through the idea of fun, good humour and enjoyment. But the connection is a fairly broad one. As an adjective, 'jolly' refers to an individual's temperament, or to his girth, or to a situation which was experienced as fun. As a verb, it has a sense of teasing, or encouraging someone for an ulterior motive ('I'll jolly him along'). The noun has the sense of an organised event – especially, as *Chambers* notes, one which someone else is paying for.

It is not obvious that these uses are all 'expressing the same concept'. There is the 'fun/enjoyment' link, but lots of other words have that too. Nor is it self-evident that an aspect of a person's character, a trip paid for by the firm and 'jolly-ing someone along' in order to achieve a particular outcome all count as 'the same concept' or 'the same meaning'. Of course, you could always make a case for it if you were so inclined. But, first, you'd have to work quite hard; and, second, it's not clear what your motive would be. Why is it so important to insist that, in all its functions, 'jolly' expresses the same concept or has the same meaning? Is it a matter of trying to make the data fit the theory? Why not just note that the word's separate functions have interestingly different (though very broadly connected) uses, and leave it at that?

This is a further intimation of a recurring theme in the book. Is it possible that the sense of a term, or the concept it expresses, depends on its grammatical function? I broached this possibility with 'chance' and 'hope' in Chapter 2. Here we can ask: does the meaning of the word 'jolly' vary (or does the concept it expresses vary) depending on whether it is acting as a noun, a verb or an adjective?

3.3 Concept analysis and mass nouns

In Section 2.4, I suggested that when concepts are referred to in the nursing literature, they are almost always identified by means of nouns or short noun phrases. For example, studies have been conducted on the concept of empowerment, the concept of resilience, the concept of clinical leadership, the concept of compassion fatigue and so on. In particular, the noun in question is virtually always a mass noun (either on its own or as part of a noun phrase). In the examples just listed, 'empowerment', 'resilience', 'fatigue' and 'leadership' are mass nouns rather than count nouns.[9]

This is partly a consequence of the syntax. If you habitually individuate concepts by means of the phrase the concept of X

where 'X' is a word or phrase without a determiner ('a' or 'the'), then that word *has* to be a mass noun.[10] If you do include the indefinite article, as in 'the concept of a nation' or 'the concept of an afterlife', then a count noun is syntactically permitted (indeed, required). But, as a matter of observed fact, this rarely happens in the nursing literature. The concept being analysed is almost always the 'concept of X', where 'X' is a mass noun (or an equivalent noun phrase).[11]

So if we were interested in 'things-that-are-jolly', and were proposing to undertake a concept analysis, it might well be described as an analysis of 'the concept of *jollity*'.

I also suggested, in Section 2.4, that identifying a concept by reference to the mass noun version of the relevant word might be too narrow, given that doing so ignores the word's inflections and derivatives. Of course, there has to be *some* way of referring to the concept being analysed. And if, conventionally, we do that by employing the mass noun, so what? It is more succinct than referring to something like:

the concept of jolly-jollies-jollity-jollify-jollification-jollily-jolliness-jolliment (including-the-various-linguistic-functions-any-of-these-words-might-have).

'The concept of jollity' is certainly more convenient than that. But the implication is that, in a concept analysis, careful note *is* taken of inflected and derivative versions of the word. One might conveniently describe the project as an analysis of 'the concept of jollity' (the argument would go), but one still pays close attention to the uses of 'jolly', 'jollies', 'jollying' and so on, as an intrinsic part of that project.

However, there is little evidence of this approach in the literature. For example, work on 'the concept of hope' in the nursing literature focuses largely on 'hope' as a mass noun, with some reference to the verb. Concept analysis studies in nursing rarely examine the details of how the inflections and derivatives of the mass noun – 'hope', 'grief', 'trust' or anything else – are used. So it is unrealistic to suggest that 'analysing the concept of X' routinely involves a study of how 'X' is used as a mass noun, count noun, adjective or verb, along with its inflection and derivatives: 'Xs', 'X-ing', 'X-ness', 'X-ful' and so on.

Rather, the assumption seems to be that an analysis of the mass noun 'X' will automatically cover these other uses. After all, the inflections/derivatives are based on the same word. They are part of the same concept. But this *is* just an assumption.[12] It's part of the standard framework. 'The concept of X' is the singularity that accounts for all uses of the word 'X' (including inflections and derivatives). Propose an analysis of X-the-mass-noun, it is assumed, and your work is done. All other possibilities are covered. But nowhere in the literature, as far as I know, is there any attempt to justify this assumption. It is an unspoken, taken-for-granted idea that has never been tested. Nor has any alternative ever been explored.

3.4 Grammar and meaning

I've been suggesting that the syntactic function of a word – whether it acts as a mass noun, count noun, adjective, verb or adverb; whether it appears in inflected/ derivative form – might affect its sense. It is not clear, for example, that there is a 'singular, unifying meaning' which hoovers up all the different jobs that 'jolly' is capable of doing. This adds another layer to what I have said already about the 'unit of meaning' not necessarily being the individual word. In Section 2.4, for example, I suggested that the constructions CHANCE TO and BY CHANCE confer two different senses on the word 'chance': in the first, 'chance' is equivalent to 'opportunity'; in the second, it is a reference to randomness, or to a lack of planning and predictability.[13] I can now add that 'chance' performs different tasks depending on whether it appears as a mass noun, count noun, adjective or verb.

(1) She had a chance to score.
(2) There's a chance that it will rain.
(3) We met by chance in Paris.
(4) Chance would be a fine thing.
(5) It was a purely chance meeting.
(6) He really chanced his arm with that shot.
(7) She chanced upon the book in Addyman's.
(8) Chances are she spotted it too.
(9) He's just a chancer.
(10) That's someone with an eye for the main chance.

(1) and (2) illustrate the difference between CHANCE TO and CHANCE THAT. In (1), 'chance' is a count noun followed by an infinitive. It is roughly synonymous with 'opportunity'. In (2) it is again a count noun, but this time followed by a noun clause. The sentence conveys the idea that it is possible that the situation referred to by the noun clause will come about. In contrast, 'chance' as a mass noun usually refers to the random, the unexpected, the unplanned, as in (3). The idea of something unexpected or random is clearly different from both the 'opportunity' sense and the 'possibility' sense, though it may be distantly related to the latter. (4) is one of the few constructions in which the mass noun is equivalent to 'opportunity'. The adjective (5) echoes the 'unplanned, random' sense of (3). With one of the verb constructions, (6), there is a shift to the idea of taking a risk in order to achieve a good outcome. In the other, (7), there is another version of the 'unplanned, random' theme – this time, however, embedded in the notion of discovery. The plural form, as in (8), reverts to the idea of probability, but with a twist: 'chances are...' is always associated with a relatively high probability that something will happen. The singular form, as in (2), merely implies that there is a possibility that it will happen. Both 'chancer' in (9) and 'the main chance' in (10) echo the sense of (1), referring to those who seek out opportunities; however, both imply that the people concerned may be unscrupulous in pursuit of their own interests.[14]

There is a wide variety of sense and reference here: bare possibility, high probability, opportunity, the unplanned, randomness, discovery, taking a risk,

selfishness, unscrupulousness. It is not that all these senses are completely unre-
lated. It is rather that it is difficult to discern a semantic 'core' in this pattern of
usage; and it is unlikely that one could formulate a definition of the 'concept of
chance' that would encompass the entire range. In any case, I am again inclined
to ask: what would motivate the attempt to formulate such a definition, other than
the assumption that there is a 'singular, unifying concept' lurking behind this variegated usage pattern, and that the concept in question can be defined? But where
does this assumption come from, and what justifies it, other than the fact that it is
so rarely questioned? Why not just study the pattern, trace out the network of use,
and leave it at that? Why insist that there must be a 'unifying something', called a
'concept', hidden beneath the network?[15]

In both 'chance' and 'jolly' examples, we see how different constructions combine with the different grammatical functions of each word to produce a specific
meaning, one which is not necessarily shared by other combinations. This is the
kind of evidence which makes the assumption that individual words are the basic
'units of meaning' look questionable. I am not, of course, claiming that this evidence is in any sense conclusive. However, evidence of the same kind will continue to pile up throughout the book.

Croft (2001) sees the view that constructions, rather than words or parts of
speech, are the basic units of meaning as nonreductionist. Though his main concern
is grammar, he argues that 'the same arguments against reductionist theories of
syntactic representation also apply to reductionist theories of ... semantic representation' (61). This again implies that we should abandon the idea that the meaning
of individual words can necessarily be defined in isolation, along with the idea that
there is always such a thing as '*the* concept of...' associated with any given word.

3.5 Verbs, prepositions and conjunctions as nouns

Early in the *Philosophical Investigations*, Wittgenstein presents us with a list of
exclamations:

Water!   Help!
Away!   Fine!
Ow!   No!

He then asks: 'Are you inclined still to call these words "names of objects"?'
(Wittgenstein 1963, §27). Here is one reaction: 'Well, obviously not. But these
are exclamations, not nouns. Nobody imagines that exclamations are the names of
anything'. This is an entirely reasonable point to make. Accordingly, my plan in
the rest of the chapter is to pursue Wittgenstein's line of thought, but using nouns
(words-acting-as-nouns) instead of exclamations. My question will be the same
as his, though. For each of the nouns I discuss, I will ask: 'Are you still inclined to
say that this word is the "name of an object", or the "name of a class of objects"?'

Given the discussion of the last three sections, I'm going to start with words
that are not usually thought of as nouns. For example, we usually think of 'say' as

a verb, 'while' as a conjunction and 'out' as an adverb or preposition. But all of them can be used as nouns, and frequently are:

(11) Let him have his say.
(12) She had an account with them for a short while.
(13) He had an out, but he wasn't going to reveal it yet.
(14) We didn't discuss the ins and outs.

So the Wittgensteinian question: in these examples, are the nouns 'say', 'while', 'out' and 'in' names of objects or classes of objects? Is there a class of 'says' that people can have, with 'his say' in (11) being one of them? Is there a class of 'whiles' of varying lengths, the example in (12) being a short one? How about a class of 'ins', a class of 'outs'? Are there perhaps two types of 'out', the one in (13) being a form of escape or avoidance, and the one in (14) being related to 'details'?

One interesting response to the Wittgensteinian question is this. Someone may point out that 'for a short while' is an adverbial phrase. You could call it an idiomatic compound adverb, more or less equivalent to 'briefly'. Perhaps we should not expect individual words in phrases of this kind to behave normally. Just because 'while' in (12) is preceded by the indefinite article and an adjective, we should not insist that it is acting as a noun. Instead, we should just see it as part of a stock phrase, and not worry too much about what part of speech it happens to be *in* that phrase. Something similar could be said about 'ins and outs'. It is an idiomatic stock phrase, which in (14) happens to be the object of a transitive verb. So let's not attach too much significance to that. See 'the ins and outs' as a syntactically unusual noun phrase, equivalent to 'the details', and don't bother unduly about which parts of speech its constituent words are.

Anyone making these points is starting to get a feel for Construction Grammar. The idea that we should take phrases like 'for a short while' or 'ins and outs' as syntactic/semantic units, and focus on what they signify *as* a unit, without obsessing over the syntax of their constituents, is already tilting in that sort of direction. There's a fair way to go before I can plausibly suggest that 'concept' is no more the name of something than 'while' in (12) is. But at least, with this kind of concession, I do have a foot in the door.

With the idea of opening the door a fraction further, let me offer a few more examples of 'other parts of speech' acting as nouns. They are not all *that* unusual.

(15) Well, he had a go.
(16) It was all of a sudden.
(17) We're having a bit of a do.
(18) They gave it the once-over.
(19) She gave him the go-ahead.
(20) I'm going to give him what-for.

As before, it is entirely possible to stick to the view that, in these examples, 'go', 'sudden', 'what for', 'once-over', 'go-ahead' and 'do' are naming words.

Personally, I think this is least convincing with 'sudden' and 'what-for'. I find it hard to imagine that there is a class of 'suddens', of which the 'a sudden' in (16) is one. Similarly, it's hard to believe that there is a class of 'what-fors', including the one in (20). Still, I accept that, for some people, there are goes, dos, once-overs and go-aheads, all of which form groups of 'things', events or actions with corresponding names. We will be returning to these disparate reactions more than once.

3.6 Complex prepositions and grammaticalisation

In the previous section, I mentioned the possibility that 'for a short while' and the 'ins and outs' might be considered as semantic/syntactic units, rather than as phrases in which 'while', 'ins' and 'outs' are functioning independently as nouns-understood-as-naming-words. There are many similar examples. Consider this brief passage from *Robinson Crusoe*:

(21) In this manner, we came in view of the entrance of a wood, through which we were to pass, at the farther side of the plain...

In this sentence, the phrase 'in view of' refers to vision. Crusoe and his companions reach a point where they can *see* the entrance to a wood. This is apparently typical of authors born before 1800 (Hoffmann 2005: 54), who use 'in view of' in a 'literal' sense to describe a situation in which a building or a feature of the landscape becomes visible. Contrast an example of the same phrase from modern English:

(22) In view of recent events, we will be changing the procedure.
(23) In view of the risk, I don't think we should do that.

Here, 'in view of' no longer refers to 'literal' seeing; nor does it refer to motion, as 'came in view' does. Its sense is closer to 'taking account of', or 'because of', or 'owing to'. It cites a/the *reason* for changing the procedure, or for 'not doing that'. In the older version of the phrase, 'view' is unmistakeably a noun, even though it occurs inside the phrase. It is the same word as 'view' in:

(24) We had a good view of the bridge.
(25) There are superb views from the top.
(26) The view from here is amazing.

In these examples, 'view' can take the indefinite article (24), or the definite article (26). It is modified by attributive adjectives (24, 25), and can be in the plural (25). None of these possibilities applies to 'view' in (22) or (23). Yet, considered in isolation, the latter is still a noun.

Back to the Wittgensteinian question. For the sake of argument, let us say that 'view' in (24), (25) and (26) is the name of a certain kind of situation, experience or relation.[16] But what about 'view' in (22) and (23)? Is it the name of anything in those examples? If so, what sort of anything?

As in Section 3.5, it is still possible to answer 'yes' to the first of these questions. (It's always possible to stick with the *noun-name-object* picture.) If you do think that 'view' as used in (22) and (23) is the name of something, then you are likely to answer the second question by saying that what it names is a sort of taking-into-account, a perspective or an assessment. Something of that kind. 'In view of...' would then be equivalent to 'from the perspective of...', or 'having made an assessment of...'; and perhaps we can be more comfortable with 'perspective' and 'assessment' as naming words than with 'view'.

Of course, I could argue against this response. I could say that it is the *whole phrase* 'in view of', not just 'view' by itself, that is the equivalent of 'taking into account'. There is a definite article in 'from the perspective of', and an indefinite article in 'having made an assessment of': neither is possible with 'in view of'. 'From the perspective of' misses the *because of* sense of 'in view of'. If points of this kind are convincing, none of the proposed equivalences is successful. However, someone who wants to stick with the *noun-name-object* picture may feel inclined to dismiss such arguments as linguistic hair-splitting. So let's change tack slightly.

'In view of' is one of a large number of COMPLEX PREPOSITIONS. That is to say, the *phrase as a whole* is regarded as syntactically equivalent to a single-word preposition like 'towards', 'for' or 'with'. They are 'treated as single units of grammar' (Hoffmann 2005: 1), even though they take the form of three or more words, usually PREPOSITION-NOUN-PREPOSITION. I say 'a large number': one dictionary of English complex prepositions lists 1,084 different constructions which take a similar form (Klégr 2002). The standard, and most accessible, work examines 30 of these complex prepositions, the ones which appear most frequently in the British National Corpus. Here are some of them (Hoffmann 2005):

In terms of	In relation to	On behalf of
In favour of	In addition to	With respect to
In spite of	In accordance with	With regard to
In view of	In line with	By virtue of
In excess of	In common with	By way of

We can ask the Wittgensteinian question of each of the nouns in these phrases. Is 'behalf' the name of something? Is 'common'? How about 'spite', 'way' and 'accordance'? Of course, 'spite' *is* the name of a motive or emotion. But this is clearly not what it means in the phrase 'in spite of' (which has a single-word equivalent: 'despite'). So if it is a name in that phrase, what sort of thing is being named?

'Behalf' is even harder to think of as a name (see Section 2.4). Is there a class of behalf-objects (called 'behalves'?) for which it is the label? It feels like a very odd idea. It's difficult to construe 'behalf' as an abstract quasi-object, because it cannot be used with a determiner. It's not possible to write 'the behalf', or 'a behalf', or 'this behalf', or 'some behalf'. The fact is that 'behalf' never appears outside the phrase 'on behalf of...' or a variation of it ('on my own behalf', 'on their behalf', 'on her behalf'). 'On behalf of' is a complex preposition, and behaves just as a single-word preposition would. Compare 'I did it on behalf of Martha' with 'I did it for Martha'. The two sentences are not synonymous, but 'on behalf of' fits the same grammatical slot as 'for'. The problem arises when we detach the noun part of the phrase, 'behalf', and treat it as a separate, disconnected noun ... and then ask what it is the name of.[17]

However, 'behalf' cannot stand, syntactically, on its own. It doesn't function as a stand-alone noun even though, if we assign it to a part-of-speech category, it's not obvious what else we can call it. At the same time, semantically, it does not appear to label a class of abstract things ('the class of behalves') or a type of abstract stuff ('samples of behalf'). Somebody committed to the *noun-name-object* picture in all cases has a bit of wriggling to do with this one.

I think the wriggling would continue with many of the nouns listed above, even though most of them do occur outside the complex prepositions they appear in (unlike 'behalf' and 'accordance'). Words such as 'regard', 'respect', 'spite', 'view', 'terms', 'virtue' and 'way' have uses outside the complex preposition, and it is possible to argue that these uses do involve naming. But their senses *inside* the construction do not coincide with their senses *outside* it; and if we ask what the 'inside' version of the noun is the name of, it's difficult to come up with a persuasive answer.

Complex prepositions of the kind studied by Hoffman are examples of something linguists refer to as 'grammaticalisation'. This is a process whereby certain words which are 'concrete', and which refer to objects, actions, events or situations, lose this 'content' – at least in a specific construction – and come to have a content-depleted syntactic function. 'View' is a good example. Originally, the phrase 'in view of' exploited the 'able to see' sense of 'view' (21). *Outside* that phrase, of course, 'view' still retains this sense: (24), (25), (26). *Inside* the phrase, however, it loses the 'able to see' meaning, and is absorbed into a complex preposition. In effect, it loses its lexical identity, and adopts a purely grammatical function as part of a larger unit. The expression often used to describe this loss of content is 'semantic bleaching' (Hopper & Traugott 2003). 'This semantic change from concrete to more abstract meanings is a typical feature of grammaticalization' (Hoffmann 2005: 54).

There is clearly a link between the idea of grammaticalisation and CxG. 'In view of' is an example of a construction which is, in itself, a basic unit of meaning. It is not a phrase whose use can be inferred by considering the 'unit-meaning' of 'view', combined with 'in' and 'of'. It cannot be 'decomposed' into its 'constituents', so its function is not derivable from the individual meaning of its elements.[18] It does not, in other words, work according to the dictionary-and-grammar-book model.

There are several other groups of grammaticalised expressions similar to these. One group consists of 'size' nouns: 'pile', 'scrap', 'whiff' and so on. In 'not a scrap of evidence', for example, 'not a scrap of' is a 'grammaticalized quantifier'

(Brems 2007: 294). The whole phrase is the equivalent of 'no': 'scrap' does not function independently as a 'naming' noun. Another group consists of 'amount' nouns: 'loads of', 'a lack of', 'a number of'. In the expression 'loads of people', the phrase 'loads of' is another grammaticalised quantifier (Brems 2010). It is the equivalent of 'many'. A third group consists of 'type' nouns: 'type' itself, 'kind', 'sort' (De Smedt et al. 2015). Grammaticalised expressions of this kind, and others like them, are all interesting. Unfortunately I don't have the space to discuss them fully.

3.7 Non-detachable nouns

At this point, we can return to the more general idea that constructions are syntactically and semantically primary, and that the 'meanings' of individual words are derivative. If that's right, complex prepositions are a special case. What is different about them is that a noun which is part of the construction has been 'bleached' of its lexical content, and now performs a purely grammatical function. The more usual case, as I suggested in Section 2.4, is that the noun is 'coerced' to have sense *A* by one construction and sense *B* by another construction. 'Chance', for example, is roughly equivalent to 'opportunity' in the CHANCE TO + INFINITIVE construction, but references possibility in the CHANCE THAT + CLAUSE construction.

The mechanism of 'coercion' is common to both examples. In a complex preposition like 'in view of', the construction coerces the noun into a semantically bleached state (a result of the grammaticalisation process). The two 'chance' constructions, by contrast, coerce the noun into one of two corresponding senses. Or a different way of putting it: some constructions coerce the noun into one sense or another; complex prepositions coerce the central noun into a 'zero' sense. The principle of coercion is the same, but the outcome varies.

With some constructions, the noun is, I will suggest, *non-detachable*. It is somewhat easier to make the case for this with complex prepositions because it is more of a stretch to argue that nouns like 'behalf', 'spite', 'sake', 'common', 'way' or 'accordance' are naming words (in the context of the constructions in which they appear). My own inclination is to say that if you disconnect 'behalf' from 'on behalf of', it is very difficult to believe that it names anything. Ditto for 'spite' detached from 'in spite of', and 'sake' detached from 'for the sake of'.[19]

Claims about the non-detachability of the noun might meet with greater resistance in some other cases. It might be tempting, for example, to say that 'way', even in 'by way of', is a naming word. And for some uses of this phrase, this is not implausible. For example:

(27) He travelled from London to Norwich by way of Colchester.

Here, one could argue that 'way' is the name of an indefinitely large class of routes, which are typically identified by mentioning a place situated somewhere between two other places. In this instance it is used to refer to one such route: the 'Colchester' route from London to Norwich. But consider now a different use:

(28)   Take, by way of example, a nurse exceptionally devoted to her patients.

In this case, it is stretching it a bit to say that 'way' is the name of anything – and quite tricky, if you do feel that way inclined, to say what kind of thing it is the name of. In (28), 'way' does not refer to a route, not even metaphorically. The best way of explaining what the phrase 'by way of' means in this example is to say that is roughly equivalent to 'as':

(29)   Take, as an example, a nurse exceptionally devoted to her patients.

But 'as' in (29) is not equivalent to 'way' in (28). Rather, it is equivalent to 'by way of' in (28). This is to explain the whole phrase, 'by way of', by substituting a single-word preposition in its place. In effect, you have replaced one (complex) preposition with another (simple) one.[20] It makes it rather difficult to believe that 'way' in (28) really is the name of something. This is another case of grammaticalisation. I would say much the same about all the complex prepositions listed in the previous section.

I have made an initial case for non-detachability with complex prepositions, because I think it's easier to see in those examples. However, I now want to go a step further and suggest that other constructions are characterised by non-detachability too. Not all constructions. Just some. Starting at the easiest end of the spectrum again, consider some examples (I apologise for the greater-than-usual Anglo-centrism, which is inevitable with idiom):

(30)   You're taking the mickey, aren't you?
(31)   For an hour, they made good headway.
(32)   I picked up a few odds and ends.
(33)   I'm afraid he's kicked the bucket.
(34)   They gave him short shrift.
(35)   He really bore the brunt of it.
(36)   We've left it in abeyance.
(37)   It will stand you in good stead.
(38)   He was released on his own recognisance.

It's a trifle optimistic, I think, to suggest that the nouns in these constructions are naming words. What do they name? What class of thing is 'mickey' the name of (and how, or where, do you 'take' it)? How about 'stead'? What kinds of things are 'abeyances' and 'headways'? What sort of entity is the 'bucket' that was kicked? We can explain what 'he's kicked the bucket' means; but we do that by explaining, the *whole phrase*. So we can agree that 'he's kicked the bucket' is an idiomatic expression meaning 'he's died'. That still doesn't answer the question 'What is "bucket" in this construction the name of?'. And that's because the only possible answer is: 'In that construction, it isn't the name of anything'.

So the idea here is that some constructions include nouns which are non-detachable. They do not have an individual 'meaning' independently of the construction they are part of. They don't *name* anything. They are not 'labels' for classes of abstract objects, quasi-objects or metaphorical 'things' of any other kind. It is difficult to see how they can be slotted into the 'objects' line of the 'naming diagram' (Figure 3.1), taking the place of cats.

3.8 'Concept' as a non-detachable noun

I have grounded the initial case for non-detachability at the simple end of the spectrum: idioms; verbs, conjunctions and adverbs functioning as nouns; complex prepositions; 'size' nouns, 'amount' nouns, 'type' nouns. But where else would I start? If I am trying to persuade you that some nouns don't name anything, and I'm anticipating resistance, then I'll obviously begin with the cases that are easiest to see and least likely to provoke an argument.

However, I'm now going to fast-forward a couple of chapters, and plant a suggestion that will probably meet with more resistance than the non-detachability of 'behalf', 'sake', 'mickey', 'loads' or 'a sudden'. It's this: suppose that, in some constructions, 'concept' is a non-detachable noun. For example:

(39) Patients need to understand the concept of risk.
(40) I'm trying to grasp the concept of a marionette sex scene.
(41) Hospitals are starting to apply the concept of futile treatment.
(42) You don't possess the concept of a negative number by having debts.

The suggestion is that expressions such as 'understand the concept of X', 'possess the concept of X', 'grasp the concept of X' and 'acquire the concept of X' are basic units-of-meaning from which the noun 'concept' cannot be detached.[21] They are not *exactly* like 'take the mickey', or 'on behalf of', or 'leave in abeyance', or 'a type of'; but those examples can stand as models for one of the arguments in Chapter 5. And if 'mickey' and 'type' are not, in their respective constructions, the names of anything, then I will want to say the same about 'concept'. As a non-detachable noun, and in 'the concept of...' constructions illustrated by (39) to (42), there is nothing that it names.[22]

To many readers, this will seem far-fetched, too much of a leap from complex prepositions and 'taking the mickey'. It *is* a leap. As I say, I'm anticipating stuff that won't be developed fully until Chapter 5. But I want to plant the suggestion now, so you can be thinking about it. As before, it is not so much a question of trying to persuade yourself that it's true or, alternatively, simply dismissing the idea. Rather, it's a matter of getting used to the possibility, and perhaps trying it on for size.

I should add that this is not the *only* thing I will be saying about 'concept' and 'the concept of...' The 'understanding', 'applying' and 'possessing' constructions are not the only ones that 'concept' occurs in. There many more. But we have to start somewhere and, for the time being, I am doing no more than providing a brief illustration of what suggesting that 'concept' is a *non*-naming noun might imply.

3.9 The modest conclusion

This chapter's conclusions are, as I suggested at the outset, modest. The discussion has been little more than a preliminary softening-up exercise. The idea has been to plant a few seeds of doubt by suggesting that some abstract nouns might not be naming words. To this end, I've presented a number of examples for the reader's consideration, and added a further layer to the ongoing account of CxG.

However, a number of questions emerge from this chapter. What, actually, *is* a 'naming word'? What other functions do nouns (or words-acting-as-nouns) have? Perhaps some of them are grammaticalised in certain idiomatic phrases, but this surely cannot apply across the board, not even to abstract nouns. If a noun isn't naming something on a given occasion, what precisely is it doing? How do we distinguish between nouns which *are* names and those which aren't? Or between circumstances in which a certain noun *is* naming and circumstances in which it isn't? In the next chapter, I'll try to answer some of these questions.

Notes

1 Matthews uses this expression on several occasions, for example pages 6, 14, 98. However, his example of 'reading off' is different from mine.
2 'It's probably ... correct to describe the simple notion that noun phrases refer to objects in the world as a notion of folk semantics' (Azzouni 2013: 351).
3 The family of philosophical ideas supporting the *noun-name-object* picture is described succinctly in Baker and Hacker (2005: 4–6).
4 In the nursing literature, it is generally assumed that 'hope' is the name of an *inner something*; that is, something in the mind. ('Cake' is the name of something in the tin; 'hope' is the name of something in the mind.) In Chapters 8–10, I'll suggest that this assumption is inconsistent with how the word 'hope' is actually used.
5 The full story is, inevitably, far more complex than this. See Tomasello (2003), especially Chapter 3, and Diessel (2013).
6 Baz (2017: 148) points out that most empirical studies of first language acquisition focus on 'words denoting middle-sized observable objects'. So there is virtually no evidence about how words which don't fit that category (abstract nouns, for example) are learned – unless, as he says, 'one *presupposes* that all words function in more or less the same way and are acquired in more or less the same way'.
7 'The allocation of a word to one of the standardly recognized lexical categories, such as noun, verb, or adjective ... is grossly inadequate as a guide to the word's use in the language' (Taylor 2012: 280–1).
8 Croft's technical account refers to the 'functions of reference, predication and modification' (Croft 2000: 87). These correspond – in English, and only roughly – to the noun function, verb function and adjective/adverb function respectively.
9 This does not apply to philosophy and psychology. These disciplines talk routinely about the concept DOG, or the concept WATER, or the concept CHAIR (using the typographical device mentioned in Section 1.7). However, philosophers generally undertake analyses of concepts such as KNOWLEDGE or HOPE. Interestingly, though, it is the verbal forms they focus on. The analysis begins with a sentence schema such as 'A knows that p', or 'A hopes that p'; and the idea is to specify the conditions that must obtain if a sentence of that form is to be true. The concept is identified through the mass noun; but the analysis is of the verb.
10 Or possibly the other way round. It's not that the absence of a determiner requires the 'selection' of a mass noun. It's rather that, if there is no determiner between 'of' and

the noun following it – 'bowl of water', 'concept of hope' – then the noun is classified as having a mass noun function. In this regard, it's worth adding that some writers in linguistics suggest that many nouns, and possibly the majority, can be both mass and count (Kiss et al. 2017). These are 'dual-life' nouns. 'Hope' is one example. See Section 8.1 for more.

11 As observed earlier, where 'X' is a noun phrase, it usually consists of a mass noun preceded by an adjective (or a noun acting as an adjective). For example: clinical leadership, compassion fatigue, moral distress, job satisfaction.

12 Construction Grammar stands this assumption on its head, acknowledging that 'inflected forms may develop some independence with regard to their respective meanings' (Hilpert 2014: 70).

13 I am here making use of the typographical convention introduced in Section 1.10.

14 It is not unusual for morphological variations to be associated with semantic differences. For instance, the singular/plural difference, illustrated here by 'chance' and 'chances', can be found with several other words. One example is 'spectacle' and 'spectacles'. The singular refers to a visually striking scene. The plural is usually used to refer to a pair of glasses (although it can, of course, refer to spectacular scenes). Other examples include: 'custom'/'customs', 'manner'/'manners', 'expense'/'expenses' and 'wood'/'woods'. Similarly with the difference between noun and adjective, particularly when the adjective takes a slightly modified form. For example, 'fishy' can mean smelling or tasting like fish; but more than half the examples in COCA mean 'suspicious'. These examples are interesting given that 'hope', 'hopes' and 'hopeful' exhibit comparable differences, as we will see in Part II.

15 'I'm saying that these phenomena have no one thing in common which makes us use the same word for all, – but that they are related to one another in many different ways' (Wittgenstein 1963, §65). Kuusela's discussion is useful: 'The different components or facets [of a word] need not be reducible to some single basic linguistic function … Rather, to understand the word's use, and the concept its use overall makes up, we need to comprehend the word's use more widely' (Kuusela 2019: 158–9). Notice, in particular, Kuusela's understanding of 'concept' as a reference to the word's overall pattern of use, and compare this idea to my Second Picture (Figure 2.1).

16 Even in these examples, 'view' counts as an abstract noun. So its ontology is somewhat in doubt. 'Situation, experience or relation' will do to be going on with. I don't think a lot hangs on the point.

17 In effect, an expression like 'on behalf of' functions as a single word rather than three. If 'for' in 'I did it for Martha' is a single-word preposition, then why not 'onbehalfof' in 'I did it onbehalfof Martha'? This gives us a way of understanding the non-detachability of 'behalf'.

18 So, again, we can think of it as a single word: 'Inviewof recent events…', which is akin to: 'Given recent events…'

19 Dennett (2010) describes expressions such as 'on behalf of' and 'for the sake of' as *fused*, and argues that 'behalf' and 'sake' are *non-referential*. He goes on to ask whether some 'mental entity' words are non-referential in a comparable way, and explores the implications of 'treating all sentences containing mental entity terms as tentatively fused' (16). If one considers the many formulaic expressions that include the word 'mind' – to say nothing of other 'mental' terms – it becomes apparent that this idea cannot be dismissed out of hand: 'make up one's mind', 'all in the mind', 'keep in mind', 'bear in mind', 'state of mind', 'to my mind', 'peace of mind', 'bring to mind', 'cross one's mind', 'an open mind', 'a piece of my mind', 'half a mind' and a lot more. My 'non-detachable' is not quite the same as Dennett's 'non-referential'; but I will, in effect, be suggesting that the expression 'the concept of…' is fused.

20 This is another example of three words functioning as a single word: 'Bywayof example…', This is equivalent to: 'As an example…', or even 'For example…'.

21 Austin (1961) is characteristically wry about the acquiring/possession metaphor, noting that a concept is often treated 'as an article of property, a pretty straightforward piece of goods, which comes into my "possession" … whether I do possess it or not is, apparently, ascertained simply by making an inventory of the "furniture" in my mind' (10). As Austin implies, it's very tempting to take the verbs 'possessing', 'having' and 'acquiring' too literally. 'She has acquired the concept', in certain contexts, is a useful and accurate thing to say. But its usefulness doesn't mean that there is a *something* she has *obtained*. It's the pictures associated with the physical acts of grasping, possessing, acquiring and so on that mislead. I'll say a lot more about this in Chapters 5 and 6.

22 Playing with the idea in notes 17 to 20, and in order to dramatise the 'non-detachability' idea, I might suggest that we understand 'the concept of risk' as 'theconceptof risk'. It is, in Dennett's terms, fused. There is a very similar, but slightly different, way of looking at it. We can think of the expression 'the concept of' as an example of formulaic language: a 'prefabricated' expression, retrieved from memory as a unit rather than being constructed, on each occasion, from its 'constituents'. It is generally agreed that there are thousands of such prefabricated strings in English. See Wray (2002), Chapter 1.

References

Aarts, B. (2011). *Oxford Modern English Grammar*. Oxford: Oxford University Press.

Austin, J. L. (1961). *Philosophical Papers*. Oxford: Clarendon Press.

Azzouni, J. (2013). *Semantic Perception: How the Illusion of a Common Language Arises and Persists*. New York: Oxford University Press.

Baker, G. P., & Hacker, P. M. S. (2005). *Wittgenstein: Understanding and Meaning. Volume 1 of An Analytical Commentary on the Philosophical Investigations: Part I - Essays*. 2nd ed. Extensively Revised by P. M. S. Hacker. Oxford: Blackwell Publishing.

Barsalou, L. W., Wilson, C. D., & Hasenkamp, W. (2010). On the vices of nominalization and the virtues of contextualizing. In B. Mesquita, L. F. Barrett, & E. R. Smith (Eds.), *The Mind in Context* (pp. 334–360). New York: The Guilford Press.

Baz, A. (2017). *The Crisis of Method in Contemporary Analytic Philosophy*. Oxford: Oxford University Press.

Bloom, P. (2000). *How Children Learn the Meaning of Words*. Cambridge, MA: The MIT Press.

Brems, L. (2007). The grammaticalization of small size nouns: Reconsidering frequency and analogy. *Journal of English Linguistics*, *35*, 293–324.

Brems, L. (2010). Size noun constructions as collocationally constrained constructions: Lexical and grammaticalized uses. *English Language and Linguistics*, *14*(1), 83–109.

Croft, W. A. (2000). Parts of speech as language universals and as language-particular categories. In P. M. Vogel & B. Comrie (Eds.), *Approaches to the Typology of Word Classes* (pp. 65–102). Berlin: Mouton de Gruyter.

Croft, W. A. (2001). *Radical Construction Grammar: Syntactic Theory in Typological Perspective*. Oxford: Oxford University Press.

De Smedt, L., Brems, L., & Davidse, K. (2015). NP-internal functions and extended uses of the 'type' nouns kind, sort, and type: towards a comprehensive, corpus-based description. In R. Facchinetti (Ed.), *Corpus Linguistics 25 Years On* (pp. 225–255). Leiden: Brill.

Dennett, D. C. (2010). *Content and Consciousness: Routledge Classics*. Abingdon, UK: Routledge.

Diessel, H. (2013). Construction grammar and first language acquisition. In G. Trousdale & T. Hoffman (Eds.), *The Oxford Handbook of Construction Grammar* (pp. 347–364). New York: Oxford University Press.

Hilpert, M. (2014). *Construction Grammar and Its Application to English*. Edinburgh: Edinburgh University Press.

Hoffmann, S. (2005). *Grammaticalization and English Complex Prepositions: A Corpus-Based Study*. Abingdon, UK: Routledge.

Hopper, P. J., & Traugott, E. C. (2003). *Grammaticalization*. 2nd ed. Cambridge, UK: Cambridge University Press.

Kiss, T., Pelletier, F. J., Husić, H., & Poppek, J. (2017). Issues of mass and count: Dealing with 'dual life' nouns. In *Proceedings of the 6th Joint Conference on Lexical and Computational Semantics* (pp. 189–198). Vancouver: Association for Computational Linguistics.

Klégr, A. (2002). *English Complex Prepositions of the Type 'In Spite Of' and Analogous Sequences*. Prague: The Karolinum Press.

Kuusela, O. (2019). *Wittgenstein on Logic as the Method of Philosophy: Re-examining the Roots and Development of Analytic Philosophy*. Oxford: Oxford University Press.

Matthews, R. J. (2007). *The Measure of Mind: Propositional Attitudes and Their Attribution*. New York: Oxford University Press.

Piccin, T. B., & Waxman, S. R. (2007). Why nouns trump verbs in word learning: New evidence from children and adults in the Human Simulation Paradigm. *Language Learning and Development*, *3*(4), 295–323.

Rosch, E., & Mervis, C. B. (1975). Family resemblances: Studies in the internal structure of categories. *Cognitive Psychology*, *7*(4), 573–605.

Taylor, J. R. (2012). *The Mental Corpus: How Language is Represented in the Mind*. Oxford: Oxford University Press.

Tomasello, M. (2003). *Constructing a Language: A Usage-Based Theory of Language Acquisition*. Cambridge, MA: Harvard University Press.

Walker, L. O., & Avant, K. C. (2005). *Strategies for Theory Construction in Nursing*. 4th ed. Upper Saddle River, NJ: Prentice Hall.

Wittgenstein, L. (1963). *Philosophical Investigations*. Oxford: Basil Blackwell.

Wray, A. (2002). *Formulaic Language and the Lexicon*. Cambridge, UK: Cambridge University Press.

4   Referring without identifying or describing

So far, I have been suggesting that not all nouns are naming words; or, to put it more precisely, I've been suggesting that, when *some* words function as a noun, they do not necessarily 'name' anything. Whether they do or not may depend, and often does depend, on what construction they occur in. 'Behalf' is never a name (or so I argued). In contrast, 'view' can be construed as naming something in a sentence such as 'There is a terrific view up here'; but it does not name anything in a sentence such as: 'In view of recent events, I have decided not to go'. However, I have not as yet been particularly clear about what *counts* as 'naming'; nor have I said much about what else a noun can be employed to do when it is not 'naming' anything. In this chapter, I try to rectify both deficits.

4.1 The terminology

The title of this chapter mentions three terms, and it is essential to understand what I intend by each of them, since they refer to different activities. I think my use of these words corresponds, very roughly, to general usage (but not necessarily to philosophical usage: I'll say more about that later). However, if you have any doubts on that score, treat my account as a series of stipulations.

I'll introduce the sense I give to the key terms by means of some simple scenarios.

[1] A What shall we call it?
    B How about a 'flask-tie'?
    A Good idea!

A and B have just invented a device which is basically a tie with a hidden pouch. It holds liquid that can be drunk through a straw. They decide to call it a 'flask-tie'. This is a case of *naming*: suggesting a label for a previously unnamed category of items.[1] However, see scenario [3].

[2] A What is that?
    B It's a fossa.

Here, we can assume that A is pointing to an animal he is unfamiliar with. B identifies it as a fossa (an animal indigenous to Madagascar). This is a case of *identifying*: saying what species the animal belongs to by using the name of that species. However, see scenario [3].

[3] A Name that tune!
   B Over The Rainbow.

A and B are playing a game, in which contestants are invited to recall the name of a tune. However, they are not asked to 'name' the tune in the sense of scenario [1]. A is not saying: 'Think of a name for this tune'. He is saying: 'What is the name/title of this tune?' 'Name' is ambiguous as a verb. It can mean thinking of a name for something, or identifying something. Either inventing a name, or retrieving it. This, then, is another case of *identifying*. Scenarios [2] and [3] are the same, except that in scenario [3] the item is said to be 'named' not 'identified'.

[4] A So describe a fossa to me...?
   B It looks like a cat, but it's related to the mongoose family. It's like a small cougar, but with a slender body, and has a mongoose-like head, but with a short muzzle and large ears. Indigenous to Madagascar.

B describes a fossa, as requested. In doing so, she describes its appearance, and makes a broad reference to the taxonomy. This, then, is a case of *describing*. It's important to recognise that, by itself, the word 'fossa' does not describe the species. It is just the name of it. It is, if you like, a label. 'Fossa' does not 'mean' the description B gives, or any description like it.[2]

[5] A Look at that!
   B Good lord. What is it?

A is presumably pointing to something, or in some other way drawing B's attention to it. This is a case of *demonstrative reference*. A does the same, of course, in scenario [2]. In both cases, A is referring to an (as yet unidentified) object by gesturing (perhaps) and using a demonstrative ('that!'). Neither A nor B identifies the object; nor do they describe it.

[6] A What do you want?
   B My coat, my handbag, my phone, and my umbrella.

Here, in answer to A's question, B specifies the items that she wants to retrieve from her room. This is a case of *identifying reference*.

[7] A What do you want?
   B My things.

Same scenario, except that B now refers to the items she wants to retrieve, but does not identify/specify them. The reference is, of course, extremely vague; but, in context, the sort of thing she has in mind will usually be clear. Here, a hotel guest seeking access to her room before going out for the day is likely to be thinking of items such as those mentioned in scenario [6], and will be understood in that way.[3] This is another case of referring, but to something not present, and without identifying, specifying or itemising. I will refer to this as *non-identifying reference*, or sometimes *vague reference*.

[8] A I've just come across a new word: 'fossa'. What does it mean?
    B Ah, that's the name of an animal indigenous to Madagascar. Related to the
    mongoose family.

As in scenario [4], B describes fossae, but more sketchily. Her main point is that 'fossa' is the name of a particular kind of animal. Instead of '… is the name of …', she could have used the word '*denotes*': 'Ah, that word denotes an animal indigenous to Madagascar…'. Either way, B says something about *what the word does*. It names, or denotes, a species. So this illustrates *denotation*.

4.2 Different activities

The significance of this set of distinctions is as follows. Identifying, referring and describing – as I will be using the words – are different activities. You can *refer* without describing or identifying ('He wants his stuff'). You can *describe* without identifying ('It is green with a big tail'). You can *identify* without describing ('It is a peacock'). In the latter two examples, there's also some referring going on ('it'), since the fact that referring and describing are different activities does not mean they can't be combined.

   The primary use I will make of these distinctions is to draw attention to the possibility that we can refer to something *without identifying or describing it*. This is what I am calling 'non-identifying reference' or 'vague reference'; and it is an extremely useful thing to be able to do (for reasons that will emerge later). Some nouns, such as 'thing' and 'stuff', are especially good it; but other nouns, which also straddle the boundary between 'abstract' and 'concrete', can be used in the same way. In Section 4.7, I will discuss a number of nouns that can do this 'referring-without-identifying' job. As for 'thing', I'll say more about it in Section 4.4. Then, in Chapter 5, I will suggest that the noun 'concept' can, and often does, perform the same task.

Reader: Just a minute. Could we go back to scenario 4? The word doesn't describe?
Me: Correct. 'Fossa' is the name, the label, for that species. It doesn't describe it.
Reader: You can get away with that because it's an animal many people have never heard of. But how about 'brick'? Surely that describes something. It describes an object as having a certain size, shape and hardness, made of clay, used to build houses. That's what 'brick' *means*.

Me: Okay, you can describe bricks because you're familiar with them. But that doesn't entail that this description is what 'brick' *means*. 'Brick' doesn't mean anything. It's just a label. It denotes, but it doesn't describe.

Reader: Well, sorry, but that's not what the dictionary says. It *defines* 'brick' as: 'baked clay; a shaped block of burned clay, generally rectangular'.

Me: Well, it has been argued that a dictionary definition of 'X' is just a subset of all the things we know about Xs. It doesn't pinpoint some 'intrinsic meaning' which is separate from, and prior to, our general knowledge of Xs.[4]

Reader: But that's what dictionaries are for! To tell you what words *mean*.

Me: Okay, then, think of my definitions as stipulations. I'm using 'identify', 'refer' and 'describe' in such a way as to make identifying, referring and describing different activities.

The point at issue here is whether the 'meaning' of a common noun is to be understood as a description. *Reader* thinks it is. In most of the conversations I've had, she also thinks that what the noun denotes is (as it were) a consequence of this description. 'Brick' denotes the things it does denote as a *consequence* of the description which is its meaning. The description is a 'sense', which (metaphorically) hunts down all the things that can be described in that way; and it is those things which the word 'brick' denotes. 'Brick' denotes this class of things only *because* the description-which-is-its meaning identifies (points to, can be used to recognise) the things in question.

On my account, 'brick' denotes directly, all by itself (subject to the proviso in the next section). It is the name of a class of objects, a label, in the same way that 'Donald Trump' is the name of an individual. It does not *incorporate* a description-which-is-its-meaning any more than 'Donald Trump' does. There are, of course, numerous descriptions of Donald Trump; but these descriptions are not part of what the name 'Donald Trump' *means*. They are just different things that can be said about Donald Trump.[5]

4.3 Denoting

Of the five terms illustrated in Section 4.1, four refer to things *people* do. The one exception is 'denote', which is something a *word* 'does'. (I'll explain the inverted commas around 'does' in a minute.) People use words, including nouns, to name things, identify things, refer to things and describe things. This is why I used scenarios in Section 4.1. In those scenarios, A and B *do* things, and they do them with words. They name the invention, identify the tune, describe the fossa, refer to their property, draw attention to a particular object, specify what's wanted and so on.

'Denote' is different. Grammatically, it is not something a person does, although it *depends* on things people do. Once the invention has been named, 'flask-tie' denotes that particular kind of object. 'Fossa' denotes the species of cat-mongoose, although someone had to name the species first. 'Coat' denotes an item of clothing, 'umbrella' denotes a device for keeping the rain off... and so on. Any word, 'X', can only denote an object, or class of objects, once it has been agreed that 'X' will serve as the name of that object/class of objects. The word's ability to 'denote' entirely depends on this kind of prior agreement.[6]

This dependence on human activity is why I put inverted commas around 'does' a couple of paragraphs back. 'Denote' is what some words 'do', but only because of previous namings, baptisms, agreements, conventions and (often) the complicated history associated with them. Words *denote* in the way that a fence *separates* two plots of land, a clock *keeps* time and a red traffic light *requires* you to stop. These things are what the fence 'does', what the clock 'does' and what the traffic light 'does'. It is perfectly understandable, correct and idiomatic to say that what the fence *does* is to separate my garden from my neighbour's. But this 'doing' is possible only because the fence was erected (with something like that intention). In the same way, what 'flask-tie' *does* is denote the tie-cum-pouch because the inventors gave it that name, and what 'fossa' *does* is denote the cougar-mongoose because Malagasy-speaking people decided to call it that.

In contrast, raining is what the weather does, growing is what plants do, flying is what birds, bats and insects do. None of these depend on prior human activity. So we have to be careful about the difference between what a river does (flow) and what the word 'fossa' does (denote). Saying that denoting is what 'fossa' does, 'coat' does and 'umbrella' does is fine. It's correct, straightforward and idiomatic. But it does not mean that these words are, so to speak, independent 'agents'. Unlike trees, birds and weather, what they 'do' is a consequence of human decision making.

These observations suggest a modification to what, in Chapter 3, I called the 'naming diagram' (Figure 3.1). In that diagram, the relation between the word and the object was represented as 'name', 'refer to' or 'identify', since these are the terms used by dictionaries to express what a noun does. In view of the discussion we've just had, we could substitute 'denote' for all of these, and reserve 'identify' and 'refer to' for what it is *people* do *with* words.

For the most part, I will pursue the same policy with 'name'. However, it is idiomatic – and certainly not incorrect – to use 'name' in the way that I'm suggesting we use 'denote'. Many dictionaries do it, and so do writers in linguistics. I am just being cautious about the difference between the *noun-object relation* and the *things people do when they use nouns*. In particular, I want to keep 'refer to' for what people do. I will often use 'name' (the verb) or 'is the name of' instead of 'denote'; but readers should bear in mind the terminological stipulations of this section.

Changing the terminology, and using 'denote' to specify the noun-object relation, does not answer any questions or solve any problems. Everything else, up to the point we've reached so far, stays as it is. It's still an open question as to whether abstract nouns denote objects (or quasi-objects) of some kind; and, if some of them do, which ones. It's still true that some nouns don't denote anything ('behalf', 'sake'), and that many nouns that do denote can also be used in non-denoting ways ('bucket', 'view'). Wittgenstein's question still hovers: 'For some words – let's say "X" ,"Y" or "Z" – are you still inclined to say that they are the names of objects? Are you still inclined to say that they *denote* things?' The question continues its hovering throughout this chapter.

4.4 'Thing'

Let's go back to the idea that we can *refer without identifying or describing*: that is, 'non-identifying reference'. This was illustrated in Section 4.1 by scenario [7], the contrast being with scenario [6] in particular. I will be arguing (Section 4.7) that many abstract nouns can be used to realise this possibility; but here I will suggest that some words are, so to speak, specialists. The function of referring-without-identifying-or-describing is especially associated with a group of nouns which are, in Fronek's (1982: 633) terms, 'capable of a considerable degree of *desemantization*' (akin to grammaticalisation, discussed in the last chapter). Included in this group are words such as 'stuff', 'matter', 'business' and 'affair'; but the paradigmatic example is the one used in scenario [7]: 'thing'.

Scenario [7] is based on an episode of *Fawlty Towers* in which Mr and Mrs White, who are guests at the hotel, want to go out for the day, and are attempting to gain access to their room so they can retrieve some of their possessions. The manager, Basil Fawlty, for reasons of his own, is trying to prevent them.

(1)   Look, Fawlty, we want our things!

In this example, 'things' refers to an unspecified set of objects of the kind you might want to take with you when you're staying at a hotel, but going out for the day. We have a very broad sense of what these objects might be, although in this context it would be pointless and pedantic to list them. The details are irrelevant. This is one type of non-identifying reference. As we shall see, there are several more.

One might imagine, given the apparently 'neuter' sense of 'thing', that the word is typically applied in situations where the thing concerned is inanimate. However, as Fronek (1982) points out, the 'thing' or 'things' referred to can also be human, plant, animal, stuff, events or various kinds of abstraction. They 'can refer to almost any category' (Fronek 1982: 636).

(2)   What creepy things they are!
(3)   She became an expert at disarming the things.
(4)   The thing was undrinkable.
(5)   The whole thing fell flat.
(6)   I find the thing extinct.
(7)   The thing is too fantastic!
(8)   Poor old thing.

Here, (2) refers to cats, (3) to triffids, (4) to a cocktail, (5) to a party, (6) to 'proper English pantomime', (7) to a theory and (8) to Ronald Reagan.

There are numerous contexts in which 'thing' or 'things' typically appears and, correspondingly, a range of subtly different functions they can have. I will briefly describe some of the most significant. (I should add that these contexts and functions are not mutually exclusive. There is some degree of overlap.)

4.4.1 Demonstrative reference

(9)   What is that thing?
(10) Take that thing with you!
(11) This thing had begun to well up inside me.
(12) This thing is bigger than both of us.

In (9) and (10), there is something physical in the vicinity, probably (but not necessarily) inanimate. In (10) especially, the use of 'thing' has an aversive or disparaging subtext, but in neither case is the 'thing' identified or described. Similarly with (11) and (12). In (11), the 'thing' is presumably a sensation or an emotion, not a physical object. With (12), we can assume that the 'thing' is a relationship, or something else which binds people together. We can assume this mainly because most adults are familiar with the construction; it is not because the 'thing' has been explicitly identified. However, we are also aware that the construction can be used ironically or satirically, precisely because it is so familiar. If it *is* used that way, 'thing' might be a reference to something else entirely. In all cases, 'thing' is a noun which refers but does not identify or describe.

4.4.2 Anaphoric and cataphoric reference

In anaphoric reference, a word is used to refer back to some other word, expression or idea which has been used/mentioned previously in the text. Examples:

(13) Ronald did not answer. *He* looked shaken.
(14) Maxie wants to play hide and seek. *It* is *his* favourite game.
(15) Climb Everest? *That* is a ludicrous idea.

Pronouns ('he', 'it', 'her') and demonstratives ('that', 'this') are commonly used in anaphoric reference. In (13), 'he' refers back to 'Ronald' in the first sentence. In (14), 'it' refers back to 'hide and seek'. In these examples, the anaphoric pronoun refers to something which is, broadly speaking, an individual: a person in one case, a game in the other. (15) is slightly different: 'That' refers back, not to 'Everest' or 'climb', but to the idea of climbing Everest: the *proposal* that Everest should be climbed.

'Thing' is another word that can be used anaphorically. Indeed, this is how it is used in examples (2) to (8). With (2), there has been previous reference to cats; with (6) there has been previous reference to proper English pantomime; and so on. In each case, the thing referred to has been identified previously. But 'thing' itself does not identify. It piggy-backs on the context provided by the earlier mentions, and thereby refers-without-identifying.

Cataphoric reference is, essentially, the inverse of anaphoric reference. The referring term precedes the identification of what is being referred to.

(16) When *she* felt hungry, Samira ate a sandwich.
(17) *It* will be a problem, though, getting him to agree.
(18) *That*'s what I've been saying. Climbing Everest isn't possible.

'Thing' can be used this way too:

(19) The thing is, I really want to go.
(20) Such things don't happen. People aren't raised from the dead.
(21) The thing was done. Tony had finally put the shelves up.

In these examples, 'thing' refers to something only identified subsequently: a desire, a phenomenon, a job. As with previous examples, it can refer (ontologically speaking) to many different types of thing: 'almost any category', as Fronek says. So far, we've had people, personal possessions, animals, plants, drinks, gatherings, cultural forms, theories, psychological states, hypothetical events and household tasks. The range of stuff that can be referred to without being identified, using 'thing', is very wide. You can see why it's such an incredibly useful and ubiquitous word.

4.4.3 Exophoric reference

With this class of uses, we move to examples where the thing referred to by 'thing' is not identified at all, whether beforehand (anaphoric) or afterwards (cataphoric). Rather, the reader/listener is obliged to infer, from the context, what kind of thing is being referred to. This use is more common with the plural than with the singular. We have already had one example:

(1) Look, Fawlty, we want our things!

Mr and Mrs White never specify what 'things' they want to retrieve. But, in the context of hotel guests going out for the day, it is not difficult to imagine what they might have in mind: coat, handbag, phone, keys, wallet. Further examples:

(22) Economically, things are starting to improve.
(23) In training, we're doing things differently now.
(24) Things have got much better since the divorce.

In examples like this, 'things' refers to 'some general unspecified aspects of people's life, environment, nature, and even the world in general' (Fronek

1982: 641–2). However, in most cases the context will provide a clue to what is intended. 'Things' in (22) might include business confidence, unemployment figures, prices, rates of interest; while in (23) it could refer to fitness regimes, skill and speed drills, the practising of 'plays', tactics.

I commented earlier on the wide (ontological) range of things that 'thing' can refer to. In the context of demonstrative, anaphoric and cataphoric reference, the distribution rate is usually 1:1. Any *one* use of 'thing' will refer to just *one* category. (2) refers to an animal; (5) refers to a type of social gathering; (6) refers to a cultural form; (11) refers to a psychological state. However, in the case of exophoric reference involving 'things', a single use may *itself* incorporate reference to a range of ontologically diverse items. In (24), for example, 'things' might refer to the speaker's financial situation, his health, his relationship with his former partner, his relationship with his current partner, his state of mind, his social activities, his stress levels, and more. It might refer to all these things, or a subset. But these are the *kind* of things that might be implicated. As with the other examples, the specific details don't matter. The point is that, in this use, 'things' can encompass considerable ontological diversity within a single reference.

There are several reasons why 'things' may be preferred to the specifying of what a speaker has in mind. In most cases – as in (22) to (24) – itemisation is unnecessary. A general, non-specific sense is all that is required to make the point, and further details would be tedious, irrelevant or pedantic. In other cases, the speaker may wish to avoid greater explicitness, preferring to keep the matter vague. The question does not affect the main point, which is that 'thing' and 'things' permit reference without identification.

4.4.4 A placeholder word

There is a class of words recognised in linguistics to which the term 'placeholder' is applied (Channell 1994, Drave 2000). Placeholder words constitute a class within the broader category of 'vague language' (Channell 1994, Cutting 2007), a designation that includes: number approximations ('20 or 30', 'under a hundred'); vague quantifiers ('several', 'loads of'); damping-down modifiers ('kind of', 'a bit'); and phrases called general extenders ('and so on', 'or something like that'), which appear at the end of sentences (Overstreet 1999). The two most common placeholder nouns are 'thing' and 'stuff'.[7]

Placeholders are generic, semantically depleted words which stand in place of more specific terms. They are used in a variety of related and overlapping circumstances:

- When the speaker cannot recall (or does not know) the correct expression.
- Where, in context, precise identification is unnecessary/pedantic.
- When there is no recognised name for what is being referred to.
- To create an ad hoc category for which there is no recognised term.
- When a 'dummy' noun has to be paired with an adjective.

'Thing' exercises all these functions. In most cases, exercising them involves reference to a single item, or a class of items, without identifying or describing them. Consider some examples:

(25) But there's this cow thing. You can catch whatsit if you eat beef.
(26) I'll just get my gardening things.
(27) One good thing about the future: the beer tasted better.
(28) He bought some things to take on a camping trip.

(25) is an example of the first function, assuming that, in saying 'this cow thing', the speaker is referring to BSE (and that, in saying 'whatsit', he is referring to CJD). In each case, the condition in question is referred to but not named. In (26), 'things' refers to clothing and/or equipment suitable for gardening. It would be pedantic/pointless to insist that the speaker should actually say 'gardening clothes', or specify the tools concerned. By contrast, it is not clear what word might be used instead of 'thing' in (27). Of course, we could say 'one aspect of', or 'one facet of', instead of 'one thing about'. But these words are as semantically depleted as 'thing'; and, in this context, far less idiomatic.

In a similar way, there is no word which denotes 'things to take on a camping trip', as in (28). This is an example of an *ad hoc category* (Barsalou 1983). Other examples might be: 'things that babies often do', and 'places to look for antique desks'. Ad hoc categories are created to be used in specialised contexts in order to refer to types-of-things which have no agreed name. 'Things' is often used in the construction of such categories ('things to sell at a car boot sale'). So, again, it refers without identifying or describing. Ad hoc categories have a significant stepping-stone role in this chapter and the next, so it will be useful to keep them in mind.

4.5 Ontological diversity

'Thing' is an indispensable word. It is difficult to imagine an extended English conversation that does not include it. It is also a noun, or at least its primary syntactic function is that of a noun. Even though it is an indispensable noun, however, it does not name anything. Indeed, it is indispensable *because* it does not name anything. Freed of denotational commitments, it can refer to virtually anything, in virtually any ontological category. At the same time, it is a syntactic wild card, able to fill noun-shaped slots in a large range of constructions, pair itself with demonstratives, create ad hoc categories, serve as a quasi-pronoun in anaphoric and cataphoric reference, act as a generic go-to noun when you can't think of the right word or when precision is unnecessary, and in several other respects do duty as an essential placeholder word.

As a noun which refers but does not name, 'thing' is different from the nouns discussed in the previous chapter, such as 'behalf', 'sake', 'spite', 'mickey', the 'view' of 'in view of', and the 'bucket' of 'kick the bucket'. Like 'thing', these nouns don't *name* anything. On the other hand, they're not used to *refer* either.

This suggests that non-naming nouns are not all of the same kind. It also implies that they abstain from naming (so to speak) in different ways, and that they may have other functions instead. 'Thing' has one such function. It can be used to refer without identifying or describing.

Let me now make a suggestion about *one* way in which we can think about the idea of a concept (I stress 'one' because there are others, as will become clear in the next chapter). The suggestion is this: to talk about 'the concept of X' is a way of referring to certain things without identifying or describing them. In that respect, *some* uses of 'concept' are not unlike *some* uses of 'thing'.

Here is a way of thinking about the relation between 'thing' and 'concept'. In Section 4.4, I introduced Barsalou's notion of *ad hoc categories*: 'things to take on a camping trip', for example. Gentner and Kurtz (2005) point out that a variation on this theme is the notion of *thematic groupings*. As an example, they suggest: *things associated with going to a movie* (12). This would include tickets, booking, programme, the show time, film theatre, travel, popcorn, British Board of Film Classification (MPAA ratings) and more. This type of ad hoc category differs from other kinds in the following way. 'Things to take on a camping trip' covers a wide variety of objects, but they are all *physical* objects. 'Things associated with going to a movie' does include physical objects, but the phrase takes advantage of the ability 'thing' has to refer to things in different ontological categories simultaneously. It includes the film classification, the programme, show times, travelling and so on. 'Things associated with going to a movie' refers to things which are ontologically diverse. And it does so without identifying or itemising any of them.

So here's another suggestion, a follow-up to the earlier one. When we talk about *the concept of X*, what we are talking about, very roughly, is: *things associated with the use of the word 'X'*.

This suggestion will have to be elaborated and qualified, and in Chapter 5 it will be. But the claim is that 'the concept of X' is akin to a 'thematic grouping' (in Gentner and Kurtz's terms). It refers to the relevant 'things' without identifying, specifying or describing them. In this respect, *things associated with the use of the word 'X'* is a sort of *preliminary* extension of the Second Picture (Figure 2.1), reproduced here as Figure 4.1.

4.6 The uses of 'football'

It might be objected that ad hoc categories ('things to take on a camping trip') and thematic groupings ('things associated with going to a movie') are themselves a little ad hoc. They are idiomatic phrases, certainly, but there's surely a limit to what they can tell us, precisely because they are so colloquial. The idea that they can help us to understand what concepts are seems a little far-fetched.

To begin the process of suggesting that it's not as far-fetched as all that, let's start with 'football'.

(29) This is the football I gave my daughter for her birthday.
(30) Lucy is out playing football.

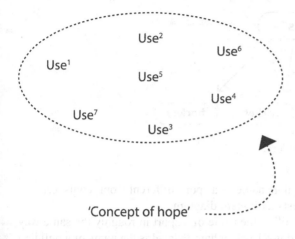

'Concept of hope'

Second Picture

Dashed arrow to be read as 'vaguely refers to'
'Concept of hope' is a linguistic expression

Figure 4.1 Uses of 'hope' and the concept of hope.

(31) What time is the football on?

(32) A matter of life and death? Football is much more serious than that![8]

(33) On the question of racism, football has got to get its act together.

In (29), 'football' is a concrete count noun. It could be slipped into the naming diagram instead of 'cat' (Figure 4.2).

(30) is a bit trickier. 'Lucy is out playing football' is obviously not the same as 'Lucy is out playing *with a* football'. In the latter example, 'football' is used in the same way as it is in (29). But it isn't used that way in (30), and consequently it doesn't fit the 'football' version of the naming diagram. Still, we can perhaps treat

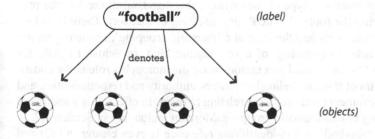

Figure 4.2 'Football' as a naming word.

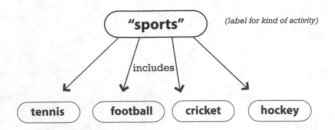

Figure 4.3 'Sports' as a naming word.

'football' in (30) as the (singular) name of a sport, different from tennis, cricket, hockey and so on. This suggests a different diagram.

In Figure 4.3, then, 'Football' is the name of a sport in roughly the same way that 'Lassie' is the name of a dog, 'Buckingham Palace' is the name of a building and 'Glittertind' is the name of a mountain.

In (31), however, 'football' is used differently again. In this case, it is a count noun rather than a proper name. But it's clearly not a count noun in the way that it is in (29), and the original naming diagram does not fit. In British English, this sentence would almost certainly be used in connection with a television pro-gramme, broadcasting live commentary on a particular game, or perhaps provid-ing highlights of all the games played that day. Here, then, 'the football' is not a physical object, and not the name of a sport. It is a way of referring to a kind of television show covering football matches. The person referring to 'the football' in (31) is referring to a nexus of things bound into this concept: television as a medium, the television schedule, the game itself, the commentary, punditry in the studio, interviews.

At this point, I want to say, 'football' stops denoting anything, and instead starts referring to a cluster of items like these, none of which need be specified because both speaker and audience know the kind of thing being referred to. This is very similar to the use of expressions like 'things associated with going to a movie'; and the items referred to by 'the football' in (31) are just as ontologically diverse as the things 'associated with going to a movie' are.

Another way of thinking about (31) involves a sort of ellipsis. In this example, 'the football' is used as a type of metonym, a shorthand substitute for 'the pro-gramme covering the football match', or something of that sort. There is a close link between metonymy and the idea of a 'thematic grouping', as metonyms are often used to refer to groupings of a very similar kind. In British English, for example, 'The Crown' is used as a metonym for the monarch's role in the consti-tution and affairs of state, including her powers, authority and responsibilities, and the various instruments and protocols relating to them. In effect, it is a shorthand way of referring to *that* thematic grouping. More on metonymy in Section 4.7.

The use of 'football' in non-identifying reference is even clearer in (32) and (33). In neither case does it denote anything, and in both cases it refers to a wide range of ontologically diverse things. However, the range of things referred to is not the same in the two cases. Example (32) is often assumed to be a joke, but it makes a serious point. 'Football' here does refer to the sport itself; but more importantly it refers beyond that to the *role* of football – and particularly the role of individual football clubs – in the life of families and communities.

> Football is like a religion to its devotees. It binds and divides, shapes and delimits, providing a critical identity for a given group and individuals. The scarf, the ground, the songs and the ritual activity have a sacred quality about them; football is at least *like* a secular religion here.
>
> (Taylor & Taylor 1997: 39)

This is precisely what the manager of Liverpool FC was getting at.

The range of things referred to in (33) overlaps with this, but does not exactly coincide with it. In this case, there is, additionally, reference to organisations: the clubs again, but also the governing bodies at various levels, professional associations, legal and ethical issues, the policing of racist abuse, the nature of sanctions against individuals, clubs and national institutions, the way in which policy is agreed and more. If 'football' has got to get its act together, this is not the name of any particular organisation; it is rather a non-identifying, non-specifying reference to all these things, loosely lassoed together. As with (31), 'football' in this example has a metonymic function.

A few footnotes to this discussion. First, 'football' is apparently a 'dual-life' noun (see Note 10 of the last chapter). It can be either a count noun (29, 31) or a mass noun (32, 33). It can even be a proper name (30). As interestingly, there is a question as to whether it is (adopting the usual terms) a 'concrete noun' or an 'abstract noun'. In (29), it is obviously concrete. It could be concrete in (30) and (31) as well, but less obviously. In (32) and (33), it seems undeniably abstract. This is slightly unexpected because nouns are usually regarded as *either* concrete *or* abstract. On this evidence – admittedly, it's only one word – it might not be a simple dichotomy.[9]

Second, the interesting characteristic of the use of 'football' in (32) and (33) is that it appears not to denote, but instead refers to a large, ill-defined and ontologically diverse assortment of things, without identifying or specifying any of them. As with 'Look, Fawlty, we want our things!', the kind of 'things' being referred to is inferable from the context; and *in* that context will normally be understood – in very general terms – by both speaker and hearer. In this respect, 'football' in (32) and (33) is a sort of one-word thematic grouping, akin to 'things associated with going to a movie'. A way of making roughly the same point is to suggest that, in those examples, 'football' functions as a metonym.

Third, if this is right, referring-without-identifying-or-describing is not restricted to one-off, specialist words like 'thing'. It may be possible with other, less specialist nouns. (It might even be possible with a word like 'concept'.)

Fourth, just to follow that one up, I think it *is* possible with other nouns, and not just 'football' (after all, 'football' does not sound like the kind of 'special' word that has a property no other noun possesses: it seems remarkably ordinary). There are, in fact, other nouns which can be used, and are used, in the same way. Not surprisingly, they can all be count *or* mass, concrete *or* abstract. Some of them, like 'Football' can even be proper names (or something very like proper names). Such words include 'property', 'pen', 'society', 'character', 'memory', 'context' and many more.[10]

Finally, this section has provided further (modest) evidence that the sense of individual words is modulated by grammatical structures and functions. We have already seen (in Chapter 3) that constructions confer different 'meanings' on constituent words; and we have noted that 'inflected forms may develop some independence with regard to their respective meanings' (Hilpert 2014: 70). Here, there is an indication that the mass-noun version of dual-life nouns can represent a switch from *denoting* to *non-identifying reference*. A mass noun/abstract noun is sometimes assigned a referring-without-identifying, metonymic role, irrespective of its functions when acting as a count noun or concrete noun. Chapter 9 will suggest that this is true of the noun 'hope'.

4.7 Metonymy and thematic groupings

In the next chapter, I will use thematic groupings and one form of metonymy as 'objects of comparison' in Wittgenstein's sense. I'll argue that the use of the expression 'the concept of X' can be triangulated by three objects of comparison: *metonymy, thematic groupings* and *domain nouns*.[11] In closing this chapter, I want to prepare the ground for this triangulation by saying a bit more about the first two.

The literature on metonymy includes several attempts to formulate a typology of metonymic expression. These typologies use various criteria to identify different types of metonymy, but here I am interested in one criterion in particular.[12] This is the criterion of 'boundedness' (Peirsman & Geeraerts 2006). Have a look at the following examples:

(34)   I don't think the suits upstairs are going to like that.
(35)   You know something? I need new wheels.
(36)   The pen is mightier than the sword.

In (34), the word 'suits' is a metonymic substitute for 'managers', the people in charge. In the parlance of the metonymy literature, 'suits' is the *source*, and the managers are the *target* (Ruiz de Mendoza Ibáñez & Diez Verlasco 2002). The metonym depends on a well-known stereotype of what managers typically wear (and hints at an equally stereotypical state of mind). Adopting the language of Peirsman and Geeraerts (2006), both source and target are 'bounded'. They refer to a particular form of clothing and a particular type of person/role, respectively. We have something rather similar with (35). 'New wheels' is a metonymic substitute for 'a new car'. Again, both source ('wheels') and target ('car') are bounded, in the sense that 'car' refers to a particular type of machine, while 'wheels' refers to a particular type of car-component. In these examples, both source and target are physical objects.

Contrast these two with (36). There are two metonyms here, 'pen' and 'sword'. The source, in each case, is bounded (and refers to a physical object). But what of the targets? 'Pen' is rather like 'football' in (32) and (33). We think of 'pen' as being a 'concrete' noun, denoting a type of writing implement, just as we think of a 'football' as a 'concrete' noun denoting a type of spherical object. In (36), however, 'pen' is referring to something much wider than that. It is a metonym for... well, at this point the matter becomes a little indeterminate. Literature of various kinds, but also works of science, philosophy, theology and so on. An interest in ideas, and the sense of a commitment to studying, writing, reading and the kind of life that goes with them. Perhaps a suggestion of communication, given the contrast with 'the sword', and an ability to persuade through writing. Stuff like that, ontologically diverse. Compared to 'suits' and 'wheels', the target of 'pen' is far more diffuse. It is, in Peirsman and Geeraerts terms, '*unbounded*'. We have a sense of the diverse kinds of thing that the speaker/writer has in mind, and can give examples (as I have just done). But there is no definitive list – and, in context, no need for one.

The target of 'sword' is equally unbounded. It refers to conflict in various forms, from war and other forms of physical aggression, to (depending on context) other less violent types of coercion. It stands, metonymically, for any attempt to impose your will, your ideas, your preferences, through force rather than by peaceful or consensual means. As with 'pen' we have a general sense of what is meant, but there is no definitive list.

What I take from this discussion is that some metonyms have *unbounded targets*, which included diffuse and *ontologically diverse* elements. They *refer vaguely* to those elements, but *do not specify or identify* any of them. They trade on the *background knowledge* that both speaker and hearer possess.

The significance of background knowledge is emphasised in the metonymy literature, and in cognitive linguistics. Lemmens (2016: 92), for example, argues that

> the meaning of words such as *weekend, workday* or *school night* can only be understood in reference to the typical (culture-specific) organisation of our time in weeks consisting of days during which we work ... or go to school, and days when we do not, and the social practices that come with that distinction.

Hanks (2013: 38) refers to the 'interrelationship between knowledge of a language and knowledge of the world', with the latter providing a repository of 'facts about the world associated with lexical items'. The shorthand of metonymy can only work if the audience already has the relevant cultural/historical knowledge. In (32), for example, the audience must understand the role that football plays in the lives of some individuals and communities; and in (33) they must know in a general way that the sport is subject to institutional governance.

As indicated earlier (Note 4), many authors accept this corollary: understanding any form of speech or writing requires 'encyclopaedic knowledge' in addition to familiarity with the words. Geeraerts (2006: 5), for example, suggests that: 'Linguistic meaning is not separate from other forms of knowledge of the world that we have, and in that sense it is encyclopedic and non-autonomous: it involves knowledge of the world'. Rayo's 'grab-bag' model of language mastery implies that: 'With each expression of the basic lexicon, the subject associates a 'grab bag' of mental items: memories, mental images, pieces of encyclopedic information, pieces of anecdotal information, mental maps, and so forth' (Rayo 2013: 647). As a bare minimum, 'cognitive linguistics … rejects a strict dichotomy between linguistic and encyclopaedic knowledge' (Lemmens 2016: 92). More ambitiously: 'the meaning of words is encyclopedic: everything you know about the concept is part of its meaning' (Croft 2006: 270).

Background knowledge is also required for an understanding of thematic groupings. You know what is being referred to by an expression such as 'things associated with going to a movie', but not because the relevant items are specified, or somehow 'built into' the 'descriptive content' of the phrase. Reference-without-identification is common to both thematic groupings and metonymy. So is the implicit appeal to 'encyclopaedic information' from the grab-bag. In fact, this theme has been with us since the beginning of the chapter. It was there in 'Look, Fawlty, we want our things!', which can only be fully understood if the audience is familiar with what it's like to stay in a hotel, and with what you are likely to need if you are going out for the day.

Metonymy, thematic groupings and desemanticised words capable of exophoric reference (like 'things') have both these characteristics in common: *non-identifying reference*, and the *encyclopaedic knowledge* required to understand what it is they are referring to. They have a third characteristic, too. The cluster of 'things' they refer to can be *ontologically diverse* (they can also be ontologically homogeneous).

These knowledge clusters are known by a variety of terms: *scripts* (Schank 1990), *cognitive domains* (Langacker 1987), *frames* (Fillmore 1985) and *idealised cognitive models* (Lakoff 1987). It is true that these expressions do not all refer to exactly the same kind of idea, and that they are applied in different kinds of context. But they're all ways of gesturing towards concatenations of knowledge which support inference-from-speech-or-writing. For example, 'scripts' apply to episodes in which there is a narrative element or sequence of events. Schank's example is the 'restaurant script', which incorporates culture-specific knowledge of what happens when you visit a restaurant. In this context, one could refer to the thematic grouping 'things associated with going to a restaurant', except that 'script' has a stronger sense of sequence.

In the next chapter, we will explore the idealised cognitive models related to 'concept', and the frames which support the idea of 'understanding the concept of X'. Something like that, at any rate. But first, a brief anticipatory word.

4.8 'Consoct'

Consider the thematic grouping 'things associated with going to a restaurant'. 'Things associated with' is a phrase. Presumably, this is a linguistic accident.

However, suppose there was a single word that meant 'things associated with' when combined with a preposition (the preposition doesn't have to be 'with'). Let's say the preposition 'of', and let's say the single word 'consoct'.[13] Then, instead of 'things associated with going to a movie', we would have the expression: 'the consoct of going to a movie'.

You can probably see where I might be thinking of going with this. 'Consoct' immediately changes the grammar. It introduces what appears to be a substantive noun (so it's different from the desemanticised 'things'). If we had such a noun, and always *had* had it, would we be inclined to ask about the *nature* of consocts? Would we think that the word 'consoct' *denotes* a certain kind of thing? Perhaps an abstract object, or a mental particular? Would we imagine that consocts had a structure, and could be constituents of thoughts or propositions? Might we suggest that they are the building blocks of theories?

'Consoct' is a Wittgenstein-esque invention.[14] 'Concept' is not. But we are now homing in on concepts, and the kind of discourse that goes with them.

Notes

1 Flask-ties do exist, and are available for sale online. An ideal gift!
2 *Reader* takes issue with this claim in Section 4.2.
3 This example is based on an episode of the 1970s UK comedy series *Fawlty Towers*. I will come back to it in Section 4.4.
4 The claim that there is no significant distinction between linguistic knowledge and encyclopaedic knowledge is associated with cognitive linguistics (Peeters 2000). Since lexical concepts are an integral part of human cognition in general, there is no *sui generis* lexical knowledge of the kind supposedly found in a dictionary. A dictionary 'definition' is merely a subset of the information that can be found in an encyclopaedia. According to Lakoff (1987), for example, the distinction between 'definitional knowledge' of words and encyclopaedic knowledge of what the words refer to is purely 'technical'. More on this topic in Section 4.7.
5 It is impossible to discuss this topic without mentioning the literature on philosophy of language, particularly the debate about reference since Kripke (1980). As I have already noted, my own use of 'refer' is not identical with its technical use in that debate. I have distinguished between referring as something people do, and denoting as something words 'do'; and my use of 'refer' is intended to reflect its colloquial sense. In philosophy of language, by contrast, it is widely assumed that there is a class of 'referring expressions'. These are not expressions that can be *used* to refer; rather, they are expressions which (it is argued) *themselves* refer.
   There are, however, philosophers who don't subscribe to this view. Strawson (1950: 326) starts his classic paper by saying: 'Referring is not something an expression does; it is something that someone can use an expression to do'. More recently, Bach has used the expression 'linguistification' to refer to the 'numerous cases in which philosophers have attributed to linguistic expressions properties that are actually characteristic of people in using these expressions' (Bach 2013: 1). Some people use a knife and fork to eat with; but it's the people doing the eating, not the knife and fork. Similarly, we sometimes use words to refer to things; but *we* are doing the referring, not the words. The words are implements – tools, as Wittgenstein would say – just as the knife and fork are.
6 On the significance of convention in naming things – individuals, groups or properties – see Millikan (2017), Chapter 2.

7 Fronek (1982) is the classic study of 'thing'. Drave (2000) does something comparable with 'stuff'. Other useful discussions are: Jucker et al. (2003), Koester (2007), Martinez & Pertejo (2015). Labrador (2012) is an interesting examination of the difficulties that 'thing' creates in translating between English and Spanish.

8 This is based on a statement attributed to Bill Shankly, the manager of Liverpool F.C., 1959–1974. There are different versions, but here's one: 'Some people believe football is a matter of life and death. I can assure you, it is much, much more important than that'.

9 In recent years there has been a surge of interest in 'abstract concepts' in disciplines such as linguistics, developmental science and neuroscience. Recent evidence suggests 'that abstract and concrete items are not completely distinct in the brain. Rather, they appear as a continuum' (Buccino et al. 2019: 1391). This could imply that 'the concrete versus abstract distinction between concepts is no longer useful' (Barsalou et al. 2018: 1). In which case, it might be argued that 'studying concepts in the context of situated action is necessary for establishing complete accounts of them … continuing to study concepts in isolation is likely to provide relatively incomplete and distorted accounts' (ibid.).

10 Like 'football', these words can all shift up or down through the gears (so to speak), from a 'micro' level (football as a thing you kick around) to a macro level (football as community and tradition). There is a parallel here, I suspect, to the way scientific terms have their senses 'tweaked' as they move between different levels and scales. See, for example, Wilson's (2017) discussion of 'force' and 'temperature' in physics (26–30). If you're wondering about 'pen', we'll get to it in Section 4.7.

11 I have not mentioned domain nouns yet, but I will explain them in the next chapter. For 'objects of comparison', see Wittgenstein (1963: §130–1) and Kuusela's (2008) illuminating discussion, especially Chapter 3. I will say more about this idea myself in Chapter 7.

12 For an excellent introduction to the metonymy literature, see Littlemore (2015).

13 This is an anglicised contraction of 'consociata', which is (roughly) Latin for 'associated things'.

14 For what I take to be a justification of this claim, see Kuusela (2008), Chapter 7.

References

Bach, K. (2013). The lure of linguistification. In C. Penco & F. Domaneschi (Eds.), *What Is Said and What Is Not* (pp. 87–98). Stanford, CA: CSLI Publications.

Barsalou, L. W. (1983). Ad hoc categories. *Memory and Cognition, 11*(3), 211–227.

Barsalou, L. W., Dutriaux, L., & Scheepers, C. (2018). Moving beyond the distinction between concrete and abstract concepts. *Philosophical Transactions of the Royal Society B: Biological Sciences, 373*(1752), https://doi.org/10.1098/rstb.2017.0144.

Buccino, G., Colagè, I., Silipo, F., & D'Ambrosio, P. (2019). The concreteness of abstract language: An ancient issue and a new perspective. *Brain Structure and Function, 224*, 1385–1401.

Channell, J. (1994). *Vague Language*. Oxford: Oxford University Press.

Croft, W. A. (2006). Metonymy: The role of domains in the interpretation of metaphors and metonymies. In D. Geeraerts (Ed.), *Cognitive Linguistics: Basic Readings* (pp. 269–302). Berlin: Mouton de Gruyter.

Cutting, J. (Ed.). (2007). *Vague Language Explored*. Basingstoke, UK: Palgrave Macmillan.

Drave, N. (2000). Vaguely speaking: A corpus approach to vague language in intercultural conversations. In P. Peters, P. Collins, & A. Smith (Eds.), *Language and Computers: New Frontiers of Corpus Research. Papers from the Twenty-First International*

Conference of English Language Research and Computerised Corpora (pp. 25–40). Amsterdam: Rodopi.

Fillmore, C. (1985). Frames and the semantics of understanding. *Quaderni di Semantica, 6*, 222–254.

Fronek, J. (1982). *Thing* as a function word. *Linguistics, 20*, 633–654.

Geeraerts, D. (2006). Introduction: A rough guide to cognitive linguistics. In D. Geeraerts (Ed.), *Cognitive Linguistics: Basic Readings* (pp. 1–28). Berlin: Mouton de Gruyter.

Gentner, D., & Kurtz, K. J. (2005). Relational categories. In W.-K. Ahn, R. L. Goldstone, B. C. Love, A. B. Markman, & P. Wolff (Eds.), *Categorization Inside and Outside the Laboratory* (pp. 151–175). Washington, DC: American Psychological Association.

Hanks, P. (2013). *Lexical Analysis: Norms and Exploitations*. Cambridge, MA: The MIT Press.

Hilpert, M. (2014). *Construction Grammar and Its Application to English*. Edinburgh: Edinburgh University Press.

Jucker, A., Smith, S., & Lüdge, T. (2003). Interactive aspects of vagueness in conversation. *Journal of Pragmatics, 37*, 1737–1769.

Koester, A. (2007). 'About twelve thousand or so': Vagueness in North American and UK offices. In J. Cutting (Ed.), *Vague Language Explored* (pp. 40–61). London: Palgrave Macmillan.

Kripke, S. A. (1980). *Naming and Necessity*. Oxford: Basil Blackwell.

Kuusela, O. (2008). *The Struggle against Dogmatism: Wittgenstein and the Concept of Philosophy*. Cambridge, MA: Harvard University Press.

Labrador, B. (2012). 'The amazing thing about this love story': A corpus-based study of thing as a function word in English and lo-nominalizations in Spanish. *Varieng, 12*, http://www.helsinki.fi/varieng/series/volumes/12/labrador/.

Lakoff, G. (1987). *Women, Fire, and Dangerous Things: What Categories Reveal about the Mind*. Chicago, IL: University of Chicago Press.

Langacker, R. W. (1987). *Foundations of Cognitive Grammar, Vol. I: Theoretical Prerequisites*. Stanford, CA: Stanford University Press.

Lemmens, M. (2016). Cognitive semantics. In N. Riemer (Ed.), *Routledge Handbook of Semantics* (pp. 90–105). Abingdon, UK: Routledge.

Littlemore, J. (2015). *Metonymy: Hidden Shortcuts in Language, Thought and Communication*. Cambridge, UK: Cambridge University Press.

Martinez, I. M. P., & Pertejo, P. N. (2015). "Go up to Miss Thingy", "He's probably like a whatsit or something". Placeholders in focus. The difference in use between teenagers and adults in spoken English. *Pragmatics, 25*(3), 425–451.

Millikan, R. G. (2017). *Beyond Concepts: Unicepts, Language, and Natural Information*. New York: Oxford University Press.

Overstreet, M. (1999). *Whales, Candlelight, and Stuff Like That: General Extenders in English Discourse*. New York: Oxford University Press.

Peeters, B. (2000). Setting the scene: Some recent milestones in the lexicon-encyclopedia debate. In B. Peeters (Ed.), *The Lexicon-Encyclopedia Interface* (pp. 1–52). Oxford: Elsevier.

Peirsman, Y., & Geeraerts, D. (2006). Metonymy as a prototypical category. *Cognitive Linguistics, 17*(3), 269–316.

Rayo, A. (2013). A plea for semantic localism. *Noûs, 47*(4), 647–679.

Ruiz de Mendoza Ibáñez, F. J., & Diez Verlasco, O. I. (2002). Patterns of conceptual interaction. In R. Dirven & R. Porings (Eds.), *Metaphor and Metonymy in Comparison and Contrast* (pp. 489–532). Berlin: Mouton de Gruyter.

Schank, R. C. (1990). *Tell Me a Story: Narrative and Intelligence*. Evanston, IL: Northwestern University Press.

Strawson, P. F. (1950). On referring. *Mind*, *59*(235), 320–344.

Taylor, M., & Taylor, R. (1997). Something for the weekend, sir? Leisure, ecstasy and identity in football and contemporary religion. *Leisure Studies*, *16*(1), 37–49.

Wilson, M. (2017). *Physics Avoidance: Essays in Conceptual Strategy*. Oxford: Oxford University Press.

Wittgenstein, L. (1963). *Philosophical Investigations*. Oxford: Basil Blackwell.

5 'The concept of...'

I ended the last chapter with 'consoct', and many readers will have thought: 'Yeah, right'. 'Consoct' is an invented word which I imagined as an alternative way of expressing the idea of a thematic grouping. Instead of 'things associated with going to a movie', we could refer to 'the consoct of going to a movie'. *The consoct of* instead of *things associated with*. That we are familiar with the latter and suspicious of the former I described as a linguistic accident. It could have been the other way round. 'Yeah, right. Inventing words to fit your thesis. Classy'.

5.1 The world of...

So here's the punch line. We do, in fact, have expressions which are very similar to 'the consoct of'. The best example is 'the world of'. Have a look at these examples:

(1) She had fond memories of her foray into the world of fashion.
(2) A majority expressed no desire to return to the world of work.
(3) There's continuing drama in the world of sport this week.
(4) My reason for being: to inhabit the world of books on a full-time basis.

In these examples, it seems a bit strained to regard 'world' as the name of anything. They are not like:

(5) Pluto is a frozen world.
(6) The world is undergoing rapid climate change.

In (5), 'world' is a near-synonym of 'planet'. In (6), 'the world' refers to a very particular planet, and is used as the equivalent of a proper name. We could substitute 'Earth' for 'the world' in this example: we couldn't do that with (1) to (4). Different again are:

(7) You mean the world to me.
(8) It will do him a world of good.
(9) That's going to make a world of difference.

(10)   You're entering a world of pain.

In these examples, the 'world' phrase is grammaticalised, and belongs in the same category as 'amount nouns', mentioned in Section 3.6. Indeed, 'a world of' in these constructions is broadly synonymous with 'a lot of' and 'loads of'. The difference is that 'a world of' suggests something rather more than 'a lot of', and implies that the 'good' (or the 'difference', or the 'pain') in question ramifies more widely than we would usually infer from 'a lot of'.

It's far easier to see 'the world of X' in (1) to (4) as referring to a large, ill-defined, ontologically diverse assortment of things. 'The world of sport' refers to items such as various sports; people who play them; the organisation of competitions; the individuals, clubs and nations that play in those competitions; the companies that sponsor them; rules, laws and referees; spectators, journalists, broadcasters; and so on.

Similarly, 'the world of books' refers to writers, readers, publishers, book sellers; libraries; the books themselves; commissioning, editing and publishing; the collection of antiquarian and rare books; book signings, festivals… in fact, almost anything to do with books at all. 'Anything to do with books'. That's quite close to 'things associated with going to a movie'. It's another 'thematic grouping' phrase.

However, we can't *quite* substitute 'anything to do with' for 'the world of' in (4):

(4*)   My reason for being: to inhabit anything to do with books on a full-time basis.

So 'world' is doing *something* over and above pointing to a thematic grouping; just as, in (1), 'the world of fashion' is not synonymous with 'anything to do with fashion'. In all these examples, 'the world of' suggests a kind of integration. The diverse items referred to are not just a random collection. In a certain, unspecified way they – loosely – hang together. In 'the world of fashion', we imagine people knowing each other, friendships and rivalries, shows, creativity, the economics, the politics, the implied sense of things working in generally understood ways. This is the difference between 'the world of' and 'things having to do with'. The former implies a kind of overall cohesiveness in a way the latter doesn't. It says slightly more than 'things associated with'. If we abbreviate 'thematic grouping' to TG, then I want to say that 'the world of' is *a TG+ expression*.

The shift to TG+, with 'the world of', changes the grammar. You can do things with the noun that you can't do with 'things associated with' or 'anything to do with'. 'The world of X' becomes a quasi-place.

In (1), it's a place you can have *forays into*.
In (2), it's a place you can *return to* (or not).
In (3), it's a place *where* drama can *happen*.
In (4), it's a place you can *inhabit*.

None of this would be possible with the TG constructions 'things associated with' and 'anything to do with'. By replacing the TG phrase with a word which (when acting as a concrete count noun) denotes a kind of place, we create syntactic options that didn't exist before. In doing so, we open up the possibility of statements about forays, returns, happenings and inhabitings. This can be understood as one of the 'metaphors we live by' (Lakoff & Johnson 1980), the introduction of the noun phrase 'the world of' creating a *metaphorical location*, where before there was only a loose assortment of 'things associated with', and a more limited range of syntactic options. The alternative grammar permits new things to be said, and provides a shorthand way of conveying information that might otherwise be verbose or clumsy.

However, 'the world of fashion' still has this in common with 'things associated with fashion': they are both ways of referring to an ill-defined assortment of things, without identifying any of them. The shift to 'the world of' retains this non-identifying reference function, but adds a triad of features:

- A sense of cohesiveness
- A different grammar
- A metaphorical location

These features are, of course, linked. The cohesiveness goes with the location: a 'place' is thought of as externally bounded and internally organised in a way that things 'associated with' are clearly not. So in referring to 'the world of fashion', for example, we are implying that this 'world', in a rough-and-ready sense, hangs together. And the location is a consequence of the introduction of a word whose count-noun function names something which occupies a position in physical space. The ontologically diverse items, loosely lassoed together by 'associated with', have become – with the grammatical switch – a syntactic singularity. Plural 'things' have been transposed into a singular 'world'.

There are a few other nouns (not very many) which, like 'world', are capable of forming what I will call *TG+ constructions*. I will refer to them as *TG+ nouns*. In each case, this triad of categories makes an appearance, though the third does not necessarily take the form of a metaphorical location (however, it does always suggest a kind of 'boundedness'). TG+ constructions have the following syntax:

The + N1 + *of* + N2

where N1 is a noun and N2 is a different noun.[1] In 'the world of fashion', for example, N1 is 'world' and N2 is 'fashion'. In these constructions, it is N1 that allows the different grammar, creates a metaphorical location and implies a cohesiveness lacking in the TG phrase. In TG+ constructions, N1 is always an abstract noun, or at least a noun exercising its abstract function. N2 is always a mass noun, or sometimes a plural. With that bare-bones framework established, we can take a quick look at three examples.

5.2 Three more TG+ nouns

There is, as I have said, a small number of words that can exercise the same TG+ function as 'world'. They include 'culture', 'role', 'context', 'field', 'problem' and 'question'. In this section, I will discuss three of them: 'role', 'culture' and 'problem'. I should emphasise, that these words are not *always* used in TG+ constructions (any more than 'world' is). Even when they appear as N1 in a construction of the form < *The* + N1 + *of* + N2 >, they are not necessarily functioning as TG+ nouns. Here, as elsewhere, we have to resist the craving for generality.

Consider the following examples:

(11)   The transformation in the role of women is the biggest event in our lifetime.
(12)   Feminism has created chaos and confusion regarding the role of women.

(11) and (12) both illustrate a metaphorical extension of 'role' as an actor might use it ('It's the role of a lifetime'). Crudely, they are both TG+ versions of a TG expression such as 'things associated with being a woman'. The 'role of' refers to a complex network of relationships, norms, expectations, institutional possibilities and impediments, control over one's own body, sexuality, women in the family, women's work (paid and unpaid) and legislation, as well as the social, economic and political ramifications of all of these. Condensing this extensive concatenation of factors into 'the role' makes it possible to refer to all of them in a broad, lassoing gesture, and creates a series of grammatical options not available to the TG phrase.

So the grammatical element of the triad (Section 5.1) is present, but so are the other two elements. As with 'the world of', 'the role of' implies a kind of cohesiveness. In (11), this is a sociological idea, 'role' implying that the lassoed factors are, at least to some degree, inter-related, and that the transformation has been, very roughly, across the board. In (12), however, it has a prescriptive ring to it. The 'role' of women is, by implication, an integrated set of requirements – a 'role', or a framework of 'roles' – which 'feminism' has (it is said) 'disrupted'. The 'role' is, in some sense, ordained, whether theologically, biologically or historically. The 'chaos and confusion' is a result of this framework being infringed.

Similarly, where 'world' creates a metaphorical place, 'role' creates a different type of boundedness: a metaphorical text, a kind of 'script', in which what women are supposed to do, or expected to do, is defined.[2] The metaphor suggests that a woman's place in the order of things is described (or prescribed) by this text. In (11), it is implied that the 'script' is subject to change, and that change can be welcomed. In (12), it is implied that radical change is unwelcome. The use of a noun in the TG+ phrase changes the grammatical options, metaphorically creates a text and implies a particular kind of cohesiveness.

It is interesting to contrast the implications of 'the role of women' with 'the world of women'. 'World of' suggests a cohesiveness which is, at least partly, organised from *within*. It is something understood most fully by women – or, generalising, by 'insiders'. 'Role of' suggests something organised from *without*: a set of expectations or requirements imposed by a particular society. Both imply cohesiveness, but they do so in different ways.

(13)   They are victims of the culture of poverty.

(14)   The people are tired of the culture of corruption.

In (13) and (14), the three elements of the TG+ triad turn up again. 'The culture of poverty' refers to the ways in which, allegedly, poverty is reproduced despite attempts to alleviate it.[3] The TG phrase might be something like: 'things which help to sustain poverty'. Substituting 'the culture of' alters the grammar, creates a metaphorical community, and implies a form of cohesiveness which arises from the values and behaviour of that community's members. It is not simply a question of being poor; it is also a question of peer relationships, socialisation, education, aspirations, ways of thinking and feeling. This is another ontologically diverse 'thematic grouping', referred to by a single word which, simultaneously, confers upon it a sense of internal cohesiveness.

Similarly, in (14) the people are tired of the 'culture of corruption', not just corruption. This once again suggests a structured set of beliefs, values, norms, practices and relationships, which is (in some sense) self-reproducing. As with 'culture of poverty', 'culture of corruption' metaphorically implies 'difficult to eradicate' precisely because it refers to a cohesive structure with its own internal organisation. It does so without identifying any of the elements which belong to the 'thematic grouping', and without specifying the manner in which they are supposedly related.

(15)   We are failing to deal with the problem of poverty.

(16)   The report sheds more light on the problem of sexual assault.

In (15) 'the problem of poverty' is not just a reference to the fact that poverty exists; and, in (16), 'the problem of sexual assault' does not just refer to the fact that sexual assault occurs. In both cases, a far wider range of issues and circumstances is alluded to. In one case: the various forms poverty takes, its causes, its demographic distribution and its effects on health, education and access to services. In the other case, definitions of sexual assault, reporting and under-reporting, the response of the police and legal system, demographic distribution, consequences for physical and mental health, and more. 'The problem of' provides a succinct way of referring to (but sometimes avoiding) all this, without the need to itemise everything that might be relevant.

As I have already suggested, the number of TG+ nouns is relatively small. In Section 5.6, however, I'll suggest that another noun can be added to the list: 'concept'.

5.3 Types of cohesiveness

So TG+ constructions are a variant of Gentner and Kurtz's (2005) 'thematic groupings', with something added. That 'something' is a set of three related features: a sense of cohesiveness, a different grammar and a 'boundedness' metaphor. Before proceeding, I need to say more about cohesiveness. Consider the following TG+ expressions:

- The world of science
- The culture of science
- The role of science
- The context of science

If we start from a TG baseline of 'things associated with science', each of these expressions adds a type of cohesiveness. They are not all the same type, because the emphasis varies: each TG+ phrase conjures up a subtly different kind of cohesive organisation, with the ontologically diverse 'elements' of science being implicitly arranged in different ways. In every example, there is a slightly different permutation of 'things associated with', and they orbit around a different centre.

'The world of science' is a *professional environment*, peopled with individual scientists and institutions. It is where you can pursue a calling or a career. It embodies certain options and various structures. It is a place through which the individual can move, adopt goals, find a trajectory.

'The culture of science' is a *form of life*, a set of beliefs, attitudes and practices. These are present in 'the world of science', but here they take centre stage. The 'culture' refers to scientific methods, principles, values. It is less an environment to move in, more a way of doing things.

'The role of science' is a *functional* expression. It refers to the institutions and achievements of science, and implies that they make (or should make) a contribution to something: 'society', policy making, the improvement of people's lives, the development of useful technology.

'The context of science' is a *background* for something else. Its cohesiveness is now its difference from other possible contexts, the fact that it is not fashion, sport or literature. Again, the elements in the other TG+ expressions haven't gone away. It's just that the boundedness of a 'context' is different from the boundedness of a 'world', 'role' or 'culture'.

We could repeat this exercise with other N2-terms. 'Education', for example: 'the world of education', 'the culture of education', 'the role of education', 'the context of education'. The key point is that every N1 term of a TG+ expression implies a certain cohesiveness in the domain it refers to, but it's a different kind of cohesiveness in each case. I'll return to this idea in Section 5.6.

5.4 Domain nouns

One reason why there are not very many TG+ nouns is that some nouns, acting as mass nouns, can do the job themselves with no help from a TG+ phrase. The noun 'football', for example, discussed in the last chapter, performs the function in sentences such as:

(17)   A matter of life and death? Football is much more serious than that!
(18)   On the question of racism, football has got to get its act together.

These, I said, are unbounded metonyms, 'football' in each case being used to refer to something like a 'world'. Indeed, 'the world of football' could be substituted for 'football' in both (17) and (18), and the sense would not alter dramatically, though the sharpness would be lost. So in this case, and in several others, an unbounded metonym is the rough equivalent of a TG+ expression. Consider also:

(19) The Hugo Boss Prize is art's greatest accolade.
(20) Society insists that women do ridiculous things to look good.

In these examples, 'society' and 'art' refer to something like a 'world' without needing to be part of a TG+ expression. We could substitute '...is the world of art's greatest accolade' in (19), and not change the sense; but there is no need to do so because 'art' is the kind of noun which, like 'football', can do the job by itself.[4] In (20), by contrast, it is difficult to think of a TG+ expression that could be substituted for 'society', at least not without a significant change in meaning. In this case, 'society' itself performs the TG+ function in a way that an expression of the form $< The + N1 + of + N2 >$ seems unable to do.

I propose to call nouns like 'society', 'art' and 'football' *domain nouns*. More precisely, I would say that they are nouns which can have a 'domain function' (in addition to several other functions). But it will be convenient, often, to refer simply to 'domain nouns'.[5] When acting as a domain noun, a word has a TG+ function, in that it refers vaguely to an ontologically diverse domain of things, without identifying any of them. In this respect, domain nouns are like metonyms with unbounded targets ('the pen', 'the sword'); but they are not genuinely metonymic, because there is no source-and-target relation involved. A domain noun is a rough equivalent of a TG+ expression of the form $< The + N1 + of + N2 >$. Sometimes, there will be a TG+ expression which is an alternative to the stand-alone noun. But in other cases, the domain noun will not have a TG+ expression equivalent at all ('society').

Domain nouns (or nouns exploiting their domain function) can be used in the same way that metonyms, TG expressions and TG+ expressions can: to refer to ontologically diverse domains of things without identifying, specifying or describing them. They appear again in Part II, especially Chapters 9 and 11.

5.5 Non-identifying reference constructions

In this section, I will briefly review the five constructions which, in this chapter and the last, have turned out to be examples of non-identifying reference: ad hoc categories, thematic groupings, domain nouns, TG+ expressions and unbounded metonyms. In all cases, it is the default option I describe. Inevitably, there are exceptions.

5.5.1 Ad hoc category

Consider the grammar of Barsalou's examples: 'things to take on a camping trip'; 'places to look for antique desks'; 'things that babies do'; 'ways to make friends'. They consist of a category noun (CN) – 'things', 'places' and 'ways' – followed by a clause. The domain of items is ontologically uniform. In Barsalou's examples, the domains are physical objects, places, activities and methods; but there is no obvious limit to the nouns that could function as CNs; for example: 'emotions on being told your father has been arrested'; 'flavours to include in a new range of crisps'. Still, the ad hoc categories that interest me here are those in which the CN is a desemanticised noun like 'things' and 'stuff'. In this form of ad hoc category, the reference is necessarily *exophoric* (Section 4.4.3), given that the items referred to are not identified.

5.5.2 *Thematic grouping*

Following Gentner and Kurtz (2005), I introduced thematic groupings as a variant of ad hoc categories. The main parallel is obvious. An example of an ad hoc category: 'things to take on a camping trip'. An example of a thematic grouping: 'things associated with going to a movie'. In both cases, we have an expression whose grammar is < *things* + CLAUSE >. As we have just seen, however, the CN of an ad hoc category can be any one of a wide range of nouns. In a thematic grouping, by contrast, the CN must be a desemanticised word like 'things' or 'stuff'. The main reason for this is that the domain referred to by a TG is not limited to a single ontological category, and only desemanticised nouns can refer to that kind of diversity. Like ad hoc categories, TGs permit exophoric reference (although 'things' is capable of exophoric reference all by itself: 'Look, Fawlty, we want our things!').

5.5.3 *TG+ construction*

This construction was introduced as a grammatical almost-alternative to a thematic grouping. Instead of 'things associated with N', we could have a construction of the form < The N1 of N2 >, where N1 is one of a limited number of TG+ nouns, including 'world', 'role' and 'culture'. A TG+ expression refers to an ontologically diverse domain of things associated with the N2 in question. The reason why this is an *almost*-alternative to a thematic grouping is that the N1, in each case, has a kind of integrative function. 'The world of fashion' is not just a bunch of 'things associated with'. It implies a kind of cohesiveness. As with thematic groupings and ad hoc categories, the TG+ construction permits exophoric reference.

5.5.4 *Unbounded metonym*

As noted in Section 4.7, an unbounded metonym is one in which the 'target' (what is being referred to) is an ill-defined, ontologically diverse domain. In 'The pen is mightier than the sword', both 'pen' and 'sword' represent unbounded metonyms. In any particular example, the domain is metonym-specific: it is determined by the metonym itself, supported by relevant background knowledge. The grammar is straightforward: either < DETERMINER + COUNT NOUN > or < MASS NOUN >. 'The pen' (in 'The pen is mightier than...') is an example of the former. 'Football' (in 'Football must get its house in order') is an example of the latter. In both cases, the reference is exophoric. This is, in fact, the primary function of an unbounded metonym.

5.5.5 Domain nouns

Nouns capable of exercising a domain function ('art', 'society') also permit exophoric, non-identifying reference to domains which are ontologically diverse. Like all the other constructions mentioned in this section, they presuppose various clusters of background knowledge: frames, cognitive domains, scripts, idealised cognitive models (Section 4.7).

In summary, exophoric, non-identifying reference to ontologically diverse domains is not an uncommon function. English affords a number of different ways of achieving it. However, in the present context it is the TG+ option that I am particularly interested in.

5.6 'The concept of' as a TG+ construction

In Section 5.3, I discussed four TG+ expressions, each of which affords a distinct type of cohesiveness: 'the world of science', 'the culture of science', 'the role of science' and 'the context of science'. My suggestion in this section is that 'the concept of science' is another TG+ expression, akin to these four, but providing another form of cohesiveness. I will also suggest that, in general, 'the concept of X' is, or *can be*, a TG+ expression, non-identifyingly referring to an ontologically diverse domain, and hinting at cohesiveness of a particular kind.

So imagine, just as an exercise, that 'the concept of science' *is* a TG+ construction (some of the time, at least).[6] In other words, it is an expression referring, non-identifyingly, to things associated with science. The things in question are of a certain kind. They include ways in which science is understood, thought about, talked about, philosophised about. They also include ways of thinking about disciplines regarded as 'scientific'; for example, their aims and methods, the relations between them, and the ways in which scientific disciplines differ from non-scientific ones. We can add institutions and conventional forms of communication, insofar as these are implicated in the way science is practised, or the ways science is understood as being practised. To the extent that we can accept all this, we have another ontologically diverse array of 'things' being referred to, in the vaguest possible manner, without any of them being identified by the expression itself.

The triad of features described in Section 5.1 is present here. Obviously, there is a convenient grammar. A singular noun, 'concept', and a short noun phrase are easier to deal with than an inchoate list of 'associated things'. There is, additionally, a sense of cohesiveness, one which is distinct from 'world of...', 'culture of...' and 'role of...'. In this case, the domain 'hangs together' in the sense that, implicitly, science has a kind of integration. The expression implies that different scientific disciplines can be treated as if they resemble each other in significant respects. Whatever it is that physicists and chemists do, there is *something* about it that makes it comparable with what astronomers and biologists do (although exactly what this something is remains open for debate). Consequently, it makes rough-and-ready sense that we can have a philosophy of science, a sociology of science, a history of science and so on.

The boundedness metaphor is not a location but an object. This 'object' has been with us since the start of the book: the idea that a concept is an object of some kind, whether a mental particular (Fodor 1998) or an abstract entity (Rosen 2017). As I observed in Section 2.1, the metaphor is particularly salient in the nursing literature: a concept has an 'internal structure' and can be broken 'into its simpler elements'. It is possible to identify a concept's constituent components (Rodgers et al. 2018), and 'to "get inside" it, and see how it works' (Walker and Avant 2005).

Two additional notes. The first is retrospective, and picks up an earlier point. If the TG+ construction account is right, then we can't complete sentences beginning 'Concepts are…'. Nor can we answer the question: 'What is a concept?' Concepts are… what? They aren't anything. But we *can* say what the word 'concept' does; and we can say what an expression of the form 'the concept of X' does. ('An expression of this form refers to a TG+ grouping in a cognitive domain, without identifying any of the ontologically diverse elements in that grouping.' At least, that's the short version.) 'Concept', it turns out, is an extremely useful word… but it doesn't name anything. Concepts are not objects of any kind.

The second note is prospective, and anticipates part of the discussion in Chapter 7, where I talk about *meaning*. There are similarities between 'the concept of X' and 'the meaning of "X"'; but they are not identical.[7] The idea, found in some writers (for example: Peacocke 1992, Horwich 1998), that 'concepts *are* meanings' is, I think, actively misleading, and looks like an attempt to find *something* that concepts can be said 'to be'. Still, 'concept' and 'meaning' do have one thing in common. 'Meaning' is another useful, in fact indispensable, noun. But, like 'concept', it does not name anything (see Section 7.5).

5.7 Concept possession

In this section, I'm going to discuss the relation between 'the concept of X' and the idea that people can 'possess the concept of X'. This relation has provoked much rumbling and grumbling in philosophy, and I'll have to say a bit about that (although I'll say more in the next chapter). A useful place to start is with Jerry Fodor.

According to Fodor (1998, 2004), the current philosophical fashion is to say that *having the concept X* takes priority over *being the concept X*. We begin by analysing what it is for someone to *have* a concept. After that, what it is for something to *be* a concept is derivative. Briefly: 'Concept *X* is just *whatever it is that having the concept X consists in having*' (Fodor 1998: 2). Fodor rejects this fashion wholesale. He thinks that it's associated with a form of pragmatism, and he won't have any truck with *that*. It entails that concepts are just 'constructs', and involves 'the reduction of concepts ... to epistemic capacities' (4). Instead, Fodor reverts to what he calls the classical view: that the analysis of *concepts* comes first, and the 'having concepts' part comes later. Once we know what a concept *is*, we will know what it means to *possess* one. And, in Fodor's view, concepts are mental particulars. They are part of the fixtures and fittings of the mind, not some derivative logical invention.[8]

One of Fodor's premises ('I suppose all this to be truistic') is:

> It's a general truth that if you know *what an X is*, then you also know *what it is to have an X*. And ditto the other way round ... [T]he link between "is an X" and "has an X" is conceptual; fix one and you thereby fix the other.
>
> (Fodor 1998: 2; italics original)

I think this 'truism' is problematic. It is based on the assumption that X is an object of some kind. To adapt one of Fodor's own examples: if you know what a pumpkin is, then you know what it is to have a pumpkin. Conversely, if you know what it is to have a pumpkin, then – *ipso facto* – you know what a pumpkin is. 'Having' appears to be a kind of possessing, almost a kind of ownership.

As reported in Chapter 3, this is something Austin (1961: 10) comments on. He says that a concept is often treated 'as an article of property, a pretty straightforward piece of goods, which comes into my "possession" ... whether I do possess it or not is, apparently, ascertained simply by making an inventory of the "furniture" in my mind'. Austin is sceptical about all this. So am I.

'Have' is a complex verb.[9] It can certainly signify possession, or something akin to it:

(21) I have an 1825 edition at home.
(22) He has a bad temper.
(23) You have a choice of colours.
(24) She is having half a slice of cake.

It is, of course, used as an ancillary verb ('they have found the gold'); and it can be part of a 'light verb construction' (Shahrokny-Prehn & Höche 2011). This expression refers to a group of common transitive verbs which take as their object a noun which can also be used as a verb. For example:

(25) Let's have a listen to your chest.
(26) You don't mind me having a smoke?

In addition, there are various idiomatic uses which are difficult to classify:

(27) They're having an absolute ball.
(28) He has a mind to shoot you.
(29) I've half a mind to resign.
(30) Actually, I do have time to devote to this.

(31)   Do you have a minute?

Fodor's 'truism' about the link between 'is an X' and 'has an X' is implicitly modelled on examples like (21) to (24). It's not clear that the same truism applies to examples like (27) to (31). If you know what a ball is, do you also know what it is to have a ball? It has nothing to do with spherical objects or formal dances. We can ask similar questions all the way down the list. If you know what a mind is, must you know what 'has a mind to' means? If you know what 'having half a mind to' is, do you know what half a mind is? If you know what it is to 'have time', do you thereby know what *time* is? If you know what a minute is, do you know what it is to 'have a minute'? In none of these cases does Fodor's 'truism' work. 'Having a minute' is not like having an 1825 edition. 'Having half a mind' is not like having half a slice. 'Having time' is not like having a bad temper. Nor does it imply that you understand what time *is*.[10]

These are all examples consistent with Construction Grammar, but clearly inconsistent with the idea of 'compositionality', which Fodor regards as non-negotiable somewhere along the line.[11] In Fodor's view, concepts are *objects* of a certain type (mental particulars); so, for him, it makes sense to say that they are the *constituents* of something (thoughts). It also makes sense to assume that, if we talk about 'having the concept of X', this is broadly the same kind of 'having' as we find in examples (21) to (24). And this is, of course, the assumption that supports Fodor's 'truism'. For Fodor, the statement 'Concepts are...' *can* be completed, and the question 'What are concepts?' can be answered. Concepts are mental particulars. They are, at any rate, *something*.

The alternative picture I am presenting does not take concepts to be objects at all. It doesn't have a view about the relation of *what the concept X is* and *having the concept X*. Because concepts are not objects, it doesn't make sense to ask what the concept X *is*; and if we talk about 'having the concept X', it is not the kind of 'having' involved in 'having the 1825 edition' or 'having a temper'. Instead, the alternative picture deals in linguistic constructions, and asks what we do with them. It asks how the expression 'the concept of X', is used, and what it means to say that someone 'has the concept of X'. It claims that both of these expressions are TG+ constructions (at least some of the time).

5.8   The TG+ account of concepts and concept possession

So here is a rough-and-ready version of what these expressions do (according to the alternative picture):

'*The concept of X*   To talk about 'the concept of X' is to refer very vaguely to an ontologically diverse domain of things without identifying them. This domain includes: how X is understood, thought about, discussed; how the word 'X' is used; how items labelled as X are differentiated from items that aren't. In referring to 'the concept' of X, a sense of cohesiveness is implied, suggesting that these ways of thinking and understanding 'hang together';

that they are, in some ill-defined way, integrated. While this type of exophoric reference is very useful, the introduction of a noun into the grammar risks encouraging the belief that 'concept' refers to an object.

'*She possesses the concept of X.*' To make this claim is to refer vaguely to an ontologically diverse domain of things without identifying them. The domain includes: the fact that she recognises examples of X, and labels them appropriately; her ability to distinguish, in practice, between things that are X and things that aren't; her knowledge of basic facts about items labelled as X; the fact that she knows how Xs can be used, or what their significance is. Again, there is an implied cohesiveness about the items in this domain. This is inherited, in part, from 'the concept of X'; but it also suggests that her references to 'X' and examples of X are consistent. As before, the introduction into the grammar of a 'having' verb combined with a noun encourages the belief that 'concept' refers to an object that has been 'acquired'.

I need to emphasise a number of things about these statements. First, they are *not* definitions. The first one is not a definition of 'the concept of X', and the second is not a definition of 'possessing the concept of X'. TG+ constructions don't define. They non-identifyingly refer to a thematic grouping (plus a sense of cohesiveness, even if this is vague, implicit and unevidenced).

Second, and relatedly, neither expression has a definitive list of items associated with it. The whole point of non-identifying reference is to *not* specify, to *not* itemise. It comes with a kind of 'general extender' tag line: 'and that sort of thing'.[12] Nor is there any boundary or boundary criterion. Again, the point is that *what* is inside the boundary (and what isn't) remains only loosely indicated – a broad, almost arm-waving gesture. It is not carefully specified.

Third, neither statement takes priority over the other. This is in reference to Fodor's attack on 'concept Pragmatism', which (he argues) takes 'having a concept' to be prior to 'being a concept'. The question of priority only makes sense if something is being defined. You define one thing, and then the definition of another thing is derived from *that*. If X takes ontological priority over Y, then Y is just a construct derived from the definition of X. It is derivative. However, since the two statements above do not define anything, there is no question of one of them being 'prior' to the other.

Fourth – but this is just a corollary of what I've said so far – the two statements do not *identify* concepts with abilities. The idea that concepts *are* abilities is a minority view in philosophy, one shared by Price (1953), Geach (1957) and Kenny (2010). Geach suggests that concepts 'are capacities exercised in acts of judgement' (7). However, the view I've outlined does not claim that concepts *are* abilities. It claims that concepts *aren't anything*, including abilities. On this view, as soon as you start to say 'Concepts are…', you're basically on the wrong track. As soon as you ask 'What are concepts?', you're asking to be misled. The alternative I have been proposing is that we should stop trying to explain what concepts are, or what kind of state 'having a concept' is. Rather, we should look at what function the two TG+ expressions above have. In both cases, the short answer is:

non-identifying reference to a whole load of stuff. (Look, Fawlty, we want our things!)

The concepts-as-abilities view is one for which I have a lot of sympathy, but it's not one I hold. I will say a bit more in Section 5.10 and the next chapter.

5.9 'Concept' as a placeholder word

Philosophers and psychologists talk routinely about 'having', 'possessing' and 'acquiring' the concept of X, but these expressions turn up very rarely in common parlance. In fact, 'possess the concept of' and 'acquire the concept of' don't appear in COCA at all. 'Has', 'have' and 'had' appear only a handful of times. Given that 'have/posses/acquire the concept' is an expression employed almost exclusively in academic contexts, it's tempting to suppose that they are used as technical terms. This is one reason why Chapter 6 is devoted to examining what philosophers and psychologists have said on the matter.[13]

In COCA, the words which precede 'concept' fall mainly into two groups: verbs and adjectives. In this section, I will consider adjectives (turning to verbs in the next). The most common adjectives are 'new', 'whole', 'basic', 'original', 'important', 'key'. 'New' and 'whole' are by far the most frequent. 'Basic' is by some distance third. Take a look at some examples:

(32)   Women as police detectives was an unfamiliar concept.

(33)   Looking at each other while talking. It's a new concept!

(34)   The key concept is becoming a 'missional' church, he said.

(35)   The whole concept of a new year's resolution has never appealed to me.

(36)   Anthropologically, monogamy is a tricky concept.

(37)   That's the basic concept. He wants them to look at the art, not read the label.

In Section 4.4.4, I discussed the use of 'thing' as a placeholder word (Channell 1994, Drave 2000). As I noted then, placeholders are generic, semantically depleted words which stand in place of more specific terms. They are used in a variety of related circumstances: for example, when the speaker cannot recall the correct expression, or where precise identification is unnecessary.

There is another interesting use: where English grammar requires a noun to be paired with an adjective; for example, 'the important thing is to leave'. In English, 'it is desirable to present such adjectives as a part of a nominalized construction' (Fronek 1982: 649). Many other languages do not need a noun in the equivalent constructions. For example, an Italian translation of 'the important thing is to leave' might be 'l'importante è partire', in which there is no equivalent of 'thing'. English does not permit 'the important is to leave', so inserts a 'dummy' noun after the adjective: 'the important thing'. 'Concept' can be used in a similar way. It has the 'dummy noun' function in (32) to (34): 'an unfamiliar concept', 'the key concept'. In some instances, it can even be replaced by 'thing': 'It's a new thing!' (in 33). Or it can be omitted altogether, adjusting the syntax accordingly: 'Looking at each other while talking. It's new!'[14]

In examples (35) to (37), 'concept' is being used as a placeholder in the absence of a more precise term, or where searching for one is unnecessary. (37), for instance, refers to the philosophy of Albert Barnes (of the Barnes Foundation in Philadelphia). Indeed, one might replace 'concept' with 'philosophy' here, or 'idea', or 'principle'. None of these terms is especially precise in this context, but it's not clear what expression would be.[15] 'Concept' is a readily available, go-to noun of first resort in such circumstances.

'Concept', like 'thing', is frequently used as a placeholder word; and, like 'thing', it can also be used in the formulation of ad hoc categories and thematic groupings. Ultimately, it can take a step further and perform as the head noun in TG+ constructions, something 'thing' can't do. But their functions overlap; and, to that extent, they are linguistically related.

5.10 Understanding and grasping concepts

The most common verbs preceding 'the concept of' in COCA are 'understand', 'introduce', 'grasp', 'use', 'develop', 'embrace' (and their inflected forms). A few examples:

(38) Experts say that children grasp the concept of money as early as age three.
(39) Patients need to understand the concept of risk.
(40) Educational leaders must embrace the concept of tradition.
(41) Oberg introduced the concept of culture shock.

Here, I am particularly interested in 'understand' and 'grasp'. Let's consider (38). What is 'the concept of money', and what counts as 'grasping' it? The sentence is taken from a CNN article on 'helping your kids become financially independent', so we should not expect precise accounts of developmental psychology; and it turns out that the situation is far more complicated than the CNN piece implies (for a helpful review, see Webley 2005).

Older studies, conducted in the Piagetian framework, identified various 'stages' in children's learning. For example, there is an early stage at which they can discriminate between money and other objects, but they have only a vague awareness of its function, and cannot distinguish between different coins. Since this stage typically occurs at ages three to four, it presumably counts as 'grasping the concept of money' according to the CNN 'experts'. Then there is the stage at which they have a notion that money can buy things, but they think that any coin can buy anything. At some point, they recognise that notes are more valuable than coins, but only in the vaguest way. Later, they begin to understand that there is a scale of 'value', and that sometimes you might not have enough money for certain things. When this awareness begins to sharpen, they initially believe that one must tender the exact amount (in other words, they do not understand 'change'). At a later stage, they realise that change can be given. Throughout this period, there is no sense that money can be earned, or any thought as to where it comes from. It is only around ages seven to eight that children come to recognise that it is a form of remuneration.

More recent studies have placed greater emphasis on variations within age groups, and the significance of social and economic context. But even this brief (and over-simplifying) account provides a sense of the sheer range of things children learn over a period of time. If 'the concept of money' is an object of some kind (mental particular, abstract entity), at what point is it 'acquired' or 'grasped'? Is being able to distinguish between coins – as physical objects – and bricks, crayons or toys sufficient? If not, at what point do you draw a firm line and say: '*Now* she has acquired it'? There appears to be no definitive threshold, not one for which a conclusive argument can be provided. What there is instead is a series of things children learn… gradually, slowly, bit by bit.

This brings us back to the idea of concepts-as-abilities (mentioned in Section 5.8). The child's learning about money can be represented as the acquisition of a set of abilities: distinguishing, understanding, recognising and so on. Which particular permutation of these abilities counts as 'having the concept'? The question barely makes sense. Any proposal about the 'concept threshold' is going to be arbitrary; and if you say that *every* relevant ability must be present, you give yourself another threshold problem. What counts as 'relevant'? How do you draw the line? Where do you stop? How do you tell where 'the concept of money' leaves off and the 'the concept of economics', say, begins?

My own suggestion about how we should construe 'the concept of money' doesn't have these problems. The whole point of a TG+ construction is that it refers to ill-defined items in the vaguest possible terms. In this case, 'the concept of money' refers to various abilities people have, to various things they can do, know about, talk about, distinguish, recognise, understand. This array of stuff comes with a built-in *and-that-sort-of-thing* coda. There is no specific content and no defined boundary. It is, as I have said before, the linguistic equivalent of a broad, arm-waving gesture. The noun used to box all this, 'concept', lends it an implied cohesiveness: a range of abilities and understandings that all, broadly, fit together. What particular thing, or permutation of things, you have in mind when you talk about 'the concept of money', or when you claim that Linden 'has acquired the concept of money', doesn't really matter. People have a general sense of what you're referring to. In certain circumstances, they will want to ask about some of the details ('What exactly is it that Linden can do? What exactly is it he understands?'). But the details are often not important.

5.11 Conclusion

'Concept' is surprisingly like 'thing', which I discussed in the last chapter. It is very commonly used as a placeholder word, and permits expressions which refer to thematic groupings. However, there are also two important differences. First, 'concept' can act as the head noun in TG+ expressions, suggesting a form of cohesiveness; 'thing' can't. Second, and relatedly, 'concept' is used to refer to discursive and linguistic domains; 'thing' is generic. Both words, however, belong to a family of devices in English which can exophorically refer to ontologically diverse domains of things without identifying, specifying or describing them. In that sense, they are both examples of 'vague language' (Channell 1994).

I can't imagine that the reader will be entirely happy with this line of thought. Certainly, she won't be fully persuaded. Nurses (not to mention philosophers and psychologists) believe that there *are* concepts, and that they explain our cognitive abilities. In their view, concepts are mental items or abstract objects. They have structures, attributes and boundaries; they are components of thoughts or propositions. In the next chapter, therefore, I will consider the reasons why people think there *must* be concepts.

Notes

1 Or, for both N1 and N2, a short noun phase ('the secret world of military science'). I do not mean to imply that *all* constructions of this form display the three characteristics. For example, 'the cup of tea' doesn't display them. But TG+ constructions *do* have them. One difference is that, in TG+ constructions, N1 is always an abstract noun.

2 Etymologically, 'role' is from the French *rôle*, originally the roll of paper on which the actor's part was written.

3 'Allegedly' because the 'culture of poverty' idea (Lewis 1966) was strongly criticised, and scholars who espoused it were accused of blaming the victim. 'Contemporary researchers rarely claim that culture will perpetuate itself for multiple generations regardless of structural changes' (Small et al. 2010: 8).

4 Metaphorical. I'm talking as if words were independent agents, and as if nouns like 'art' and 'football' have certain properties which make them 'able' to do this 'job'. What I mean is that they are sometimes *used* in this way.

5 In Chapter 9, I will suggest that 'hope' is sometimes a domain noun. This doesn't mean it can't have other functions. In fact, it has *many* other functions.

6 We will see in Section 5.9 that 'the concept of...' is not always a TG+ construction.

7 Briefly: to ask about the meaning of the word 'X' is usually to ask for either a definition or a synopsis of its use. To ask about the concept of X is usually to ask what accounts, understandings and theories of X there are.

8 Fodor starts from disputed premises and, not surprisingly, some philosophers think his position is 'a deeply mistaken one' (Levine & Bickhard 1999: 6). There is a good symposium on Fodor's account of concepts, beginning with Fodor (2004), in *Mind & Language*, Volume 19(1). I'll refer to him again in Chapter 6.

9 '*Have* is a ubiquitous verb in English. To examine all its different uses and functions would require several bulky volumes' (Wierzbicka 1988: 295). Of course, it can also be a noun: 'the haves and the have-nots'.

10 This is another example of Wittgenstein's observation: 'When words in our ordinary language have prima facie analogous grammars we are inclined to try to interpret them analogously; i.e. we try to make the analogy hold throughout'. See Section 2.3, and Chapter 1 of Kuusela (2008).

11 'Compositionality'. This is the idea that the meaning of a sentence, or a thought, is derived from the meaning of its constituents, and can *only* be so derived. It's related to the dictionary-plus-grammar model. Fodor takes compositionality to be a 'non-negotiable' requirement of any account of thought or language. 'As between the two, at least one of thought and language must be compositional' (Fodor 2001). Since he acknowledges that not all language is compositional, it follows that thought *must* be. 'An account of concept possession that is incompatible with the compositionality of thought is, ipso facto, out of the running' (Fodor 2004: 37).

12 For a study of general extenders – 'and so on', 'and so forth', 'and that sort of thing', 'and stuff like that' – see Overstreet (1999).
13 There are very few attempts to compare the philosophical and psychological uses of 'concept' with its ordinary use. An interesting example is Slaney and Racine (2011), which concludes that the 'meaning of the term' in psychology and philosophy is 'quite mysterious'.
14 In an interesting footnote, Fodor (2008: 29) acknowledges that 'a case could be made that concepts like EVENT, AGENT, CAUSE, ACTION, THING… function as place-holders for bone fide predicates. Quite plausibly, to say "He flew out the window; what an odd THING to HAPPEN!" is just to say "He flew out the window; how odd!".' It's ironic that he didn't consider the possibility that CONCEPT, or 'concept', might (sometimes) function in the same way.
15 As I noted in Section 4.4.4, the functions of placeholder words overlap. As here. There is not much to choose – in (37), for example – between saying that 'concept' is a dummy noun paired with 'basic', and saying that is being used in the absence of a more precise term.

References

Austin, J. L. (1961). *Philosophical Papers*. Oxford: Clarendon Press.

Channell, J. (1994). *Vague Language*. Oxford: Oxford University Press.

Drave, N. (2000). Vaguely speaking: A corpus approach to vague language in intercultural conversations. In P. Peters, P. Collins, & A. Smith (Eds.), *Language and Computers: New Frontiers of Corpus Research. Papers from the Twenty-First International Conference of English Language Research and Computerised Corpora* (pp. 25–40). Amsterdam: Rodopi.

Fodor, J. (1998). *Concepts: Where Cognitive Science Went Wrong*. New York: Oxford University Press.

Fodor, J. (2001). Language, thought and compositionality. *Royal Institute of Philosophy Supplements, 48*, 227–242.

Fodor, J. (2004). Having concepts: A brief refutation of the twentieth century. *Mind and Language, 19*, 29–47.

Fodor, J. (2008). *LOT 2: The Language of Thought Revisited*. Oxford: Clarendon Press.

Fronek, J. (1982). *Thing* as a function word. *Linguistics, 20*, 633–654.

Geach, P. T. (1957). *Mental Acts*. London: Routledge and Keegan Paul.

Gentner, D., & Kurtz, K. J. (2005). Relational categories. In W.-K. Ahn, R. L. Goldstone, B. C. Love, A. B. Markman, & P. Wolff (Eds.), *Categorization Inside and Outside the Laboratory* (pp. 151–175). Washington, DC: American Psychological Association.

Horwich, P. (1998). *Meaning*. Oxford: Clarendon Press.

Kenny, A. (2010). Concepts, brains, and behaviour. *Grazer Philosophische Studien, 81*(1), 105–113.

Kuusela, O. (2008). *The Struggle Against Dogmatism: Wittgenstein and the Concept of Philosophy*. Cambridge, MA: Harvard University Press.

Lakoff, G., & Johnson, M. (1980). *Metaphors We Live By*. Chicago, IL: University of Chicago Press.

Levine, A., & Bickhard, M. H. (1999). Concepts: Where Fodor went wrong. *Philosophical Psychology, 12*(1), 5–23.

Lewis, O. (1966). *La Vida: A Puerto Rican Family in the Culture of Poverty*. New York: Random House.

Overstreet, M. (1999). *Whales, Candlelight, and Stuff Like that: General Extenders in English Discourse*. New York: Oxford University Press.

Peacocke, C. (1992). *A Study of Concepts*. Cambridge, MA: MIT Press.

Price, H. H. (1953). *Thinking and Experience*. London: Hutchinson.

Rodgers, B. L., Jacelon, C. S., & Knafl, K. A. (2018). Concept analysis and the advance of nursing knowledge: state of the science. *Journal of Nursing Scholarship, 50*, 451–459.

Rosen, G. (2017). Abstract objects. *Stanford Encyclopedia of Philosophy*, https://seop.illc.uva.nl/index.html.

Shahrokny-Prehn, A., & Höche, S. (2011). Rising through the registers: A corpus-based account of the stylistic constraints of light verb constructions. *Corpus, 10*, 239–257.

Slaney, K. L., & Racine, T. P. (2011). On the ambiguity of concept use in psychology. Is the concept 'concept' a useful concept? *Journal of Theoretical and Philosophical Psychology, 31*, 73–89.

Small, M. L., Harding, D. J., & Lamont, M. (2010). Reconsidering culture and poverty. *Annals of the American Academy of Political and Social Science, 629*(1), 6–27.

Walker, L. O., & Avant, K. C. (2005). *Strategies for Theory Construction in Nursing*. 4th ed. Upper Saddle River, NJ: Prentice Hall.

Webley, P. (2005). Children's understanding of economics. In M. Barrett & E. Buchanon-Barrow (Eds.), *Children's Understanding of Society* (pp. 43–67). Hove, UK: Psychology Press.

Wierzbicka, A. (1988). *The Semantics of Grammar*. Amsterdam: John Benjamins.

6 Must there be concepts?

The most familiar reaction to the suggestion that 'there are no such things as concepts' is that it's wrong. More emphatically: it *must* be wrong. There *have* to be concepts. It's not possible that there aren't. The reasons vary, but the emphasis is always the same. Underlying the italics is a series of indispensability arguments. 'Reference to concepts is unavoidable. Concepts are indispensable. They must exist because, if they did not, we wouldn't be able to categorise things, or have thoughts, or formulate beliefs, or make judgments'. Suggesting that there are no such things is a bit like suggesting that there is no such thing as oxygen. 'No oxygen' means no combustion, no breathing, no water. 'No concepts' looks just as radical.

So in this chapter, I'll consider reasons why 'there must be concepts'. The discussion will take us into areas of philosophy and psychology, although I don't have the space to consider everything that might count as a 'theory of concepts'.[1] Instead, I'll concentrate on the ontology of concepts – the kind of things they are supposed to be – and on the functions they're alleged to have.

6.1 Indispensability arguments

First, I will say something more general about indispensability arguments. They are roughly of the form: 'Reference to Xs is indispensable; therefore, there must be Xs'. They are familiar from debates between Platonists and nominalists about the existence of abstract entities (Cowling 2017), and they often refer to indispensability in scientific theories. For example, one argument is to the effect that 'mathematical talk' is indispensable in the sciences; therefore, the corresponding mathematical objects (numbers, functions and so on) must exist. A comparable argument for the existence of concepts might suggest that 'concept talk' – reference to concepts – is indispensable in philosophy and cognitive science; so concepts must exist. For if we cannot avoid referring to concepts, there must be such things as concepts to refer to.

However, the argument is not as compelling as it might seem. There are too many counter-examples. 'A great deal of scientific language indispensably involves what many practitioners in the field will describe as things that don't exist' (Azzouni 2017: 107). One frequently cited example is Melia's (1995):

(1) The average star has 2.4 planets.

Reference to averages (and other statistical ideas) is indispensable in many sciences, given that there is no convenient way of presenting the same information without using expressions which include the term 'average' or one of its equivalents. However, few people would infer, on these grounds, that 'averages exist'. It's not even clear what that means other than something like: 'certain calculations are routine and necessary'. Astronomers don't believe that something called 'the average star' exists; nor do they think that any star has 2.4 planets. So the truth of (1) presumably does *not* entail an ontological commitment to averages, or to the existence of 'the average star'.[2]

It's not just averages. Across the sciences, including biology, sociology and economics, there are many other idealised 'entities' and 'calculated nonentities' (as Azzouni calls them): point masses, weightless inextensible cords, frictionless planes, isolated populations, perfectly rational agents and plenty more. References to non-existent things are imported into mathematical equations to make them solvable. For example, centres of mass are used to describe the motion of galaxies, despite the fact that these 'centres' are not in (and not part of) any of the objects concerned. Assumptions known to be false are made about materials in fluid dynamics and mechanics. It is 'the supposed structural postulations of these materials – that they contain such-and-such kinds of entities as *parts* – that are falsely mathematicised in this way' (Azzouni 2017: 111). These entities are represented as parts of pieces of wood, bodies of water or steel beams undergoing stress. But they don't exist.

Of course, these are all examples of indispensable-but-non-existent things which we *know* don't exist. Mentioning them is intended to suggest that, on its own, the argument 'Reference to X is indispensable, so Xs must exist' doesn't work. However, there are also examples of indispensable-things which some people think exist, while others don't. Numbers are a case in point. No-one doubts their indispensability; but is that sufficient to establish their existence? Some think it is (Tennant 1997, Colyvan 2003). Others think it isn't. Many of the latter group argue that numbers are non-existent (Azzouni 2010, Dorr 2008). Azzouni claims that it is possible to make true statements about things 'that don't exist in any sense at all'. He is talking about mathematical objects; but I could say something similar about concepts: 'It can be true to state that someone possesses the concept of X, even though concepts don't exist'.

The examples cited above show that, if that claim were true, 'concept' would not be a unique case. The indispensability of reference to X does not, in general, entail the existence of Xs. It may be the case *both* that the word 'concept' is indispensable *and* that there are no such things as concepts. Later, I will turn to some examples of what indispensability arguments for concepts look like.

6.2 The ontology of concepts

But first a broad-brush look at the ontological options. As I have suggested in earlier chapters, there are three different views (or types of view) about what concepts *are*:

- Mental somethings
- Abstract objects
- Cognitive abilities

According to Margolis and Laurence (2007), there are two 'dominant frameworks'. One of them proposes that concepts are *mental representations*; the other proposes that they are *abstract objects*. In this section I will discuss the two dominant options. In Sections 6.3 to 6.5, I will assess some typical indispensability arguments. In Section 6.6, I'll say something about the idea that concepts are abilities.

6.2.1 Mental representations

In low resolution, the idea here is that concepts are mental phenomena. They are items which are, quite literally, present in the mind. 'Concepts are particular entities or goings-on in the mind or in the head of individuals' (Glock 2010: 117). They are implicated in the having of thoughts, the holding of beliefs, the making of judgments. Indeed, as I will explain further in a moment, they are usually said to be the *constituents* of beliefs, thoughts and/or judgments. 'Concepts are the basic timber of our mental lives … Concepts are constituents of thoughts' (Prinz 2002: 1, 2). 'Concepts are the glue that holds our mental world together' (Murphy 2004: 1).

There is, in this low-resolution talk, a distinct sense of 'gizmo'-ness, to use Wilson's (2006) word.[3] It's true that, in general terms, a 'mental phenomenon' might be an object, state or process. However, the not untypical reference to 'entities', 'constituents' and 'glue' suggests that the standard framework is lurking in the bushes. 'Concept' is a noun, and nouns are naming words, so 'concept' must be the name of *something*, or some *thing*. Concepts are, as it were, installations in the head. They are a kind of gizmo, without which your mind wouldn't work – just as, without spark plugs, your car won't start.

Moreover, like spark plugs, concepts are not only essential constituents; they also have constituents of their own. They are made of other concepts, smaller gizmos. They have a structure. Or at least some of them have. Others may be 'atoms': basic-level, non-splittable concepts which can be combined to make more complex concepts; and these in turn can be combined to make even more complex concepts, and so on. Ultimately, a group of concepts (whatever their level of complexity) can be combined to form a thought – or a belief, or a judgment, or some other propositional attitude – in roughly the same way that a group of components can be combined to make a car.

In slightly higher resolution, concepts are mental representations. That is to say, they represent things. The concept DOG, for example, represents dogs.[4] In this respect, the concept/thing relation is parallel to the word/thing relation. The word 'dog' also represents dogs, but it does so in a different medium, so to speak. 'Dog' is a *linguistic* representation; DOG is a *mental* representation. And the parallels don't stop there. The way in which concepts can be combined to form a thought is parallel to the way in which words can be combined to form a sentence. 'The dog ate its dinner' is a sentence which has words as its constituents. THE DOG ATE ITS DINNER is a thought which has concepts as its constituents. If you express the thought in words, it is (in effect) 'translated' into the sentence.

So concepts and words are both representational, and they can both be combined (into thoughts and sentences, respectively). But how much further do the parallels go? For example, does thought have a grammar in the same way language does? On the face of it, THE DOG ATE ITS DINNER has the same syntax as the sentence 'The dog ate its dinner'. But does that expression – 'THE DOG ATE ITS DINNER' – accurately represent the thought itself, or is it merely a convenient way of *referring* to it, using English as a resource?

The answers to this question can get very complicated very quickly. According to Margolis and Laurence (2007), 'the internal system of representation has a language-like syntax and a compositional semantics and, to that extent, amounts to a language of thought' (562); and they refer to 'the analogy with natural language syntax'. This claim is based on a version of the Representational Theory of the Mind (RTM) associated with Fodor (1975, 2008), and it appears to suggest that mental representations, in the form of thoughts, *do* have a syntax. But notice 'language-like' and 'analogy'. So, yes, we're justified in referring to a 'Language of Thought' (LOT); but, no, its syntax is not the same as English syntax (or the syntax of any other language).[5]

What is it to 'have' a concept according to the 'mental representation' view? Fodor's view of this, as we saw in Section 5.7, is fairly straightforward. It's ordinary 'having'. To have a concept is not massively different from having a pumpkin. Having or possessing a concept means… it has been installed. You've acquired it. The mental-particular-which-is-the-concept is permanently resident in your mind. I suspect there is a broad consensus about this view. As far as I'm aware, no-one who thinks concepts are mental representations has seriously challenged it. (Exactly *how* you acquire concepts is more controversial.[6] Fortunately, we do not need to resolve that issue here.)

6.2.2 Abstract objects

The idea of concepts as mental representations was motivated by the 'cognitive revolution' (Ramsey 2007) and Turing's suggestion that cognitive processes are computations (Fodor 2008). In contrast, the idea of concepts as abstract objects goes back to the older tradition associated with Gottlob Frege. On the low-resolution view, concepts aren't in the head. They are, in some sense, *external* to the mind, not resident within it. For Frege, this externality is literal, and is comparable to the externality of things in the physical world. Physical objects exist independently of the mind; so do concepts. Physical objects are not mental phenomena; neither are concepts. The difference is, concepts are not in space-time, and cannot be seen, heard, touched or manipulated. In this respect, they are like numbers and other abstract entities: things which are neither mental nor physical, but have a different kind of existence altogether.

For this reason, Frege talks about a 'third realm'. Some entities, he suggests,

> are neither things in the external world nor ideas. A third realm must be recognised. Anything belonging to this realm has it in common with ideas that it cannot be perceived by the senses, but has it in common with things that it does not need an owner so as to belong to the contents of consciousness.
>
> (Frege 1984: 363)

The first realm consists of physical objects; the second realm consists of mental phenomena; and the third realm consists of abstract entities.[7]

Despite the differences between them, there are parallels between concepts-as-mental-representations (CMRs) and concepts-as-abstract-objects (CAOs). In both cases, they are the constituents of something. CMRs are the constituents of thoughts. CAOs are the constituents of propositions. It's just that CMRs and thoughts are part of the second realm, while CAOs and propositions are part of the third realm. In one case, we're talking about mental structures; in the other we're talking about abstract structures.

But what *is* a proposition? I'll suggest that, roughly, it is what a sentence expresses, or the statement that it makes. Consequently, two different sentences can express the same proposition. For example, suppose I say: 'The dog is small!', and a French speaker says: 'Le chien est petit!'. The words are not identical, but the two sentences express the same proposition. For this reason, propositions are often held to be *the things which are true or false*, not sentences. As far as truth and falsity are concerned, 'The dog is small' and 'Le chien est petit' are not separate things, both of which happen to be true (or not). Rather, they express a single proposition; and it is the *proposition* – not the sentence which expresses it – that is true or false. And the proposition, like the concepts it consists of, is an abstract entity.

So there is a mirror image here. According to one theory, concepts are mental representations, and are constituents of thoughts. According to the other, concepts are abstract objects, and are constituents of propositions ('larger' abstract objects, as it were). In both cases, the constituents can be 'combined' in order to create something more complex: a thought in one case, a proposition in the other.

In higher resolution, the complexities start again. For example, what do CAO theorists have to say about the ideas in our heads? Do they deny their existence? Well, no. They think 'there are things in our heads that *correspond* to concepts; but on their view, the things in our heads aren't concepts; they're *mental representations* of concepts' (Balaguer 2016: 2370). CMR theorists think that mental representations *are* concepts; CAO theorists think that they *represent* concepts. So it does start to get a trifle messy. Again, however, we don't have to resolve these 'high-resolution' issues here. My aim is only to provide a quick sketch of what the 'abstract object' view of concepts involves.

6.3 'If we didn't have concepts, we couldn't...'

So let's return to the indispensability arguments for the existence of concepts. 'Reference to concepts is indispensable; therefore, concepts must exist'. I have already suggested (Section 6.1) that this is not a valid inference. There are too many counter-examples, too many things we refer to indispensably that are *known* not to exist. So it is possible to accept the premise – reference to concepts is indispensable – but not accept the conclusion. This is basically my position. I'm happy to accept that 'concept' is, for all practical purposes, an indispensable word; but I don't think it follows that concepts exist.

However, this is obviously not the end of the matter. Can't the premise be beefed up a bit? Suppose we say *why* reference to concepts is indispensable? Suppose we point to the things that would be impossible if we didn't have concepts? This, of course, is what many of the indispensability arguments look like. 'If we didn't have concepts we couldn't categorise things'. 'If we didn't have concepts, we couldn't have thoughts'. Psychologists tend to adopt the 'we couldn't categorise' line (Murphy 2004); philosophers go for the 'we couldn't have thoughts' line (Prinz 2002). In this section, then, I will respond to arguments which take this general form: 'If we didn't have concepts, we couldn't...'

There is another argument about the relation between thought and concepts that I will have to consider. Prinz (2002), for example, makes two claims: 'Without concepts there would be no thoughts' (1), and 'concepts are constituents of thoughts' (2). These claims are not the same, given that the first might be true even if the second isn't. Both claims are made routinely in the literature (for example: Crane 1990, Fodor 1994, Carey 2004, Weiskopf 2010, Carston 2012, Bloch-Mullins 2015), although they are not always distinguished from each other. In this section, I'll deal with the first. In Section 6.5, I'll look at the second.

Let's imagine, then, that you, the reader, want to argue like this.

> If there are no such things as concepts, how can I have thoughts, make judgments, or entertain beliefs? If I don't have the concept of a squirrel, how can I have thoughts about squirrels? Isn't it just obvious that I can't have the thought that squirrels eat nuts if I don't have the concepts SQUIRREL, EAT and NUT?

So here's the good news. I'm happy to agree that you can't have thoughts about squirrels if you don't have the concept of a squirrel.

The crucial point is this: I have not denied that it makes sense to say that someone 'has the concept of X' (Sections 5.7 and 5.8). The question is: if you make this claim, what exactly are you saying? On the view outlined in Chapter 5, you are saying that the person concerned has various understandings and abilities. Crudely, she understands what Xs are, knows some basic facts about them and can correctly identify an X when she sees one. In making this claim, you are *referring* to these understandings and abilities, but you're not *identifying* any of them. Nor are you implying that 'having the concept of X' can be *defined* as having this or that particular ability. The reference to 'having the concept' is, very roughly, of the form: 'You know the sort of thing I mean, Fawlty'.

Given this view, the claim that 'you can't have thoughts about squirrels if you don't have the concept of a squirrel' is perfectly correct. You can't have thoughts about squirrels if you don't have various abilities and understandings ('I'm not going to identify them, but you know the sorts of thing I mean'). So on that point, there is a meeting of minds between me and you-the-reader.

The difference is this. *You* assume that 'concept' is detachable (to use the term adopted in Section 3.7). If someone 'has the concept SQUIRREL', then there is something – a concept – that they *have*. You infer that the concept SQUIRREL is a mental gizmo that has to have been installed (if thoughts about squirrels are to be possible). Alternatively, you infer that the concept SQUIRREL is an abstract entity that has to be 'grasped' (before you can have squirrel-related thoughts). If Judy has the concept of SQUIRREL, there is a particular *thing* that she 'grasps' or 'possesses'. The only question left hanging is: exactly what kind of thing is it? The abstract entity or the mental gizmo?

I, in contrast, am untroubled by such questions. The view I have outlined has no such implications. I can agree that Judy 'has the concept SQUIRREL'; but I don't infer that there must (therefore) be a *something*, a 'concept', that she possesses.

This is a reprise of Section 5.7. 'If you know what it is to have an X, then you must know what an X is' – Fodor's truism – is the assumption which lurks underneath the debates about what concepts are, and motivates the idea that they must be *something*. The grammar of 'have the concept of X' is assimilated to the grammar of other 'having' constructions: 'I have the 1825 edition', 'you have a choice of colours', 'she is having half a slice of cake'. In such cases, there really is an edition I have, a choice you have and a slice of cake she is having. These nouns *are* detachable. 'Concept', on the view sketched here, isn't.

As Wittgenstein (1964: 7) observes: 'When words in our ordinary language have prima facie analogous grammars, we are inclined to try and interpret them analogously; i.e. we try to make the analogy hold throughout' (see Section 2.3). On the view outlined in Chapter 5, 'having the concept SQUIRREL' cannot be interpreted analogously to 'having the 1825 edition' or 'having half a slice of cake'. Unlike 'edition' and 'slice of cake', 'concept' is non-detachable. We can agree that Judy *has the concept*; but that doesn't mean that we can start looking for *an object which she has*.

Reader: But if someone has something, then there must be *something* that she has, something she possesses. There has to be a gizmo, as you put it, *somewhere*.

Me: Well, referring back to the discussion in 5.7, not necessarily. 'Having a look', 'has the time', 'have a say', 'have half a mind', 'has the last laugh', 'has the makings', 'having a ball', 'has 2.4 planets', 'having kittens'. Good luck with finding the thing possessed in any of those examples.

Reader: Even if I give you some of those, we can surely distinguish between idioms like that and cases in which there really is something possessed. To use your own examples – the 1825 edition, or a slice of cake.

Me: Yes, but on what basis? Okay, you want to say that 'have the concept SQUIR-REL' is more like 'have the 1825 edition' than 'have the time'. But isn't that because you're *already* convinced that concepts are objects of some kind?

Reader: Put it this way: a list of 'having' idioms isn't going to persuade me that they're not.

Me: It's not meant to. At this point in the discussion, I'm considering indispensability arguments. Specifically: 'You can't have thoughts about squirrels if you don't have the concept SQUIRREL'. And I'm saying: that's true. But I'm also saying: I don't think that 'having the concept' entails that there is a something that you have. The 'having' idioms show that there are linguistic precedents for that. They suggest that Fodor's truism… isn't.

The other versions of the 'If we didn't have concepts, we couldn't…' argument can be met with exactly the same response. For example: 'If we didn't have concepts, we couldn't categorise things; we couldn't identify squirrels *as* squirrels'. Agreed. If we didn't have certain abilities and understandings, we could not recognise squirrels as squirrels. But even if it's true to say that you 'have the concept of a squirrel', it does not follow that there is a particular *something* (namely a concept) that you *possess*.

6.4 A grammatical remark

'We couldn't categorise without concepts'. I think this is what Wittgenstein calls a grammatical remark or a grammatical statement (Wittgenstein 1964: 30, 54). When using this expression, Wittgenstein has in mind what he calls 'depth grammar' (1963: §664). He does not mean syntax, or 'surface grammar', rules for the correct arrangement of words.[8] One simple example of a 'grammatical statement' is: 'One plays patience by oneself' (1963: §248). This is not an interesting empirical claim, much less an interesting metaphysical one. It is simply a reminder that the word 'patience' is reserved for solitaire games. It is a 'grammatical remark'.

Wittgenstein's point is that similar claims are made in philosophy, but we mistake them for interesting claims about the world. In *PI* §248, he is comparing 'One plays patience by oneself' to 'Sensations are private'. This is often taken to be a significant statement about the *nature* of sensations, such as pain. Sensations are private because (for example) only *you* can know you are in pain. A sensation is an inner, private thing that no-one else has access to. And this tells us something interesting about the difference between pains and visible parts of the body.

However, comparing 'Sensations are private' to 'One plays patience by oneself' suggests a different picture. It implies that it is the equivalent of something like: 'You can't have another person's pain'. But, in that case, the metaphysical interest evaporates, because this is on a par with: 'You can't have another person's elbows', or 'You cannot smile somebody else's smile'. These are things that 'belong' to one person, but can't also belong to another. They are not, so to speak, transferable. I can't give someone my smile in the way that I can give them my car keys.[9]

In this sense, then, elbows are private, and smiles are private (and, of course, many other things too). It's not just sensations. So if Wittgenstein's comparison is valid, 'Sensations are private' says no more about the nature of sensations than 'Elbows are private' says about the nature of elbows. It is a 'grammatical statement'.

What are the implications of construing 'We could not categorise without concepts' as a grammatical remark in the same vein? Here's another analogy. Consider the claim: 'You cannot understand words such as "plaise", "fraise" and "chaise" if you don't have French'. This again is a grammatical comment. Understanding words like these (and many more) is *part of what is involved in* 'having French', 'being able to speak French', 'knowing French'. If we say that someone 'has French', or can 'speak French', what we mean is, precisely, that they understand words of this kind. Nobody thinks 'French' is a sort of module that has to be installed in someone's head before they can understand 'chaise' or 'chasse'. We don't think of it as a mind-gizmo whose presence is a causal condition of understanding such words, as if it were something like the Babel fish in *The Hitchhiker's Guide to the Galaxy* (Adams 2017). Rather, learning these words (and others) *is* learning French; and 'having French', being able to speak it, *is* understanding what these words mean.

If we construe 'We could not categorise without concepts' in the same manner, we are suggesting that 'having concepts' *is* being able to categorise (among other things). Learning to identify *this* as a dog and *that* as a chair just *is* acquiring the concepts DOG and CHAIR. In making this suggestion, we're implying that concepts are not mental gizmos that have to be installed in the mind if categorising and identifying are to be possible. They are not mental objects which have to be 'acquired' so that we can combine them in thoughts, or abstract objects that have to be 'grasped' so that we can understand propositions. Just as 'she has French' or 'she can speak French' are different ways of referring to the fact that she understands words like 'chaise' and 'chasse' (among others), so 'he possesses the concept CHAIR' is just a different way of referring to the fact that he is able to identify chairs (among other things: describing them, sitting on them and so on). In both cases, we have two different ways of talking; two different ways of saying the same thing.[10]

In the case of 'concept', as well as in the case of 'French', construing matters this way involves a shift. Rather than seeing the word as referring to a bit of mental 'equipment', without which we could not do certain things, we see it as just a different way of talking about the doing-of-those-things. We drop the equipment/gizmo analogy, and no longer construe 'We could not categorise without concepts' on the model of: 'We could not see without eyes'. Instead, we construe it more on the model of: 'We could not see without vision'.

Similarly, it becomes apparent that asking the question 'How do we categorise things?', and answering 'We have concepts', is like asking 'How does opium induce sleep?' and answering 'It possesses a *virtus dormitiva*'. The expression *virtus dormitiva* ('sleep-inducing property') is used by Molière to satirise the circular explanations often used in early medicine:

> I am asked by the learned doctor the cause and reason why opium causes sleep. To which I reply: it has a sleep-inducing property, whose nature is to lull the senses to sleep.[11]

Here is a satire modelled on Molière's: 'I am asked how we are able to categorise. I reply that there are categorising objects, which I call "concepts", whose nature is to enable categorisation. Thus, we could not categorise without concepts'.

6.5 The constituents of thought

We can now turn to the second claim mentioned in Section 6.3, that 'concepts are the constituents of thought'. This appears to be a deeply entrenched assumption, as it is rarely argued for, more frequently just stated. It raises two interesting questions: first, what kind of things thoughts are (Piccinini & Scott 2006); second, what, in this context, counts as a 'constituent'. As Machery (2009: 26) observes, 'the notions of component and constituent and, *a fortiori*, metaphors like "building blocks" are typically not fully explained'. However, there is an implicit model for the relation *concept/thought* in many of these discussions – and that is the relation *word/sentence*. So I'll start with one of the commonest ways people think about thoughts and thinking, namely 'inner speech'.

6.5.1 Inner speech

Think the sentence: 'The grass is green'. That is, 'recite' the sentence in inner speech. 'Recite' isn't quite the right term. Neither is 'say', because the point is: you are not actually saying anything. It is a *bit* like speaking out loud, only without the speaking. You 'utter' the sentence 'privately'. No-one can listen in.

This is an experience (or an activity) which is very difficult to describe precisely, but it's one with which almost all of us are familiar (Hurlburt et al. 2013). It is one of the things that is described as 'thinking' or 'having a thought'. Normally, such 'thoughts' occur spontaneously; they are not 'recited' at somebody else's invitation, as in the last paragraph. Indeed, for many people 'inner speech' is almost continuous, a constant 'dialogue with oneself' which takes up a large proportion of daily mental activity. What I want to focus on here, though, is the idea of a sentence, 'spoken' as part of inner speech. Such a sentence, as with 'The grass is green', corresponds (in some sense) to what is written on the page. The words occur in that order, and the 'inner saying' has a certain duration, however short. The sentence is 'in English': the words are English, and so is the syntax. The experience, in that respect, is the same (more or less) as uttering the sentence out loud... only not.

So if you're thinking 'The grass is green' in inner speech, and if that counts as a thought you are having, what are the constituents of that thought? On the face of it, an obvious answer is: the individual words in that sentence. So: if the constituents of the thought are concepts, and if the thought *is* the sentence of inner speech, then the constituents of the thought must be the words of that sentence.

However, the idea that concepts are words of inner speech is surely much too narrow. It implies that *all* concepts take this form, and that doesn't seem very plausible. Moreover, if you think that concepts are also required for categorising and identifying things – and if concepts are words in inner speech – then, presumably, every time you identify something, you must *say* the corresponding word 'internally'. For example, every time you recognise something as a bird, you are using the concept BIRD; so you must say 'bird' to yourself in inner speech. But that, I take it, just isn't true. Indeed, it seems that it can't be true. If it were, the day would be full of inner speech along the lines of: 'Bird. Bird. Bird. Tree. Tree. Fence. Gate. Flower. Flower. Flower…' I don't know about anyone else, but my stream of inner speech does not take that form. Recognising, categorising, identifying things is just not a matter of *constantly* saying words like this to yourself.

The natural conclusion is: something's gone wrong. Equating concepts with inner speech words must be a mistake. Presumably, then, it is also a mistake to *identify* thoughts with inner speech. But this brings us back to the question: what *are* thoughts? And in what sense are concepts their constituents? At this point, both thoughts and concepts seem to recede into a mysterious background. We are, in some sense, aware of inner speech;[12] however, if an episode of inner speech is not *in itself* a thought, where has the thought disappeared to?

6.5.2 Thought and imagery

A lot of thoughts just 'present themselves'. Steph and Lewis are discussing how to arrange the furniture. Steph says: 'I've had a thought'. 'What's that?' asks Lewis. Steph replies: 'Why don't we put the chair over in that corner? And then we could move the table to the space under the window'. Is Steph claiming that when the thought 'occurred' to her, it came in that fully fledged form? Did these two sentences just appear in her mind? It's not impossible, but it's unlikely. It's certainly not a requirement of her having had the thought in the first place. Perhaps she had a sudden image of what the room would look like if the two adjustments were made. Perhaps she'd been evaluating various arrangements in her imagination, and decided that this particular one was worth trying.

Well, suppose we ask her: 'What was actually going on when you had the thought, Steph?' She says: 'This picture just appeared in my mind'. Is the picture the thought, then? Or must it be 'translated' into something sentence-like first? But, no, she says the sentence just 'arrived' when Lewis asked her what the thought was. As for the thought itself, she'd had that already, in the form of the picture. Right, so take this account seriously. If that's the thought, what are its constituents? Are we referring to parts of the picture? Sub-pictures, so to speak? The sub-picture of the chair, the sub-picture of the table, the sub-picture of the window…? Are those the constituents of her (overall) mental 'picture'?

At this point, the same doubts arise. The idea that concepts are mini-pictures is too narrow. If concepts are sub-pictures, the implication is that *all* concepts take pictorial form. Again, this does not seem very plausible. Nor is it compatible with the idea that recognising something as a bird requires the concept BIRD. If concepts *are* sub-pictures, that would mean that *every time* we categorise something as a bird, we must have a sub-picture of a bird in our minds. Every time. It would be the pictorial equivalent of saying 'Bird. Bird. Tree. Fence. Flower' to yourself continually in inner speech. Again, it looks as if something's gone wrong. Thoughts can't be pictures, concepts can't be mini-pictures.

As Glock (2006: 39) points out, Frege, Wittgenstein, Ryle and Price all argued convincingly that 'inner' words and images 'are neither necessary nor sufficient for conceptual thought, and they do not determine its content'.[13] If you *identify* thoughts with sentences of inner speech, or with mental 'pictures', and then throw in the idea that concepts are the constituents of thoughts, you arrive at some very counter-intuitive conclusions.

6.5.3 *Thought and introspection*

Rather than assuming that thoughts can be identified with internal speech or imagery, does it help if we try to work out what thoughts are by introspecting? Maybe. 'Think about what you plan to do after you have finished reading' (Schwitzgebel 2011: 128). So what happened when you read that? If you tried to comply with the suggestion, what form did the thinking take? Was there any visual imagery, or auditory imagery, or inner speech? No? What, then? If there *was* some kind of imagery or inner speech, was there anything else in addition to that? If so, what? How confident are you about your response?

Speaking for myself, I find questions of this kind virtually impossible to answer. If invited to think about what I'm planning to do when I've finished work this afternoon… there is a sort of mental wrinkle, but I cannot say precisely what form it takes. It is, at best, very fragmented. Maybe an image of the television, maybe a snippet of inner speech, maybe a brief memory of what I did after work yesterday. But as soon as I make these suggestions, I think: no, that's not really it. The point is: I don't know. My impression is that this fragmented stuff is what happens when I try to 'catch the thought in action'. If the invitation had not been issued, I would not have focused my attention on what I was doing in response to it. At some point, I might have had a fleeting thought about what I was planning to do – heaven knows in what form – without any of the fragmented bits and pieces I'm reporting on now. But, as I say, I don't know.

Of course, I can make a meal of it. I can sit here and work through imagery, inner speech and memories of previous 'finishing work' occasions. I can tell myself: 'I am now thinking about what I'm planning to do when I have finished work this afternoon'. And that's a fair description. But my sense is that none of this is necessary. When I first read Schwitzgebel's invitation, I had some sort of thought anyway, and it was brief, indeterminate, impossible to describe. A mental 'wrinkle', with maybe a brief snapshot of my kitchen... plus the background knowledge that, on this occasion, the kitchen signifies a meal. But that's the best I can do. Yes, I can deliberately go through the motions of 'Hey, this is thinking!', and work the whatever-it-is into a deliberate, extended sequence. But I'm fairly sure that something happened *before* I got round to laying it on with a trowel. What was it like? I don't know. Even the bit about the 'wrinkle' and the snapshot of the kitchen may be artefacts of trying to 'catch' the thought as it was happening.

Schwitzgebel asks whether the answer to the question 'What was the thought like?' is 'as obvious as that your desk has drawers, your shirt is yellow, your shutters cracked?' (128). My reply is: no, not remotely. But here's another question: if thoughts – or at least thoughts of this kind – are so difficult to describe, how do we know what their constituents are? Can a metaphorical 'wrinkle' and a 'maybe-snapshot' *have* constituents? And if they do, what grounds are there for thinking that those constituents are concepts?

6.5.4 Unsymbolised thought

There's an interesting idea that might help with these questions. Employing a method called Descriptive Experience Sampling (DES), Russ Hurlburt and his colleagues have identified a phenomenon they call 'unsymbolized thinking' (Hurlburt & Akhter 2008). In interviews, DES subjects provide full accounts of what their 'inner experience' was at a specific moment in their everyday lives (when a beeper went off). Hurlburt and Akhter suggest that the aim is 'to discover and describe the naturally occurring phenomena of lived experience' (1373).[14]

Unsymbolised thinking is 'the experience of an explicit, differentiated thought that does not include the experience of words, images, or any other symbols' (Hurlburt & Akhter 2008: 1364). The thoughts and thinking reported by DES subjects are fully specific *thoughts that p*, or *wonderings whether p*. Benito, for example, 'is watching two men carry a load of bricks in a construction site. He is wondering whether the men will drop the bricks'. Despite this determinate specificity, there is no imagery associated with the thought: no inner speech, no mental picture. The thought has 'no rhythm or cadence; no unfolding or sequentiality ... there is no temporal, spatial, grammatical, or otherwise formal separation' between any of the thought's 'characteristics'. The thought presents itself as a unit, a singularity, to 'the footlights of consciousness' (1366–7). It is 'directly observable', and 'does not need to be inferred'.

According to Hurlburt and Akhter, unsymbolised thought accounts for approximately a quarter of *all* lived experiences, with perhaps 70% of subjects reporting it. If this is a genuine form of thinking, it appears to be a very common one.

It is possible to be sceptical about the existence of unsymbolised thinking, and many authors have been (for example, Carruthers 1996: 242). Given the lack of properties attributed to it – no imagery, rhythm or sequentiality; no temporal, spatial or grammatical divisions – it is hard to understand in what sense unsymbolised thinking is 'directly observable'. What exactly is it that DES subjects are observing? A determinate singularity with no sensory or structural properties at all? That sounds as close to 'nothing' as it's possible to get, while still claiming that there's a something. At the same time, when reflecting on my own experience of thought (Section 6.5.3), I half-appreciate what Hurlburt is getting at. Perhaps my thought about what I was planning to do when I'd finished work was an unsymbolised one. Perhaps the metaphorical 'wrinkle' and the 'maybe-snapshot' were just artefacts – scraps resulting from my trying to pin the thought down, while simultaneously trying *not* to add gratuitous imagery to it.[15]

However, if unsymbolised thoughts exist – and a large majority of DES subjects are signed up to that – then they obviously don't have constituents. Indeed, Hurlburt and Akhter's (2008) description appears to emphasise this: an unsymbolised thought is a singularity with no sensory properties, no sequentiality, no temporal, spatial or grammatical divisions. How can anything conforming to that description have any constituents? Constituents of what? If there really are unsymbolised thoughts, then they are not thoughts for which constituents, of any kind, are conceivable. So that version of the indispensability argument – 'concepts are the constituents of thought, so concepts must exist' – collapses. If unsymbolised thoughts don't *have* constituents, then concepts can't be *that*.[16]

6.5.5 *Summary*

If episodic thoughts are identified with inner speech, or imagery, then they have constituents. However, many of the things we call thoughts are accompanied by neither. If episodic thoughts are as fragmented, indeterminate and incomplete as introspection suggests, their 'constituents' must be no less so; but it's not clear what *counts* as a 'constituent' of something fragmented, indeterminate and incomplete. Finally, if thoughts are (or can be) 'unsymbolized', then it's difficult to see how they can have constituents at all.

6.6 Concepts as abilities

The third view of the ontology of concepts (Section 6.2) is that they are cognitive abilities. For example, Geach (1957: 7) suggests that concepts 'are capacities exercised in acts of judgment'. So the concept DOG is identified with an ability, or set of abilities. These abilities might include the capacity to use the word 'dog' correctly, recognise dogs, discriminate between dogs and other animals and provide basic information about them. But it's easier to argue that *possessing* a concept can be identified with such abilities than it is to argue that the concept *itself* can be identified with them. 'That concept possession is an ability of some kind is accepted willy-nilly, even by Fodor' (Glock 2010). The disagreements only begin when you ask what the thing possessed is. Possessing a certain gizmo, or 'grasping' it, may well be associated with all kinds of abilities; but that doesn't explain the nature of the gizmo. And that's what Fodor, along with the majority of authors, is interested in: what concepts *are*.

It may not be surprising, then, that even writers who favour the idea of concepts being somehow related to abilities acknowledge that concepts cannot *be* abilities. A number of reasons are offered (for example, Glock 2010 and Hacker 2013). One is that concepts can be instantiated by things. The barking object in front of me instantiates the concept DOG. It 'satisfies' the concept, 'exemplifies' it, 'falls under' it. The same cannot be said of abilities. The object in question does not 'instantiate' an ability, or 'fall under' an ability. The ability to what? Does the object 'fall under' the ability to recognise dogs, or the ability to use the word 'dog' correctly? That doesn't appear to make any sense, and it's certainly not how we talk.

A second reason is that concepts are said to have an *extension* (the class of things they apply to) and an *intension* (the features in virtue of which members of that class are included in it). The extension of DOG is the class of dogs; its intension includes appearance, behaviour, the fact that dogs are often pets and so on. None of this applies to abilities. If I possess the concept DOG, the corresponding range of abilities has no equivalent of extension or intension.

The third reason is that concepts are supposedly constituents of thoughts (or propositions), but no-one claims that abilities have the same function. If I think 'my cheque must have bounced', what ability is a constituent of that? My ability to recognise a cheque when I see one? My ability to explain what, in this context, 'bounce' means? Why would anyone think that either of those was a constituent of the thought? Of course, I can't have the thought unless I understand what cheques are and what bouncing is; but that is a condition of the thought, not a constituent or a component of it.

These reasons are all related. They refer to the different predicates typically attached to 'concept' on the one hand, and 'ability' on the other. Concepts – philosophers say – are instantiated, have extensions and intensions and are the constituents of thought. None of these predicates are attached to 'abilities'. So 'concept' and 'abilities' (of various kinds) cannot denote the same kind of thing. But the hidden premise here is precisely that – concepts are *a kind of thing*. So, given that concepts do not share their predicates with abilities, they cannot be the kind of thing an ability is. They cannot, in other words, *be* abilities.

Drop the hidden premise, and we can say with Hacker (2013) that 'a concept is not *an* anything' (384). But it is still possible to 'possess a concept'; and 'concept possession is requisite for all but the most rudimentary forms of thinking'. This makes it possible to identify concept *possession* with cognitive and linguistic abilities (129). The problems arise if we assume that 'possessing a concept' is analogous to 'possessing a book', and that it makes sense to ask questions about the nature of the thing 'possessed'. However, as I've argued already, the grammar of 'she possesses the concept of democracy' cannot be assimilated to the grammar of 'she possesses the book by Pasternak'.

The idea that concepts are abilities has obvious points of similarity with the view I outlined in Chapter 5. However, as I argued there (in Section 5.8), it is not identical to that view. In taking *the concept of X* and *she possesses the concept of X* as TG+ constructions, I am proposing that we interpret these expressions in a certain way, and understand them as performing a certain function – non-identifying reference to a large, indeterminate, ontologically diverse domain of items. I'm not trying to *identify* difficult-to-fathom things we call 'concepts' with easier-to-fathom things called 'abilities'. I accept that describing this view as an 'abilities' theory of concepts might be a convenient shorthand; but I still want to insist that there is a difference between saying that concepts *are* something, and saying that the word 'concept' is used in certain ways and in certain constructions.

Towards the end of her discussion of Glock's (2010) argument, Saporiti (2010) makes this remark: 'The way I like to think of concepts is in terms of the use of linguistic expressions. A concept, Wittgenstein says, "is a technique of using a word"'. I think this is slightly too narrow, but I agree with the basic idea. Saporiti continues:

> Surely a view of this kind will spare us the trouble of postulating obscure entities. All we do in talking about concepts and trying to explain or clarify them is to talk about uses of linguistic expressions … In particular, this view does not postulate inner states, events or processes suited for representing concepts and thoughts … *In a sense, the proposed view does away with concepts* – it seems to deprive us of our topic. But what is at stake? What was it we wanted concepts for? Instead of concentrating on the question how to define the word 'concept' we should ask ourselves why we want to talk of concepts in addition to, and independently of, the use of words.
>
> (168: my italics)

Possessing concepts, Saporiti thinks, amounts to possessing a complex (primarily linguistic) ability. On her view, then, it makes sense to talk about 'having' or 'possessing' concepts; but it also makes sense to talk about 'doing away with' concepts themselves. This is pretty close to the case I have been trying to make here. We can legitimately say that 'Lewis possesses the concept of X', but it doesn't follow from this that there is an 'obscure entity', the concept of X, that Lewis possesses.

For me, the sense in which we can 'do away with concepts' is this: 'concept' is not a naming word. It does not denote any class of things, objects, quasi-objects, mental particulars or abstract entities. Talk about concepts is, as Saporiti suggests, an indirect form of talk about word-use (plus, on my view, a bit more). If that's right, then 'concept analysis' is – more accurately, can be superseded by – an analysis of patterns of usage. In the next chapter, we'll begin to see what that might imply.

Notes

1 This means that I won't have room to discuss the 'internal structure' of concepts, or the question as to whether some concepts are innate. For reviews of the literature on conceptual 'structure', see Machery (2009), Murphy (2004). For a review of philosophical debates about concepts, see Margolis and Laurence (2019).

2 This is another 'having' construction where you can't detach the object of the verb. Even if it is true that the average star has 2.4 planets, that doesn't mean that you can

start looking for the 2.4 planets 'it' 'possesses'. In this case, of course, you can't detach the subject of the verb either, and start looking for the average star. This is another case for which Fodor's truism (see Section 5.7) doesn't hold.

There is an interesting philosophical literature on the construction < *The average* + COUNT NOUN >. For example, Collins (2017) argues that, in the sentence 'The average American has 2.3 children', the phrase 'the average American' is a *referentially defective expression*. It does not refer to anything: there is no such thing as the average American. Nevertheless, the statement is true. It appears to follow that true statements can include noun phrases which don't refer to anything. In contrast, consider: 'The tall American has two children'. In some situations, this statement will be true, and 'the tall American' will refer to a particular individual. So it is a mistake to assume that 'the average American' can be construed by analogy with 'the tall American'.

3 Wilson uses the expression in the same context as I do. Discussing the 'classical picture' of concepts, he suggests that 'the prospective student of concepts quickly imagines that there is little to adjudicate beyond determining in what ontological dominion these gizmos properly sit' (2006: 5).

4 I am here using the convention mentioned in Section 1.7. Dogs are animals. 'Dog' is a word. DOG is a concept.

5 The existence of LOT (or 'Mentalese') is proposed on theoretical grounds, one of whose premises is that thinking must be like computation (because otherwise we could not account for it in naturalistic terms). But it is not clear what form LOT takes, or why we are not aware of it phenomenologically as a language which we routinely translate into English or some other natural language. A succinct but clear take-down of the Mentalese idea is Gauker (2018: 69–71). For reasons why it is hard to make sense of the idea that Mentalese could have a syntax, see Pessin (1995).

6 For a symposium, see Carruthers (2002) and the commentary that follows it. For a recent review of psychological studies, see Perszyk and Waxman (2018). Carey (2009) is the standard work on the origin and development of concepts.

7 Some recent writers, like Peacocke (1992), agree that concepts are abstract objects, but they reject the idea of a third realm.

8 For a fuller explanation of how Wittgenstein's notion of a 'grammatical remark' differs from what we ordinarily call a rule of grammar or syntax, see Section 7.6.

9 For excellent discussions of the grammar of 'privacy', see Hacker (1993), especially Chapters 1–2, and Fogelin (2009), Chapter 2. There are, as Hacker says (7), many threads woven into the 'private language arguments' of *Philosophical Investigations*, §§243–315. My remarks in the text don't even scratch the surface.

10 Or virtually the same thing. On a given occasion, there will usually be contextual reasons why we choose one way of talking rather than the other. See further in the text.

11 From *The Imaginary Invalid*, Molière (1673/2017).

12 I am here sidestepping a discussion about what this 'awareness' amounts to. It is almost universally assumed that inner speech either consists of, or is 'perceived' as, an auditory thing. It has an 'auditory-phonological component' in that it 'resembles, in its phenomenology, the experience of hearing someone speak' (Langland-Hassan & Vicente 2018: 4). I have never understood this. To me, inner speech does not 'resemble the experience of hearing someone speak' at all; and I suspect the 'auditory-phonological component' is illusory. We are certainly aware of 'speaking silently'; but we construe our awareness of mental events by modelling it on 'outer' perception, so we latch on to familiar examples of sensory experience in order to make sense of it. In the case of 'inner speech', the sense we latch on to is hearing.

13 'Interior monologue or mental imagery is neither necessary nor sufficient for the truth of "He is thinking (musing, reflecting)", although they may and often do accompany the thinking' (Hacker 1993: 152).

14 The paper I've cited gives the fullest account of unsymbolised thinking, and has an appendix on the DES method. There are other sources for DES, most engagingly

Hurlburt and Schwitzgebel (2007), which describes the method fully, has lots of data-plus-commentary and includes discussions between the two authors throughout. Hurlburt believes that the method makes accurate descriptions of 'inner' experience possible; Schwitzgebel is more sceptical.

15 I think Hurlburt is wrong in assuming that unsymbolised thinking must be a form of 'experience', and in arguing that unsymbolised thoughts are 'directly observable'. This is 'Cartesian theatre' stuff – in this case, a theatre in which we're apparently watching a play which has no plot and no actors. I suspect that it misrepresents what's going on.

16 Alshanetsky (2019) considers the case in which I know I've had a thought, but I don't know what it is, and must work at trying to articulate it. This is a thought I might struggle to put into words because it is opaque to me, and not necessarily because it is complex. The question is: does this thought, prior to its articulation, have constituents?

References

Adams, D. (2017). *The Hitchhiker's Guide to the Galaxy*. London: Pan Books.

Alshanetsky, E. (2019). *Articulating a Thought*. Oxford: Oxford University Press.

Azzouni, J. (2010). *Talking about Nothing: Numbers, Hallucinations and Fictions*. New York: Oxford University Press.

Azzouni, J. (2017). *Ontology Without Borders*. New York: Oxford University Press.

Balaguer, M. (2016). Conceptual analysis and x-phi. *Synthese, 193*, 2367–2388.

Bloch-Mullins, C. L. (2015). Foundational questions about concepts: context-sensitivity and embodiment. *Philosophy Compass, 10*(12), 940–952.

Carey, S. (2004). Bootstrapping and the origin of concepts. *Daedalus, 133*(1), 59–68.

Carey, S. (2009). *The Origin of Concepts*. Oxford: Oxford University Press.

Carruthers, P. (1996). *Language, Thought and Consciousness*. Cambridge, UK: Cambridge University Press.

Carruthers, P. (2002). The cognitive functions of language. *Behavioral and Brain Sciences, 25*, 657–674.

Carston, R. (2012). Word meaning and concept expressed. *The Linguistic Review, 29*(4), 607–623.

Collins, J. (2017). The semantics and ontology of *The Average American*. *Journal of Semantics, 34*(3), 373–405.

Colyvan, M. (2003). *The Indispensability of Mathematics*. New York: Oxford University Press.

Cowling, S. (2017). *Abstract Entities*. Abingdon, UK: Routledge.

Crane, T. (1990). The language of thought: no syntax without semantics. *Mind & Language, 5*(3), 187–212.

Dorr, C. (2008). There are no abstract objects. In T. Sider, J. Hawthorne, & D. Zimmerman (Eds.), *Contemporary Debates in Metaphysics* (pp. 12–64). Oxford: Blackwell Publishing.

Fodor, J. (1975). *The Language of Thought*. Cambridge, MA: Harvard University Press.

Fodor, J. (1994). Concepts: A potboiler. *Cognition, 50*, 95–113.

Fodor, J. (2008). *LOT 2: The Language of Thought Revisited*. Oxford: Clarendon Press.

Fogelin, R. J. (2009). *Taking Wittgenstein at His Word: A Textual Study*. Princeton, NJ: Princeton University Press.

Frege, G. (1984). Thoughts. In B. McGuinness (Ed.), *Gottlob Frege, Collected Papers on Mathematics, Logic, and Philosophy* (pp. 351–372). Oxford: Blackwell.

Gauker, C. (2018). Inner speech as the internalization of outer speech. In P. Langland-Hassan & A. Vicente (Eds.), *Inner Speech: New Voices* (pp. 53–77). Oxford: Oxford University Press.

Geach, P. T. (1957). *Mental Acts*. London: Routledge & Kegan Paul.

Glock, H.-J. (2006). Concepts: Representations or abilities? In E. Di Nucci & C. McHugh (Eds.), *Content, Consciousness, and Perception: Essays in Contemporary Philosophy of Mind* (pp. 36–61). Newcastle, UK: Cambridge Scholars Press.

Glock, H.-J. (2010). Concepts, abilities and propositions. *Grazer Philosophische Studien, 81*, 115–134.

Hacker, P. M. S. (1993). *Wittgenstein: Meaning and Mind. Part I: Essays (Volume 3 of an Analytical Commentary on the Philosophical Investigations)*. Oxford: Blackwell.

Hacker, P. M. S. (2013). *The Intellectual Powers: A Study of Human Nature*. Chichester, UK: John Wiley & Sons Ltd.

Hurlburt, R. T., & Akhter, S. A. (2008). Unsymbolized thinking. *Consciousness and Cognition, 17*, 1364–1374.

Hurlburt, R. T., Heavey, C. L., & Kelsey, J. M. (2013). Toward a phenomenology of inner speaking. *Consciousness and Cognition, 22*, 1477–1494.

Hurlburt, R. T., & Schwitzgebel, E. (2007). *Describing Inner Experience? Proponent Meets Skeptic*. Cambridge, MA: The MIT Press.

Langland-Hassan, P., & Vicente, A. (2018). Introduction. In P. Langland-Hassan & A. Vicente (Eds.), *Inner Speech: New Voices* (pp. 1–28). Oxford: Oxford University Press.

Machery, E. (2009). *Doing Without Concepts*. Oxford: Oxford University Press.

Margolis, E., & Laurence, S. (2007). The ontology of concepts – abstract objects or mental representations? *Nous, 41*(4), 561–593.

Margolis, E., & Laurence, S. (2019). Concepts. In E. N. Zalta (Ed.), *The Stanford Encyclopedia of Philosophy*. https://plato.stanford.edu/archives/sum2019/entries/concepts/.

Melia, J. (1995). On what there is not. *Analysis, 55*(4), 223–229.

Molière. (1673/2017). *The Imaginary Invalid*. Newton Stewart, UK: Anodos Books.

Murphy, G. L. (2004). *The Big Book of Concepts*. Cambridge, MA: MIT Press.

Peacocke, C. (1992). *A Study of Concepts*. Cambridge, MA: MIT Press.

Perszyk, D. R., & Waxman, S. R. (2018). Linking language and cognition in infancy. *Annual Review of Psychology, 69*, 231–250.

Pessin, A. (1995). Mentalese syntax: Between a rock and two hard places. *Philosophical Studies, 78*(1), 33–53.

Piccinini, G., & Scott, S. (2006). Splitting concepts. *Philosophy of Science, 73*(4), 390–409.

Prinz, J. J. (2002). *Furnishing the Mind*. Cambridge, MA: MIT Press.

Ramsey, W. M. (2007). *Representation Reconsidered*. Cambridge, UK: Cambridge University Press.

Saporiti, K. (2010). In search of concepts. *Grazer Philosophische Studien, 81*, 153–172.

Schwitzgebel, E. (2011). *Perplexities of Consciousness*. Cambridge, MA: MIT Press.

Tennant, N. (1997). On the necessary existence of numbers. *Nous, 31*(3), 307–336.

Weiskopf, D. A. (2010). The theoretical indispensability of concepts. *Behavioral and Brain Sciences, 33*(2–3), 228–229.

Wilson, M. (2006). *Wandering Significance: An Essay on Conceptual Behavior*. New York: Oxford University Press.

Wittgenstein, L. (1963). *Philosophical Investigations*. Oxford: Basil Blackwell.

Wittgenstein, L. (1964). *Preliminary Studies for the "Philosophical Investigations". Generally Known as The Blue and Brown Books*. Oxford: Basil Blackwell.

7 Wittgenstein, language and method

I closed the last chapter by quoting Saporiti (2010):

> The way I like to think of concepts is in terms of the use of linguistic expressions. A concept, Wittgenstein says, 'is a technique of using a word' … All we do in talking about concepts and trying to explain or clarify them is to talk about uses of linguistic expressions … In a sense, the proposed view does away with concepts. (168)

I take this literally. In fact, I'll go a half-step further than Saporiti, and delete 'in a sense'. Then, turning to the first sentence of this passage, we can leave out the first bit. Why should we think of concepts in terms of anything if we're going to do away with them? And that leaves us with: *the use of linguistic expressions*.

So from here on I will assume that there are no such things as concepts – not as nurses and philosophers think of them – even though the word 'concept' is useful (to the point of being indispensable).

The corollary of 'doing away with concepts': if there are no concepts, we cannot do 'concept analysis'. However, there is something we can do instead, and that is study the ways in which interesting words and expressions are *used*. This is what I will be doing with 'hope' and 'moral distress' in Part II. First, though, I want to present a number of Wittgenstein-esque observations about language, and describe some methods that can be used in the studies I have in mind.

7.1 Language as labyrinth

Language, says Wittgenstein (1963), 'is a labyrinth of paths' (§203). 'We do not *command a clear view* of the use of our words' (§122). He constantly emphasises the multiplicity, diversity and complexity of linguistic expression.

Reader: Well, yes, language is complex. Obviously. Do we really need Wittgenstein to tell us that?
Me: The problem is: people acknowledge it in the abstract, but then promptly forget it when they start talking about specifics. Remember what you said in Section 2.3:

> *Reader*: Okay, so there's all this variety in uses of the word 'hope'. But why should we *not* assume that they all express the same concept? After all, it's the same word. Why would we use that word if it didn't mean the same on each occasion…? Why would we use it if it didn't always refer to the same phenomenon, namely hope?
>
> *Me*: So on the one hand you concede 'variety in use', and agree that 'language is complex'. But on the other, in the particular case of 'hope', you argue for the sameness of meaning, the sameness of the concept, the sameness of the phenomenon.
>
> *Reader*: But there has to be sameness somewhere in language. Otherwise, it would be complete chaos, and we wouldn't be able to understand each other.
>
> *Me*: Diversity and complexity aren't *chaos*. Being suspicious of sameness assumptions when examining particular bits of language – like the uses of 'hope' – doesn't lead to a breakdown in communication. All I'm saying is: the complexity is greater than we give it credit for. Not chaotic, but labyrinthine. Language as labyrinth.

The labyrinth paragraph, §203 of the *Investigations*, continues like this: 'You approach from *one* side and know your way about; you approach the same place from another side and no longer know your way about'.[1] In everyday life, we use the word 'hope' – in all its variations and diversity – without thinking about it, and without any misunderstandings. If that's chaos, we're comfortable with it. But if we take a step backwards into philosophy, or wonder about the role of hope in health care, we end up focusing on a narrowly restrictive range of uses and forget all the others (as I will show in Chapter 11). The result is that our theories of hope are lop-sided. We imagine that we have provided an analysis of *hope* when, in fact, our accounts are based on a limited range of uses of the word 'hope'. In everyday life, we 'know our way about'; but when we start to think about 'hope' in the abstract, we manage to lose our bearings.

To pursue this example a bit further. In the health and psychology literatures, hope is almost universally assumed to be a state of mind, or a state of the person.[2] This fits, or appears to fit, numerous examples of 'hope'.

(1)   Elizabeth is hoping to unseat the incumbent.
(2)   Martha hopes to be comfortable in her post-operative body.

(1) and (2) can be read as referring to the states of mind of Elizabeth and Martha, both of whom have a 'positive' psychological orientation towards a possible future outcome. But consider these examples:

(3)   Will AJ win? Not a hope. The other guy's an expert.
(4)   Frank's got as much hope of climbing Everest as my two-year-old.

Here, there is no reference to anyone's state of mind. The speaker in (3) is clearly not saying anything about AJ's psychological orientation. Indeed, the statement could be true even if AJ says that he hopes to win. What the speaker is saying is that, in his view, the *probability* of AJ winning is zero, or very close to it. Similarly, in (4), the speaker is saying that Frank has very little *chance* of climbing Everest. Again, this statement is consistent with the possibility that Frank himself wants to climb Everest, and thinks he can. In neither case is any reference being made to the state of mind of the person concerned.

These are the sorts of example we overlook when thinking, in general terms, about hope, and in trying to determine 'what kind of thing' it is. In everyday conversation, no-one would find (3) or (4) puzzling or unexpected. However, when we philosophise they can look like annoying exceptions to our account of the 'nature of hope'. As a consequence, they may be ignored altogether, or be dismissed as 'marginal', 'secondary', 'atypical'. However, the pattern of use for 'hope', as Chapters 8–10 will demonstrate, is surprisingly complex. Can that pattern be ignored simply because it doesn't fit some taken-for-granted assumptions about what hope 'essentially' is, and *must* be: namely, an inner state of the person?

7.2 Core meaning

The 'sameness' assumptions articulated by *Reader* in Section 2.3 (and above) are one expression of what Wittgenstein (1964: 17) calls 'the craving for generality'. This is the 'tendency to look for something in common to all the entities which we commonly subsume under a general term'. At some level, in some respect, the same word must be associated with the same – well, the same *something*. The same concept, the same meaning, the same phenomenon, the same whatever-it-takes. However much variety there is in uses of the word 'hope' (or any other word) there must be some underlying sameness. Why, otherwise, would we use the same word?

This conviction is often associated with the assumption that a word will always have a 'core' meaning, which underlies all its uses. Taylor (2012: 228), for example, refers to 'the expectation that one meaning can be identified as basic'. In many cases, of course, there will also be 'extended' meanings; but these must, in some sense, be derivable from the core. The relation between 'core' and 'extended' meanings can vary. The extension might be metaphorical ('mouth of a person', 'mouth of a river'). It might be a metonym ('the sword' referring to force or conflict). It might be analogical ('throw a ball', 'throw into jail'). Moreover, initial extensions might give rise to second-order extensions, or third-order extensions. Idiomatic uses which don't fit this kind of hierarchical patterning can be regarded as the exceptions that prove the rule ('throw a party'?). Figure 7.1 is a picture of this assumption.

This picture preserves the idea of 'sameness' of meaning for the word concerned – ignoring the slightly annoying exceptions, and treating them as unfortunate anomalies that can be explained later – and thus satisfies the craving for generality. There are numerous words for which this picture might work, apart from 'mouth'. Going no further than words for body parts, we find metaphorical extensions such as 'leg' ('it cost me an arm and a leg'), 'hand' ('she had a hand in it'), 'eye' ('keep

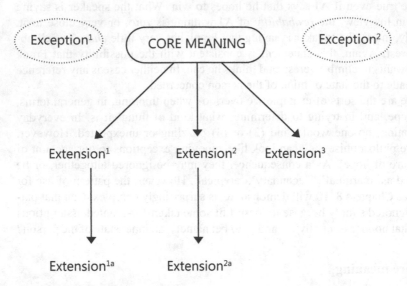

Figure 7.1 Core meaning.

an eye out'), 'ear' ('he has a tin ear'), 'nose' ('he has a nose for trouble'). There are of course many other examples that don't refer to parts of the body. Consider 'square'. This has the core sense of an enclosed geometric figure with four equal sides and four right angles; but it also has extensions, and extensions of extensions ('square' as a person, 'set square', 'square dance', 'square root', 'square eyes', 'square deal', 'square meal', 'square leg', 'all square' and so on). For nouns of this kind, and hundreds more, the 'core meaning' idea is not implausible.

But for a large range of nouns it is. Have a look at some examples.

(5)　Your book's on the table. / It's an interesting book.
(6)　He tore the newspaper in half. / The Washington Post is a newspaper.
(7)　The bank had closed. / The bank raised its interest rate.
(8)　The school is round the corner. / I'll have to talk to the school.

In each case, the noun is used in two distinct senses. The first of each pair refers to a physical object; the second doesn't. In (5), 'book' is first a physical item on the table, and second a text (this is known as the 'tome/text' distinction). In (6), 'newspaper' is first an item that can be picked up, and second a business enterprise in the field of journalism. In (7), 'bank' is first a building, and second a financial institution. In (8), 'school' is first a building (or a collection of buildings), and second a group of people staffing an educational organisation. These are all reminiscent of 'football' (Section 4.6): the thing you can kick, the game you can play, the set of institutions that must get its house in order.

The question is, for each of the examples: which is the core meaning, and which is the derived meaning? As Vicente (2018) says, 'there seems to be no reason to assume that the text (or the tome) sense of *book* is its literal meaning' (959). Similarly for the document (or journalistic enterprise) sense of 'newspaper'; the building (or institution) sense of 'bank'; and the building (or organisational) sense of 'school'. You could, of course, insist that one of them *must* be the core sense. Perhaps the tome, the document, the building. But this seems to be no more than a prejudice in favour of names for physical objects. On what basis is the 'core meaning' in these cases to be identified?

In the case of 'school', among many other words, the choice is not even a binary one. We have 'school' as building, 'school' as people, 'school' as institution, 'school' as process ('school starts at 8:30') and 'school' as experience ('next year he'll be going to school'). Which of these has the best claim to being the core sense? I think you could pick any one of them and argue that the others are derived from it. You *could*. But why would you want to? What motive would you have other than the desire to make 'school' fit a predetermined pattern?

Stock (2008: 158–60) has another interesting example: 'culture'.

(9)   I'm interested in Japanese culture.
(10) He's a bit of a culture vulture.
(11) Infanticide was practised by many early cultures.
(12) These days we've got a throw-away culture.

In (9), the reference is to the customs, beliefs and traditions of a country, implicitly conceived of as a kind of cohesive unity (recall the discussion in Sections 5.1 and 5.2). In (10), the reference is to the arts. In (11), 'culture' is roughly synonymous with 'civilisation' or 'society'. In (12), it refers to a particular form of habitual behaviour and perhaps the values that go with it. Once more, the question can be asked: which of these is the 'core meaning' of the word, and on what basis would you decide? As with 'school', you could make a case for any of them, arguing that the rest were derived. In which case, in the absence of a compelling justification, the choice seems arbitrary.

Stock is a lexicographer, and many lexicographers are sceptical about the idea of 'core' meaning. For example, Aitchison, quoted in Hanks (2013: 86), thinks that it might work for words like 'square' and 'bachelor', but for a majority of words 'it may be difficult to specify a hard core of meaning at all'. She has several reasons. First, 'it may be impossible to tell where the "true meaning" ends and encyclopaedic knowledge begins'. Second, 'words may have "fuzzy boundaries" in that there might be no clear point at which the meaning of one word ends and another begins'. Third, 'a single word may apply to a "family" of items which all overlap in meaning but which do not share any one characteristic' (ibid.).

Another lexicographer says: 'I don't believe in word senses'. This is someone who was a President of the European Association for Lexicography, and a General Editor of the Collins-Robert English/French Dictionary (B. T. Sue Atkins). She is quoted in a paper which adopts 'I don't believe in word senses' as its title (Kilgarriff 2008). So there are even compilers of dictionaries who think that the picture in Figure 7.1 works only for a limited range of words.[3]

7.3 Family resemblances

In linguistics, cases like those discussed in the previous section are said to exhibit 'inherent polysemy' (Pustejovsky 1995). This expression refers to a form of polysemy where there is an 'ambiguity available by virtue of the semantics inherent in the noun itself' (Ježek & Melloni 2011: 7). Although it is not fully clear what characteristics of a word account for this property, by implication the different 'senses' of the word have equal standing. They do not have a hierarchical 'structure', one sense being 'core', and the others being derived. They are examples of 'meaning egalitarianism', to use a phrase of Ludlow's (2014: 82). Figure 7.2 illustrates the idea, and should be contrasted with Figure 7.1.

This diagram depicts a network of uses rather than a hierarchy of senses. The dotted lines between *Uses* represent links of various kinds: similarities, analogies, overlaps, parallels. The dashed oval suggests that the pattern of *Uses* is open-ended: the range of *Uses* cannot be exhaustively defined, and there may not be complete consensus as to what counts as a *Use* and what doesn't.

This lack-of-a-core-meaning is closely related to Wittgenstein's 'family resemblances'.[4] The idea is that words can form a network, or even a chain, in such a way that, although 'adjacent' senses do have things in common, the ends of the chain (or different parts of the network) may have nothing in common at all. It's easier to illustrate this idea than to describe it. Wittgenstein's best known example is 'game' (1963: §66):

> Don't say: 'there *must* be something in common, or they would not be called "games"' – but *look and see* whether there is anything common to all. – For if you look at them you will not see something that is common to all, but similarities, relationships, and a whole series of them at that.

And he proceeds to list some of the many different kinds of thing called games.

Tomasello (2003: 54), uses 'run' as an example: '*run* as a physical activity, as the activity of operating machines, as the activity of operating a store, as the activity of standing for political office, and so on'. We can extend this:[5]

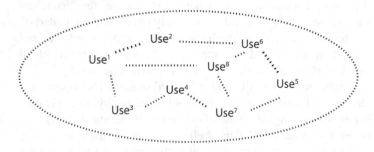

Figure 7.2 Meaning egalitarianism.

Run a race	It will run for an hour	The wheels run freely
Run circles round	My ice-cream's run	Tears run down his face
Runs through my mind	Run him through	Run a comb through your hair
It's run down	Run the tape	Two weeks left to run
I'll run it past her	Run through the script	The stockings have run
Run into debt	The food's run out	Run the paragraph on
Run up a garment	Run for office	Run to seed
Runs in the family	Running a risk	Run him down (criticise)
Running a temperature	It will run you £50	Run an organisation

With some difficulty, I've put these in a sort of order, starting with uses that are arguably variations on the idea of movement, and ending with uses which seem to have nothing in common with 'run a race' at all. You can perhaps see links between some of the phrases which are close to each other in the network: 'run into debt' and 'the food's run out', for example. But by the time you get to the end, it's hard to see a link between 'run an organisation' and 'it will run you £50', let alone between either of those and 'run a race'.[6]

Reader's question was: 'Why would we use that word if it didn't mean the same on each occasion? Why would we use it if it didn't always refer to the same phenomenon?' To which the answer seems to be: it looks as if some words *don't* always mean the same on each occasion. When we 'look and see', what we find is a very complex network of uses, some of which have nothing in common with each other at all.[7]

Just as the craving for generality might encourage someone to think that all words have a hierarchical usage pattern, corresponding to Figure 7.1, so it might lead someone else to think that all words exhibit the kind 'family resemblance' network pictured in Figure 7.2. We should beware of the temptation in both cases. For some words, it will be possible to arrange the pattern of use in a hierarchy. For other words, this won't work, and the pattern of use will be a network. For any word we find interesting, we should avoid jumping to conclusions. We can only determine what the pattern is like by examining it. As Wittgenstein (1963: §66) says: 'Don't think, but look!'.

7.4 Definitions

For any word exhibiting the family resemblance pattern, it won't be possible to formulate a 'definition' capable of capturing all cases. Consider the 'run' examples in Section 7.3. It's difficult to believe that it would be possible to construct a definition that applied to all of them. There are no features which they all have in common; nor can we identify any set of necessary and sufficient conditions that accounts for every use. Similarly for the things that we call 'games', Wittgenstein's primary example (and, as I shall suggest in Part II, for 'hope').

Wittgenstein imagines his own *Reader* responding to this. 'But if the concept "game" is uncircumscribed like that, you don't really know what you mean by a "game"'. To which Wittgenstein replies: 'When I give the description "The ground was quite covered with plants" – do you want to say I don't know what

I am talking about until I can give a definition of a plant?' (1963: §69). The point is: words do not need a definition – and they do not need a 'boundary' – in order to be useful.[8] The conviction that a definition is necessary for an 'analysis of the concept', a conviction which permeates the nursing literature, is one we can let go of. A lot of language is too labyrinthine for definitions; and we create problems for ourselves by assuming that it is simpler than in fact it is (Kuusela 2019: 128).

Nevertheless, definitions can still be helpful, as Wittgenstein suggests: 'we can draw a boundary – for a special purpose' (Wittgenstein 1963: §69). So a boundary can be drawn, a definition can be formulated, if it will be useful in a particular context. There are several kinds of usefulness that we can identify.

The first is the familiar practice of defining a term in anticipation of a discussion which requires its use. There is a spectrum of cases. At one end are '*ad hoc* definitions, set up arbitrarily to suit the purpose to hand, but claiming or implying nothing further' (Harris and Hutton 2007: 8). At the other end are more general proposals: 'I suggest that, from now on, we define "*X*" as follows…'. These are global (at least in aspiration: everyone should follow suit); but there will still be a context, implicit or explicit, in which the proposed definition is meant to apply. In all cases, the definition is *proffered*. It is not implied that this is how the term is normally used. This first category, then, is that of the *stipulative definition*.[9]

The second is where a proposal of the first kind has been accepted by a particular community, and the defined expression has become a *technical term*. This is a familiar situation in the sciences. There are, roughly, two sorts of case. One is where the defined term is already in common usage, but the scientific community draws a definitional 'boundary' round it, and employs it in a distinct manner, sometimes quite remote from its ordinary senses. An example would be the use of 'work' and 'force' in physics. A different sort of case is where the term has no prior 'common usage', but is introduced at a certain point in time. An example is 'natural selection', introduced by Darwin in 1858.

Finally, there is a useful kind of 'definition' which is very different from those described so far. Here's another of Wittgenstein's analogies:

> If we look at the actual use of a word, what we see is something constantly fluctuating. In our investigations we set over against this fluctuation something more fixed, just as one paints a stationary picture of a constantly altering landscape.
>
> (Wittgenstein 1974: 77)

The stationary picture – a painting or a photograph – misrepresents the landscape insofar as it does not convey all the variegated, irregular detail. For example, if I paint the landscape around my house, do I paint it in spring, summer, autumn, winter? At a particular time of day? From what angle? All of these options present different facets of the landscape. Each tells us something about the surroundings; but none of them can get anywhere near representing 'the whole'. It's not even clear what that would mean.

In this analogy, the landscape is language. The inconsistent, fluctuating, variegated use of certain words and expressions creates a complex pattern that cannot be represented 'as a whole'. We can't provide a complete grammar of even an apparently simple word such as 'hope', as Part II will testify. There are various strategies and devices we can adopt in order to cope with this complexity; but one of them is to create an analogue of the stationary picture. And that analogue is a definition.

Like the painting or the photograph, a definition can only present one facet of a word's 'landscape'. But it can still tell us something useful about that landscape, something that will help us to see connections, identify functions, recognise similarities and differences. A definition, or a rule, can 'capture' aspects of the 'overall' pattern of usage. The trick is to prevent oneself from falling into the trap of assuming that it can capture them all: 'one falls into dogmatism if one demands that the definition *must* hold of all the cases of the use of the word in the relevant meaning' (Kuusela 2008: 141).

A definition can also be seen as a model. It isolates 'for study, by means of simple or simplified models of language use, facets of complex uses of linguistic expression' (Kuusela 2019: 142). In Chapter 8, for example, I provide what I call the 'basic schema' of the word 'hope', used as a verb. This is intended as a model in Kuusela's sense, and it looks like a definition. Indeed, similar schemas have been proposed as *the* definition of 'hope'. But the 'basic schema' is not intended as a definition in that sense. It is no more than a starting point for understanding just one aspect of how the verb 'hope' is used. 'Inasmuch as our language is complex, I shall point out simpler structures which can be set side by side with it to see what light they shed on it' (Ambrose 1979: 46–7). The 'basic schema' is a 'simpler structure'.

7.5 Meaning as use

As I noted earlier, Wittgenstein's remarks about family resemblances do not amount to a general thesis about the nature of language. The same goes for his well-known comment about 'meaning as use': 'For a large class of cases – though not for all – in which we employ the word "meaning" it can be explained thus: the meaning of a word is its use in the language' (Wittgenstein 1963: §43).

Note the qualification: 'though not for all'. Wittgenstein does accept that some words denote physical objects – they are 'names' – and that the 'meaning' of these words is linked to the objects they denote. However, he cautions against extending this account to abstract nouns and words referring to mental states and processes. Take the word 'number', for example. Is there a class of things that 'number' denotes in the way that 'chair' denotes a class of physical objects? Well, some say 'yes'. But then they have to explain what kind of object 'number' is the name of; and this leads to the idea of 'abstract' entities. The claim is that the relation between the name and the thing is the same in both cases: 'chair' denotes *this*; and 'number' denotes *that*. However, the '*that*' is an abstract object, not a physical one.

The same comparison is made with mental states. 'Cake' denotes *this*; and 'hope' denotes *that*. As with abstract objects, the relation is the same. But the *that*, in this case, is a mental object, not a physical one. In both cases, the insistence on a *noun-name-object* picture trumps the difficulty of understanding what a non-physical object can be. 'Cake' is the name of something in the tin; 'hope' is the name of something in the mind.

The difficulty of understanding what an abstract object is partly motivates the 'meaning-as-use' idea. If we assume that the 'meaning' of a noun is always the thing it denotes, we run into trouble with words like 'number', 'hope', 'concept' and 'belief'. So Wittgenstein says: 'As a way out of the difficulty posed by this question I suggest that we do not talk about the meaning of words but rather about the use of words' (Ambrose 1979: 44). It is a proposal to drop one picture of 'meaning', and try another instead.[10]

So meaning-as-use does not constitute a 'theory of language', any more than Wittgenstein's comments about family resemblances do. It is not a principle to be applied religiously to every case; and it cannot capture every aspect of how language works. It is another 'stationary picture', another 'snapshot'. It is an alternative model to meaning-as-denotation, or 'meaning-as-list-of-concepts'.[11] It suggests a different way of thinking about the understanding of words.

When we start to think in that way, we find that, in addition to denoting objects and describing things, there is a vast range of uses to which words are put. Not all sentences can be modelled on 'the cat sat on the mat' or 'the grass is green'. The first of these sentences picks out two objects, and states the relation between them. The second names an object, and states that it has a certain property. In both cases, an object is identified, and then a description is attached to it. However, not all sentences perform this kind of identifying-and-describing task; and Wittgenstein suggests that a large proportion don't.

I observed in Section 3.5 that Wittgenstein adopts various strategies to convince us that the naming-and-describing picture accounts for only some of what we do with language. For example, he presents a list of exclamations – 'Water!', 'Ow!', 'Away!', 'Help!', 'Fine!', 'No!' – and asks: 'Are you still inclined to call these words "names of objects"?' (1963; §27). More generally, he suggests that we 'think of the tools in a tool-box' (hammer, pliers, saw, screw-driver, rule, glue-pot, chisel, spirit level, wrench), and then says: 'The functions of words are as diverse as the functions of these objects' (§11). Most of the *Investigations* is devoted to exploring the difficulties we get into if we stick with naming-and-describing as a way of understanding non-physical-object words, and to suggesting that these difficulties might be resolved if we adopt the language-as-tool-box picture.

Consider, for example, the word 'meaning' itself, one of the philosophically troublesome words.[12] Does this word name an entity, a certain kind of non-physical object? There are philosophers who say 'yes'. The most influential example is Frege, who argues that meanings – which he calls 'thoughts' – belong to the 'third realm' (see Section 6.2.2). They are 'neither things of the outer world nor ideas' (Frege 1956: 302). They form a sort of intermediate ontological layer between words and the physical world.

But the idea of this 'realm' of meaning is intrinsically peculiar. Where is it? How do we know about it? How exactly are words and meanings related? Are they somehow attached to each other? If so, in what way? It is all very mysterious. As Dummett (1973: 154) observes: 'the realm of sense is a very special region of reality; its denizens are, so to speak, things of a very special sort'. Indeed, it's not fully clear how even Frege proposes to answer such questions. Such puzzles are created by the assumption that 'meaning', as a noun, must be the name of *something*, a quasi-object which isn't physical, but which nevertheless has thing-like properties. It's just that, having made that assumption, we are confronted by apparently unresolvable problems about the precise nature of meanings, and how exactly they are related to the rest of the world. Perhaps, then, 'meaning' is not a naming word after all, even if it is a noun.

So what happens if we switch to the tool-box picture? How can we understand the use of 'meaning' on a meaning-as-use basis rather than a noun-name-object basis? The first thing to say is that there are many uses of the words 'means' and 'meaning', so there will be no single, blanket answer to this question. In Paley (2017) I explored a series of uses which occur in non-linguistic contexts. By this I mean contexts in which the word 'means' appears, but not in reference to word meaning. For example:

(13) Reducing fat in the diet means cutting the amount of animal protein.
(14) My goal is to run the marathon, which means training really hard.
(15) Tourism is down; that means fewer jobs and lower wages.
(16) Scarce ice means fewer perches for polar bears to hunt seals.

In cases of this sort, 'means' functions as an inference marker. In (13) and (14), the inference concerns the type of action necessary, given a prior condition or requirement. In (15) and (16), the inference is about cause and effect. For both types of inference, the logic is: 'If this, then that'. The word 'means' is used to mark the place at which this inference is made.

These are just two uses of 'means' as an inference marker (there are several more), and nothing has been said yet about 'meaning'.[13] So the 'tool box' exploration of 'meaning' has barely started. But, hopefully, the flavour of the project has been conveyed. No attempt is made to 'define' meaning, or to determine the 'nature of meaning'. There is no analysis of the 'concept', and no list of 'attributes'. Instead, I start with the word 'means', and start to explore *one* of its functions (that of inference marker) in *one* context. This is the switch from *analysing the concept* to the Wittgensteinian project of *examining the use*. It is, as Baz (2017: 118) suggests, 'the difference between studying a fantasy and studying something real'.

So the tool-box picture encourages us to switch from seeing philosophically troublesome words as the names of objects-of-some-kind, to seeing them instead as tools which perform certain language-related tasks. But the 'inference marker' function of 'means' is not representative of functions in general. The number of functions a word can have – in different contexts and constructions – is countless.[14]

7.6 Grammar *vs.* syntax

Wittgenstein's use of the word 'grammar' is idiosyncratic. I need to say a bit more about this. From here on, to avoid confusion, I will use 'Grammar' with upper case 'G' when I am referring to Wittgenstein's sense. In contrast, 'grammar', with lower case 'g', will mean what linguists usually mean by it. I'll try to clarify the distinction, and show how, for Wittgenstein, Grammar is a philosophical idea.[15]

In linguistics, grammar and syntax are closely related. Both refer, broadly, to the more 'formal' aspects of language, but 'syntax' has a narrower range. Crudely, grammar consists of two main divisions: one is morphology, the other is syntax. Morphology is the study of the different forms of individual words. For example, the construction of the simple past tense in English verbs (add 'ed': 'walked'); or the formation of the plural form in nouns (add 's': 'tables'). In contrast, syntax concerns how words are strung together to form sentences, for example, the construction of the English passive ('Rosie drank the Prosecco', 'the Prosecco was drunk by Rosie').

Together, then, morphology and syntax constitute grammar. What Wittgenstein means by 'Grammar' is different. It is far wider than the rules for deciding on the inflection of a word, or the rules for combining words in sentences, though there is some overlap. A first stab is to say that 'Grammar' refers to a word's pattern of usage – subject to the qualification that the 'pattern' may be of the family resemblance variety rather than the hierarchical variety.[16]

For example, to clarify the Grammar of 'hope' will not only be to note that it is both a noun and a verb; or that it has mass- and count-noun functions; or that it forms several adjectives ('hopeless', 'hopeful'). Nor will it be to say that, typically, the verb occurs in one of three constructions: 'hope that', 'hope to' and 'hope for'. Rather, it will be to examine the uses of 'hope' in different circumstances, and to study its *functions* in various constructions. For example: the difference between 'hope to' and 'hope that', between 'I hope' and 'she hopes', and between 'she hopes' and 'she is hoping'; its use with modal verbs ('can hope') and negations ('without hope', 'not hope'); its use in metonymy and ellipsis; and more (see Chapters 8–11). The concern is not for the morphology and syntax *as such*, but for the various tasks that 'hope' performs in different linguistic contexts.

Crucially, syntax is not a guide to Grammar.[17] We cannot assume that expressions with the same syntax are bound to have the same Grammar. Consider some examples we have already seen:

(17)   She's my only friend.
(18)   She's my only hope.
(19)   Is there any wine?
(20)   Is there any hope?
(21)   The tall American has two children.
(22)   The average American has two children.
(23)   Emily grasped the reins.
(24)   Emily grasped the concept.

Each pair of sentences differs by only one word, and the syntax appears identical. Yet the Grammar of the two members of the pair is different. (17) to (20) were discussed briefly in Section 2.3. The identical syntax encourages us to assume that the nouns 'friend', 'wine' and 'hope' function in the same way. In (18) 'hope' seems to play the same role as 'friend' in (17). In (20) it seems to have the same function as 'wine' in (19). So we are tempted to infer that 'hope', even though it is an abstract noun, can be treated in the same way. Given that 'friend' is the name of an object, and 'wine' is the name of a liquid, '*hope*' is presumably the name of an object (or a state, or a force, or a process) as well. However, it turns out that in sentences like (18) and (20), 'hope' does *not* have the same function as 'friend' in (17) and 'wine' in (19). It does not *name* anything. As Chapters 8–10 indicate, its Grammar is completely different .

In a similar way, (22) does not pick out a particular American and describe her/him, which is what (21) does. In fact, the expression 'the average American' is referentially defective (Collins 2017). Likewise, in (23) we can say that 'the reins' refers to something Emily has grasped; but we cannot say the same of 'the concept' in (24). Both statements might be true, but the kinds of circumstances they refer to are very different. In (23) we can infer that *there is something* Emily has grasped. 'The reins' are detachable. In (24) 'the concept' is *not* detachable. It is, in Collins' terms, a referentially defective expression.

7.7 Methods

It may be helpful to summarise some of the main aspects of Wittgenstein's perspective on language:

A. Language is a set of tools which permit us to perform various tasks in various contexts.
B. These tasks extend beyond identifying objects and describing them.
C. A word's 'meaning' is the history of its use in different constructions and countless utterances.
D. For some words, this history forms a family resemblance network.
E. We cannot make assumptions about the function of a word-in-context; we have to look.
F. There is no limit to the variability of functions which different words can have.
G. Definitions often cannot 'capture' use *in toto*, but they can be used as models or stipulations.
H. The Grammar of a word or expression does not necessarily correspond to its syntax.
I. The craving for generality leads us to think in terms of pictures applying to all cases.
J. We learn how to use words, but we don't learn how to describe that use.
K. So we forget how complex our use is, and succumb to an urge to misunderstand it.

L.   Grammar reminds us of what we have forgotten by compiling and ordering a multiplicity of examples.

In the rest of this section, I'll briefly describe some Wittgenstein-esque methods of exploration.[18] I won't illustrate them here, but I will indicate where they are used elsewhere in the book.

7.7.1 Describing the uses of words

Rather than listing the attributes of a concept (which supposedly identify the conditions for the concept's application), we describe the *uses* of a word or expression, exploring the pattern of use across the range of constructions in which the expression appears. This is not as simple as it sounds. The familiarity of a word like 'hope' does not imply that a description of its use will be plain sailing. Wittgenstein 'stresses that descriptions must be complex, accurate and detailed' (Savickey 1999: 88) because the assumptions we make about how our words are used often turn out to be mistaken, and the reader will need to check the details if she is to be persuaded that something she thought was straightforward... isn't. Wittgenstein calls this 'assembling reminders', a phrase which makes the exercise sound almost trivial. It definitely isn't. Especially as the person doing the assembling may himself labour under the misapprehension that things will be simpler than in fact they are (as I discovered with 'hope').

7.7.2 Words as tools

The investigation of an expression's pattern of use seeks to understand the jobs it is asked to do. What is of interest is the expression's function, what it achieves in various contexts. We shouldn't assume that our words necessarily 'do anything describable as "naming items in the world" in order to be fit for their different uses' (Baz 2017: 133). Nor should we assume that a word or expression only has one function. Indeed, we must expect it to have several, and be ready to examine the possibility that they vary with the constructions in which the word appears. The discussion of 'hope' in Chapters 8–10 examines the word's use in different constructions, showing how the tasks it performs vary in each of them. Snippets of this examination have already appeared in Part I.

7.7.3 Pictures

Wherever there is philosophical discussion of an expression, we can look for the pictures which underlie what is said about it. These pictures are rarely articulated explicitly, but their influence is pervasive. They are often vague, incomplete and lacking in detail. They are often no more than hazy assumptions, even though they underpin the inferences that writers make about the expression in question. We can look, in particular, for the giveaway 'must' – 'this *must* be the case' – as this is frequently a clue to a picture's influence. Pictures are deeply entrenched and, usually, they do fit a range of cases. The trick is to recognise them *as* pictures, rather than as metaphysical truths, and to acknowledge that alternative pictures are possible. Part I of this book has described the picture of concepts-as-a-type-of-object, and examined its relation to another picture: nouns-as-naming-words. In Chapter 11, I will describe a picture of hope – as an 'inner something' – that underlies recent discussions in health care.

7.7.4 Counter-pictures

You can't argue with a picture. You can't suggest that it is 'untrue' or 'inaccurate' (because it *does* fit a limited range of cases); and you can't reason anyone out of it, because few people adopt it consciously, and no-one adopts it for a reason. However, you *can* suggest that it is misleading if we try to make it fit cases beyond the limited range, and that it gives rise to unnecessary problems as a consequence. Just as usefully, you can propose a counter-picture. This is part of Wittgenstein's strategy: advising us 'to look at things like *this*, not like *that*' (Baker 2004: 137). For example, the 'meaning-as-use' idea is intended as a counter-picture to the 'words-name-objects' picture, described on the first page of *Philosophical Investigations*. In Chapter 12, I identify a picture underlying the 'moral distress' debate, and propose a counter-picture.

7.7.5 Definitions

I have discussed the use of definitions in Section 7.4, and little needs to be added here. In Chapter 8, the 'basic schema' of 'hope' is a model, an 'object of comparison', representing just one aspect of the use of 'hope' as a verb (although some uses of the count noun conform to the same schema). In Chapter 12, I discuss an expression, only recently coined, for which definitions have been proposed in the literature: 'moral distress'. Here, the investigation focuses on the political context of these definitions and what they are designed to achieve. A series of definitions is traced over time, each adding a new twist to the original idea; and I suggest that this series is best conceived as a normative project in nursing, not as an attempt to pin down a newly identified psychological state. The *function* of the expression, as evidenced by the discourse concerning how it should be defined, is therefore the central question of this chapter.

7.7.6 Questions

Wittgenstein constantly asks questions. According to Kenny (1973), the *Investigations* contains 784 of them, but most of them go unanswered because Wittgenstein's most common response to a question is to ask a different one. The *Blue Book*, for example, begins like this: 'What is the meaning of a word?' It is a question Wittgenstein does not attempt to answer. Instead, he asks another one: what are we doing when we explain the meaning of a word (Wittgenstein 1964)? Notice the form of the original question: 'What is...?' followed by a noun. In asking this type of question, we already risk falling into the trap of assuming that all nouns are naming words: 'We are up against one of the great sources of philosophical bewilderment: a substantive makes us look for a thing that corresponds to it' (Wittgenstein 1964: 1). So we should avoid trying to answer such questions. Part I has suggested that 'What are concepts?' gets us off on the wrong foot; and Part II treats 'What is moral distress?' and 'What is hope?' in the same way.

7.7.7 Particular cases

In response to general claims about a concept, Wittgenstein investigates particular cases in order to show how the craving for generality dissolves in the face of multiple uses. When we place our expressions in the context of everyday use, the temptation to postulate abstract objects and mental states recedes, given that the same expression can convey many different things. The cases examined can be real or invented. In Chapter 8, for example, I show how even a simple expression, 'I hope so', can convey two completely different kinds of information, neither of which makes any reference to an 'inner power', a 'life force', a 'theological virtue' or any of the other things hope has been defined as. In this instance, the two cases are invented, although they are based on real-life conversations. Elsewhere, in Chapter 9, I use a recent book review and an even more recent news story to examine elliptical uses of 'hope', again illustrating a different function of the word, and again including no reference to inner forces, powers or virtues.

7.7.8 Thought experiments

Wittgenstein is quite comfortable about inventing simple language-games, non-existent machines and imaginary ethnographies in order to make us think about our use of language. As Kuusela (2008: 270) notes, he even goes in for invented natural history and invented history of ideas. I haven't done anything quite like this; but I have engaged in broadly comparable thought experiments. At the end of Chapter 4, for example, I invented a word, 'consoct'. The idea was that the expression 'the consoct of X' could be understood as a possible grammatical alternative to 'things associated with X'. There is, of course, no such expression; but there is no obvious reason why it should be dismissed as impossible. There *might* have been an expression of this kind... and that possibility provided a bridge to 'the concept of X' in the following chapter.

7.7.9 Analogies

In philosophy, analogies are ubiquitous, although they are not always recognised *as* analogies. They are not necessarily misleading, and the same analogy can mislead us some of the time and prove useful at other times. However, the risk is that, if we don't realise that what we are inclined to say is based on an analogy, we may think that we are merely stating the facts, 'perceiving a state of affairs of the highest generality' (Wittgenstein 1963: §104). Even so, analogies are unavoidable, and Wittgenstein uses them prolifically. But he always points out that they *are* analogies, and employs them as prompts to ways-of-seeing: 'Look at it this way rather than that'. I have used linguistic analogies for a similar purpose: for example, the use of 'the world of X' as an analogue for 'the concept of X' in Chapter 5.

Wittgenstein's primary aim is to find ways of prompting the reader to look at things differently. He is engaged in 'a dialogue whose principal goal is to effect a change in ways of seeing things' (Baker 2004: 155). It is more a matter of persuading the reader that things *need not* be as she had said they *must* be, or that things *may* be as she had said they *could not* be (151), than of establishing this or that thesis. What the reader does with the different-way-of-seeing is, however, obviously up to her.

Notes

1 Baz (2020) says that, according to Wittgenstein, there are things about philosophically troublesome words which 'we cannot have failed to know, but which, for some reason, are hard to *see*' (36). A simple analogy: ask someone to think of words that are nouns *and* adjectives *and* verbs *and* adverbs (Section 3.2). Many people find this difficult ('hard to see'), and some are tempted to deny that there are any such words. Yet they are using them all the time ('cannot fail to know').
2 See, for example, virtually every contribution to Gallagher and Lopez (2018).
3 Hanks (2013) suggests that the question whether words 'have meaning at all' is a serious one, 'and is being asked by lexicographers' (65). His own view is that they don't, at least not in the usual sense. See Ludlow (2014) for further scepticism.
4 Closely related, but not identical. Wittgenstein contrasts the 'family resemblance' idea with the view that all the things described as 'X' must have a feature (or features) in common. Ludlow contrasts the 'meaning egalitarianism' idea with the view that, for every word, there is a 'primary' meaning. You can think that all uses of 'X' must have something in common without insisting that any one use is primary. 'School' and 'culture' from Section 7.2 might be offered as examples.
5 I'm just looking at the verb 'run' here. Including the noun would make things even more complex.
6 As always, it's possible to dig in. Some people insist that 'run' conveys the same idea in all these examples. They suggest 'movement', or 'progression from A to B' (both literal and metaphorical), or 'change', or 'sequence'. They have to work particularly hard with 'running a risk', 'run him down' (in the sense of 'criticise him'), 'runs in the family', 'running a temperature' and 'it will run you £50'.
7 Kuusela (2008: 172) says that the use of a word can certainly indicate a 'kinship' between the objects to which it is applied; but this kinship 'need not be the sharing of a common property'. Rather, it 'may connect the objects like the links of a chain, so that one is linked to another by *intermediary links*. Two neighbouring members may have common features and be similar to each other, while distant ones belong to the same family without any longer having anything in common'.
8 This point comes up again in the discussion of 'moral distress' (Section 12.1).
9 Harris and Hutton (2007), Chapter 1, is a good discussion of stipulative definition. The book as a whole is well worth reading.
10 To say that a word 'has meaning' – or to say that it 'is meaningful' – is to say only that it is used and understood. It is not to imply that there is *something*, a meaning, which the word *possesses*. So this is another case in which 'having an X' does not imply that 'there is an X' which is had (see Section 5.7).

11 Putnam (1975: 146): 'The problem in semantic theory is to get away from the picture of the meaning of a word as something like a list of concepts'. This is akin to the picture associated with concept analysis in nursing, which generally aims at a list of 'defining attributes'.

12 'Philosophically troublesome words' is Baz's (2017) expression. Some of his examples are 'know', 'cause' and 'meaning'. In Chapter 11, I will suggest that 'hope' is troublesome in a comparable way.

13 For a more detailed analysis, see Paley (2017), Chapter 5.

14 Horwich (2020) talks about Wittgenstein recognising 'the limitless variability of the functions of the different words in a language'.

15 I mentioned Wittgenstein's distinction between 'surface grammar' and 'depth grammar' (Wittgenstein 1963: §664) in Section 6.4. 'Depth grammar' is what I am here referring to as 'Grammar' with a capital 'G'. A helpful essay on the distinction is Baker (2004), Chapter 3.

16 So, recalling the Second Picture of Figure 2.1, we might say that *the Grammar of 'hope'* is equivalent to *the concept of hope*. If we did, would anyone then argue that we need to 'possess' Grammars in order to categorise? Would they wonder what kind of gizmo a Grammar was?

17 'One of Wittgenstein's central ideas is that philosophers are often misled by taking similarities in syntactic structures as indicators of a similarity in *Grammar* – that is, as Wittgenstein uses this notion, as similarities in *use*' (Fogelin 2009: 83). The capital 'G' here is mine.

18 I have learned a great deal that is relevant to this section from Baker (2004), Kuusela (2008, 2019), McGinn (2013) and Savickey (1999). I don't pretend what I say here is comprehensive. Wittgenstein uses other methods in addition to the ones I describe. I've mentioned only those used at some point in this book.

References

Ambrose, A. (Ed.). (1979). *Wittgenstein's Lectures, Cambridge, 1932–35. From the Notes of Alice Ambrose and Margaret Macdonald*. Oxford: Blackwell.

Baker, G. (2004). *Wittgenstein's Method: Neglected Aspects*. Malden, MA: Blackwell Publishing.

Baz, A. (2017). *The Crisis of Method in Contemporary Analytic Philosophy*. Oxford: Oxford University Press.

Baz, A. (2020). *The Significance of Aspect Perception: Bringing the Phenomenal World into View*. Cham, Switzerland: Springer Nature.

Collins, J. (2017). The semantics and ontology of *The Average American*. *Journal of Semantics*, *34*(3), 373–405.

Dummett, M. (1973). *Frege: Philosophy of Language*. London: Duckworth.

Fogelin, R. J. (2009). *Taking Wittgenstein at His Word: A Textual Study*. Princeton, NJ: Princeton University Press.

Frege, G. (1956). The thought: a logical inquiry. *Mind*, *65*(259), 289–311.

Gallagher, M. W., & Lopez, S. J. (Eds.). (2018). *The Oxford Handbook of Hope*. New York: Oxford University Press.

Hanks, P. (2013). *Lexical Analysis: Norms and Exploitations*. Cambridge, MA: The MIT Press.

Harris, R., & Hutton, C. (2007). *Definition in Theory and Practice*. London: Bloomsbury Academic.

Horwich, P. (2020). Wittgenstein on truth. In S. Wuppuluri & N. Da Costa (Eds.), *Wittgensteinian (adj.)* (pp. 151–162). Cham, Switzerland: Springer Nature.

Ježek, E., & Melloni, C. (2011). Nominals, polysemy, and co-predication. *Journal of Cognitive Science, 12,* 1–31.

Kenny, A. (1973). *Wittgenstein.* London: Allen Lane.

Kilgarriff, A. (2008). "I don't believe in word senses". In T. Fontenelle (Ed.), *Practical Lexicography* (pp. 135–151). Oxford: Oxford University Press.

Kuusela, O. (2008). *The Struggle Against Dogmatism: Wittgenstein and the Concept of Philosophy.* Cambridge, MA: Harvard University Press.

Kuusela, O. (2019). *Wittgenstein on Logic as the Method of Philosophy: Re-examining the Roots and Development of Analytic Philosophy.* Oxford: Oxford University Press.

Ludlow, P. (2014). *Living Words: Meaning Underdetermination and the Dynamic Lexicon.* Oxford: Oxford University Press.

McGinn, M. (2013). *The Routledge Guide to Wittgenstein's Philosophical Investigations.* Abingdon, UK: Routledge.

Paley, J. (2017). *Phenomenology as Qualitative Research: A Critical Analysis of Meaning Attribution.* Abingdon, UK: Routledge.

Pustejovsky, J. (1995). *The Generative Lexicon.* Cambridge, MA: The MIT Press.

Putnam, H. (1975). *Mind, Language and Reality.* New York: Cambridge University Press.

Saporiti, K. (2010). In search of concepts. *Grazer Philosophische Studien, 81,* 153–172.

Savickey, B. (1999). *Wittgenstein's Art of Investigation.* Abingdon, UK: Routledge.

Stock, P. F. (2008). Polysemy. In T. Fontenelle (Ed.), *Practical Lexicography* (pp. 153–160). Oxford: Oxford University Press.

Taylor, J. R. (2012). *The Mental Corpus: How Language is Represented in the Mind.* Oxford: Oxford University Press.

Tomasello, M. (2003). *Constructing a Language: A Usage-Based Theory of Language Acquisition.* Cambridge, MA: Harvard University Press.

Vicente, A. (2018). Polysemy and word meaning: an account of lexical meaning for different kinds of content words. *Philosophical Studies, 175*(4), 947–968.

Wittgenstein, L. (1963). *Philosophical Investigations.* Oxford: Basil Blackwell.

Wittgenstein, L. (1964). *Preliminary Studies for the "Philosophical Investigations". Generally Known as The Blue and Brown Books.* Oxford: Basil Blackwell.

Wittgenstein, L. (1974). *Philosophical Grammar.* Oxford: Blackwell Publishing.

Part II

Words

8 'Hope'

The basic schema

This is the first of four chapters examining the pattern of usage associated with the word 'hope', along with its inflected and derived forms.[1] In Chapters 8–10, I look at several constructions 'hope' appears in, examining its functions in different types of expression. Then, in Chapter 11, I turn to the discussions of hope in an academic context, pointing out the similarities and differences between the uses of the word 'hope', as reviewed in the preceding three chapters, and what is said about hope in nursing, psychology and philosophy. The approach draws on both Wittgenstein and Construction Grammar, using many examples adopted (or adapted) from COCA; and it is aimed at clarifying some of the things I've found puzzling about accounts of hope in the health care literature. Although I think the material in Chapters 8–10 is interesting in its own right, it is in Chapter 11 that I will draw out its implications for nursing and health care.

The pattern of use is far more complex, I think, than previous writers – across all three disciplines – have recognised; but I have tried to pursue the enquiry one step at a time, and I've organised the material in as logical a manner as I could manage. However, I make no claim to being comprehensive; indeed, that is neither an achievable, nor even an intelligible, goal.

I will begin with some simple observations, which are partly grammatical and partly terminological.

8.1 Verb, count noun, mass noun

A number of health care writers have recognised that 'hope' can function as both a verb and a noun (for example: Cutcliffe & Herth 2002, Dorcy 2010, Larsen & Stege 2010). However, I have been unable to trace any contributions to the literature which distinguish between 'hope' as a count noun and 'hope' as a mass noun.

I introduced the distinction between count and mass nouns in Section 1.9, perhaps implying that it is a hard and fast one. However, recent writers in linguistics have recognised that many nouns, possibly the majority, can be both mass and count (Koslicki 1999, Kiss et al. 2017). Clear examples of such nouns – which act as count nouns in some linguistic contexts, and mass nouns in others – include 'coffee', 'beer', 'burglary', 'space', 'medicine' and 'silence'. Consider:

(1)   There's a lot of coffee in Brazil.
(2)   He ordered a coffee and a cake.

In (1), 'coffee' is used in a 'mass noun' way, while in (2) it is used in a 'count noun' way. Arguably, nouns such as this are intrinsically neither count nor mass; but the constructions in which they appear activate one function or the other. 'Coffee', in itself, has both 'mass' and 'count' potential (Pelletier 2012); but the 'a *lot of* coffee' construction coerces the 'mass' sense, while the indefinite article in '*a* coffee' coerces the 'count' sense. The expression used to describe these nouns is 'dual-life'. So 'coffee', 'burglary', 'beer', 'medicine' and 'silence' are 'dual-life' nouns (though, according to Pelletier 2010, there's an argument for saying that, potentially, *all* nouns can be).

At any rate, 'hope' is certainly a dual-life noun. It has both mass and count uses. Some examples:

(3)   It's a forlorn hope.
(4)   I have but one hope.
(5)   All those hopes and dreams…
(6)   As darkness fell, hope faded.
(7)   I think there's a glimmer of hope.
(8)   There's not much hope of him winning.

(3), (4) and (5) are count uses; (6), (7) and (8) are mass uses. In (3), the syntactic clue is the indefinite article. We can't say 'a mud' or 'a cutlery', but we do say 'a biscuit' and 'a piano'. In (4), the clue is the adjective 'one', which cannot be applied to mass nouns ('I have but one biscuit', but not: 'I have but one mud'). In (5), it is the plural form: as already noted, mass nouns don't take plurals. In (6) the absence of any determiner (definite or indefinite article) indicates that 'hope' is being used as a mass noun. In (7), 'a glimmer of' is what is known as a 'classifier phrase' (Pelletier 2010). Phrases of this kind can be used only with mass nouns ('a blade of grass' or 'a bowl of water', but not: 'a piece of prize'). With (8), 'not much' is one of another group of expressions used only with mass nouns ('there's not much spaghetti', but not: 'there's not much piano').

So 'hope' has both mass and count noun functions, though it also has some other features not shared by all dual-life nouns. For example, like 'silence', but not like 'cutlery' or 'coffee', it functions as a verb.

It is important – for reasons that will become apparent – to keep in mind the distinction between 'hope' as a *verb*, as a *count noun*, and as a *mass noun*; and I will be referring to it throughout Chapters 8–11. Unfortunately, though, the reason why the distinction is important is not because the different functions of 'hope' map cleanly on to the three syntactic categories. It would be jolly convenient if they did, but they don't. This is part of what makes identifying the functions of 'hope' so difficult: there are no hard and fast syntactic rules to guide us.

Still, it is commonly assumed in the literature that patterns of use *do* map on to syntactic categories. It is often claimed, for example, that the noun 'hope' and the verb 'hope' have separate functions, implying a patterned difference in use (Eliott & Olver 2002, Clayton et al. 2008, Nierop-van Baalen et al. 2016). As we shall see, however, the verb, the mass noun and the count noun do not have consistently different functions. For example, the mass noun has at least one function that the verb and count noun don't have; but it has others that are shared with the count noun. It is, as I say, quite complex.

Here is a reminder of what I said about this complexity in Section 2.2. The job that 'hope' does varies in several ways, depending on: whether a positive or negative assertion is being made; whether the mood of the verb is indicative or interrogative; whether the verb is used in the first person or the third person; whether the mass noun is used with ellipsis; whether an auxiliary modal verb is used; whether the simple present or the continuous present is used; whether a personal or impersonal ('there is…') statement is being made; and several more variations. Moreover, the adjectives and adverbs have complexities of their own.

This rich variety of use has largely escaped the attention of other writers. Philosophers have focused on sentences of the form 'A hopes that X' (indicative, positive, simple present, third-person use of the *verb*). Authors in nursing and psychology try to define the *noun*, without attempting to examine its use in a variety of contexts. In both cases, the focus is on a restricted and atypical range of uses. It's as if previous writers in philosophy, psychology and nursing have inspected a couple of large trees near the road, but not noticed that they are on the edge of a dense forest. I return to this theme in Chapter 11.

8.2 The basic schema

Here, I will deal mainly with 'hope' the verb, but will make some reference to the count noun. The next chapter will focus attention on the mass noun. Let's begin with some comparisons:

I want to

I would like to

I would prefer to ⎭ … climb Ben Nevis.

I'm itching to

I hope to

These are 'wanting' 'preferential' or 'attraction' verbs.[2] This is a family of verbs, all of which suggest wanting something, preferring something or being attracted to something. They are verbs of 'favouring', and there are of course many more of them.[3]

The choice between some of these statements might be arbitrary. Does it matter whether I say 'I want to climb Ben Nevis' or 'I would like to climb Ben Nevis'? In many cases, probably not. But there are some contexts in which it might. For example, in British English, 'I would like to…' sounds a bit more polite, or perhaps more considerate, than a blunt 'I want to…'; and on some occasions that differ-ence of nuance might be significant.[4] In other cases, the nuance is more marked. 'I would prefer to…' implies that there is a choice, which may have been specified previously ('Would you prefer to climb Ben Nevis or sail on Loch Linnhe?'). 'I'm itching to…' injects a sense of urgency, the feeling of somebody who can't wait to get started. So there are *potential* nuances here – potential differences in what is implied. But whether these nuances are activated depends on context.[5]

The circumstances in which we use 'hope' are rather more specific. If hoping is a type of wanting (to put it in soundbite terms), then it is wanting of a particular kind. In imitation of a philosophical analysis, I'll suggest the following schema, which from here on I will refer to as the *basic schema*:

If it is true that 'A hopes that/to/for X', then we can generally infer that:

[a]   A would like X as an outcome.[6]
[b]   A believes that X is possible, but not certain.
[c]   A understands that various factors might prevent X.
[d]   A believes that her control over these factors is limited.

'I hope to climb Ben Nevis' implies that: (a) climbing it is definitely something I would like to do; (b) it is possible that I'll be able to climb it; (c) various factors might prevent me from doing so (the weather is not conducive; something else may have to take priority); (d) my control over these factors is limited (I might be able to organise my schedule, but there's nothing I can do about the weather).

Notice that this schema works equally well for things that I have no control over at all. 'I hope my team wins today.' (I mean: the team I support, not one I play in.) So I want my team to win; it is possible, but not certain, that they will; there are factors which could prevent this happening (they might not play very well, the other team might have a particularly good day, the referee might make poor decisions); there is nothing I can do about any of this.

There are four aspects of the basic schema that I need to make clear before we proceed.

8.2.1 The basic schema is not an analysis or a definition

The rubric says:

If it is true that 'A hopes that/to/for X', then we can generally *infer* that:

The use of 'infer' here is crucial. This is not an *analysis* of 'A hopes that/for X', of the kind associated with analytic philosophy. Rather, the schema indicates *what we can normally infer* when statements of this form are asserted.[7]

Admittedly, the schema echoes the 'standard' or 'orthodox' definition dis-cussed by philosophers. The *locus classicus* for the orthodox definition is Day (1969), together with Downie (1963). Day defines 'A hopes that X' in the follow-ing way:[8]

A wishes that X, and A thinks that X has some degree of probability, however small.

These two conditions correspond, roughly, to [a] and [b] of the basic schema. But the general consensus is that this is inadequate and a third condition is necessary. Various attempts have been made to identify this 'third condition' (for example: Bovens 1999, Pettit 2004, Meirav 2009, Martin 2014, and Segal & Textor 2015, Kwong 2019); but the debate continues.[9]

It might look as if I am attempting to join this debate by suggesting two more conditions, [c] and [d]. However, I must emphasise that, unlike these authors, I am *not* trying to formulate a 'definition of hope'; and the schema is not intended as even a sketch of a definition. Why this is so will be evident from the discussion in Section 7.4; but the impossibility of a 'definition' will, in any case, become clear as the current chapter, along with the next three, proceeds. For now, take the schema as illustrating aspects of how the verb 'hope' is used, and how various states of affairs can be inferred from these uses. In some contexts, the salient inference will involve element [a]; in others, it will involve element [b]. Less frequently, it will involve element [c] or [d]. Everything depends on the job that 'hope' is being asked to do in a given situation. The one thing we should not expect is that the job in question will always be the same.

8.2.2 'Hope' has an object

To the extent that 'hope' is an 'attraction' verb, it requires a syntactic object. There must be something that is hoped *for*. Grammatically, there are several variations on this theme. I hope *for* something, I hope *that* something, I hope *to* something. I don't hope-full-stop, so to speak. If someone says 'Penny for your thoughts...?', and I reply 'I'm hoping', the natural next question is: what are you hoping for? At which point, it would be unintelligible if I were to say: 'I'm not hoping *for* anything. I'm just hoping'. This is common to the 'attraction' verbs. You can't 'want' without wanting *something*. You can't 'desire', but not desire something. You can't 'wish', and not wish for something. It might be assumed that this is a psychological truth; but I regard it as, in Wittgenstein's terms, a grammatical remark (Section 6.4). The key point for now is that you can't do object-less hoping, any more than you can do object-less wanting.

This observation applies also to the count noun. 'My hope is that I'll get a new job'; 'the hope of finding survivors faded'; 'the hope for a truce was frustrated'; 'her one hope was that he would have a change of heart'. Indeed, the object is precisely that which individuates the hope being referred to. The hope that I'll get a new job is different from the hope that my team will win *in virtue of the fact* that the two hopes have different objects. The object is 'internal', as we might say, to that particular example of wanting. It is not an optional extra.

It's true that the object is not always specified. Ellipsis is not uncommon. However, it will be possible, in the majority of instances, to infer the object from the context. For example, a newspaper story about the case of a man who has been on death row for 11 years says this: 'All his appeals have been exhausted. His last hope lies in the courts reviewing whether recent decisions ... apply retro-actively'. In context, it is clear that the object of 'hope' is a reprieve. Similarly, in a report of a disaster: 'As darkness fell, hope faded'. Again, it is obvious that the object-hoped-for is the discovery of victims who are still alive. Of course, ellipsis also occurs with the verb, especially in answers to questions: 'Will you be able to get a new job?' 'I hope so'. (I will say a lot more about 'hope' and ellipsis in Chapter 9.)

8.2.3 The element of attention

Suppose, in a particular case, that elements [a] to [d] are all true. Might we nev-ertheless resist saying 'A *hopes* for X'? I think we might, in some circumstances. Remember that the basic schema is not intended as an analysis of 'A hopes for X'. Elements [a] to [d] are not individually necessary conditions; and they do not, together, amount to a sufficient condition.

Here's an example. Someone says to me: 'Are you hoping that your team fin-ishes in the top half of the table?' As it happens, I haven't had this thought. I hope the team does well. I certainly hope they don't get relegated. I'm sure they won't finish in the top five or six. I would *like* them to finish in the top half of the table. But until I was asked the question, I had not had the thought: 'I hope they finish in the top half'. Still, when the question is put to me, I say 'yes'.

So now we can pose another question. If, before I was asked, someone said 'JP hopes his team finishes in the top half of the table', would they be correct? I am not sure this question has a determinate answer. You can say: well, look, the following statements are all true:

[a] JP would like his team to finish in the top half of the table.
[b] JP believes that this is possible, but far from certain.
[c] JP understands that various factors might prevent this outcome.
[d] JP believes that his control over these factors is non-existent.

So JP *hopes* that his team will finish in the top half. QED. Alternatively, you could say: well, granted all that, even so, JP has not consciously had the thought 'I hope my team ... etc.' So how can you claim that he hopes for this outcome? Are you perhaps suggesting that he was unconsciously hoping that his team would finish in the top half...? Is that not a bit far-fetched? To which the reply might be: well, when he was asked whether he was hoping, he agreed that he was. So he must have been hoping *before* then; it's just that he had not thought about it explicitly.

As I say, I don't believe the question has a correct or incorrect answer. It depends on what you think the best way of describing this situation is. However, it's possible that *in certain circumstances* we might want to say that there is a fifth element of the basic schema. Something like this:

[e] A is consciously aware of elements [a] to [d] at some relevant time.

In other words, in certain situations we might want to infer element [e] along with the other four. This would mean inferring that: A is consciously aware that elements [a] to [d] are true; and/or that she pays attention to them; and/or that she has had the explicit thought 'I hope that/to/for X'.

Notice that, in this context, the implications of a first-person 'hope' statement are different from a third-person 'hope' statement. If Richard says 'I hope for outcome X', then we can infer that element [e] is true. If, however, somebody else says 'Richard hopes for outcome X', we may not be able to infer that. Richard may be in the same position as JP was before being asked whether he hoped that his team would finish in the top half of the table. He may want X, may think that it is possible... and so on; but he may not consciously have had the thought 'I hope for X'.

I will refer to element [e] again in Section 8.4, when we turn to the use of the present continuous tense: 'I am hoping' and 'she is hoping'.

8.2.4 Beliefs about possibility

Element [b] of the basic schema raises interesting questions. It is generally assumed that one can't hope for something which one believes to be impossible, or for something which one believes to be certain, or which has already been achieved. You can't hope to square the circle, or jump over the Albert Hall; nor can you hope that $2 + 2 = 4$, or that Professor Dame Donna Kinnair was confirmed as CEO of the RCN in 2019 – not, at least, if you have the usual beliefs about 2, 4, squares, circles and the Albert Hall, and not if you already know that Professor Dame Donna Kinnair *was* confirmed as the CEO of the RCN in 2019. So element [b], or its equivalents, are normally taken to mean that the individual concerned believes that the probability of the outcome is somewhere between 0 and 1.

In principle, then, hope is always possible if the probability of the desired outcome is believed to be such that $p > 0$, no matter how small p in fact is. Unless the outcome is logically or mathematically impossible, p will be finite, even if it is infinitesimally small.[10] In practice, of course, we tend not to bother with this technicality. If the probability of an outcome is very close to zero, we will usually treat it as if it *were* zero. I do not, for example, hope that Barnet, a non-league team, will win the FA Cup – even though I am a Barnet supporter – because I know that a non-league team has only won the Cup once in 150 years; and that was in 1901, long before the start of the professional era. It is not completely impossible that a non-league club could win again; but it is so unlikely that I treat it as if it *is* impossible.

However, there may be circumstances – we shall see that there are – in which a very small probability, close to zero, is not just a 'technicality'. In circumstances of that kind, we might not treat the very small probability as if it were zero, and treat it instead as something that justifies claiming that the outcome is 'still possible'. Whether someone does this, or whether they do in fact treat the very small probability as equivalent to zero, depends on a number of factors. One of them is the nature of the outcome, and how important it is to the person concerned.

Another might be their understanding, or lack of understanding, of the idea of probability itself. A third might be their appraisal of the relevant evidence, which could incline them to 'round up' or 'round down' the likelihood they assign to the outcome concerned. There are other possibilities, too, which I will discuss in Section 11.9.

For now, the main point is this: whether or not someone thinks of herself as hoping for a given outcome depends, at least in part, on how she understands 'possible' in element [b] of the basic schema. I will say more about this in Chapter 11.

8.3 'Hope' as an epistemic verb

I suggest that 'hope' belongs to another family of verbs in addition to the 'attraction' family. Consider the following statements about the prospects of Olga attending a conference:

I know that

I fear that

I understand that

I imagine that   ... Olga will attend the conference.

I hope that

I doubt that

Wierzbicka (2006) calls these expressions *epistemic verbal phrases*.[11] The effect of these phrases is to qualify the degree of assurance that the speaker can give to her audience, implicitly referring to the kind of evidence – or lack of it – that supports the assertion. In each case, by implication, the probability that Olga will attend the conference is assessed by the speaker.

'I know that...' gives full assurance: the speaker is in no doubt that Olga will come, though the basis for this confidence is unspecified. 'I fear that...' implies that her attendance is highly likely, but signals that the speaker regards this as regrettable (or signals the speaker's acknowledgement that his audience will regard it that way). 'I understand that...' is a notch or two below both 'I know that' and 'I fear that'. The speaker implies that he has reasons for thinking Olga will come, and hints that they are authoritative; but he does not assure his audience, categorically, that she will. 'I imagine that...' drops a further notch, suggesting that the speaker has general background reasons for thinking Olga will come – it's the sort of conference, perhaps, that she enjoys – but implies that he has no specific evidence that she will attend this particular gathering. 'I hope that...' suggests that it is *possible* Olga will come, but hints that there may be reasons why she won't. (Additionally, of course, it implies that the speaker would welcome her arrival, a point I'll turn to in a moment.) 'I doubt that...' suggests that it is unlikely that Olga will come, and implies that the speaker has general background reasons for thinking that she won't; nevertheless, it does not altogether rule out the possibility that she will.

In this kind of context, then, epistemic verbs calibrate the audience's expectations. They give a broad estimation of likelihood, and some of them hint at the kind of evidence the speaker has, or doesn't have, for the assertion. Some of them appear, superficially, to describe a mental state: 'imagine', 'understand', 'fear', 'hope' and 'doubt'. However, this cannot be taken too literally. There is not much to choose, for example, between 'I doubt that she will come' and 'she probably won't come'. The pragmatic force of all these statements is to suggest (broadly) the degree of probability of an outcome, given the nature of the evidence available to the speaker. It is not to describe the speaker's state of mind.[12]

For example, consider (9) and (10), where the latter is an answer to the question 'Will Olga come?':

(9) I imagine that Olga will attend the conference.
(10) I imagine so.

I've suggested that, in this context, the speaker may well have general background reasons for thinking Olga will come, and that the assertion falls well short of an assurance that she will. What it does *not* do is report an act of imagination on the speaker's part. To see this, contrast the following two statements:

(11) I imagine being married to her.
(12) I imagine what my garden will look like in the summer.

In these two cases, the speaker is presumably referring to acts of imagination, perhaps 'visual' in some sense (the garden), and/or a kind of fantasy narrative (the being married). But the same kind of activity is surely not being referred to in (9) or (10). Does the person making either of these statements *visualise* Olga attending the conference, or create an anticipatory 'inner *narrative*' in which she does? It's hard to believe that he does. And if someone insists that, for statements (9) and (10) to be true, the speaker *has to* engage in visualisation or inner narrative – otherwise the use of 'imagine' is incorrect – then I'm not sure how to respond. I can express my scepticism; I can ask whether people *really* visualise something every time they say 'I imagine so'; and I can suggest that a dogmatic assumption about meaning is being allowed to trump usage. But I can't provide a conclusive argument.

At any rate, it does not seem to me that 'I imagine' in (9) and (10) is being used to describe a mental state or process, in the way that it appears to be in (11) and (12).

I would say something similar about the following example:

(13) I fear that Olga will attend the conference.

As I have already suggested, (13) implies that Olga probably will attend, and that the speaker (or his audience) does not welcome this prospect. Still, we should not be in a hurry to ascribe actual *fear* to the speaker. It's perfectly possible to say 'I fear that she will attend', or 'I'm afraid that she will attend', and not experience any fearful emotion. This is because the statement refers (a) to the probability that Olga will attend and (b) to a negative valence associated with her coming. The word 'fear' is used *in order to convey a recognition of this valence*. It is not used to imply that the speaker is experiencing the emotion of fear. It is not, in that sense, intended to report on a particular state of mind.[13]

So what of 'hope'?

(14)   I hope that Olga will attend the conference.

In one sense, of course, 'I hope' does refer to the speaker's mental state. After all, I've already described it as a 'wanting' verb. Moreover, it's true, according to White et al. (2018), that the distinction between 'attraction' and 'epistemic' verbs – or, in their terminology, the distinction between 'preferential' and 'representational' verbs – is generally assumed to be such that the two categories are mutually exclusive. However, as they also observe, 'some verbs appear to fall into both categories' (419); and they mention 'hope' as one of these. In order to see why it is plausible to claim that 'hope' is an epistemic verb as well as an attraction verb, I will look at two syntactic markers: first, the difference between 'hope to' and 'hope that'; second, the parenthetical use of epistemic verbs.

8.3.1 *'Hope to' and 'hope that'*

It will not have escaped the reader's attention that, when 'wanting' verbs were introduced at the start of Section 8.2, the examples all involved 'hope to'. Now, in suggesting that 'hope' is an epistemic verb as well as an 'attraction' verb, I have switched to examples of 'hope that'. There is an interesting contrast between 'I hope to climb Ben Nevis', and 'I hope that Olga will attend the conference'; and this is true, even though the basic schema fits both of them.

Authors in philosophy and linguistics have explored the way in which certain syntactic differences track the distinction between 'attraction' and epistemic verbs (Stalnaker 1984, Anand & Hacquard 2013); and it is well known that the epistemic verbs tend to be associated with finite subordinate clauses ('that...'), while the 'attraction' verbs tend to be associated with non-finite subordinate clauses ('to...').

(15)   Alison thinks that he's a Marxist.
(16)   Nancy wants to go to Oxford.

This correlation has been well studied in the language acquisition literature (De Villiers & De Villiers 2000, White et al. 2018). For example, Harrigan et al. (2016) show that the difference between 'that...' clauses and 'to...' clauses affects children's understanding of 'hope'. When 'hope' is accompanied by 'that...', children assimilate it to epistemic verbs like 'think'. They assume that 'hope', like 'think', is used to report beliefs. However, when it is followed by 'to...', they assimilate it to 'attraction' verbs like 'want'. They assume that it is used to report desires and preferences. So the syntactic environment of 'hope' gives a preliminary clue as to whether, on this particular occasion, it is the 'attraction' or the 'epistemic' dimension which is most salient.

8.3.2 Parenthetical verbs

Linguists have pointed out that epistemic verbs can occur in the parenthetical, or 'S-lifting' (Ross 1973), position. Consider, for example:

(17)   Monica caught the train, I believe.
(18)   Gail is going to give a speech, I gather.

Most 'attraction' verbs cannot take the place of 'believe' in (17) or 'gather' in (18). 'Want' and 'desire' don't work here:

(19*) Monica caught the train, I want.

But 'hope' does work. It can occur in the parenthetical position, often with an interrogative intonation:

(20)   Monica caught the train, I hope?[14]

In the same way, 'I believe so', 'I understand so' and 'I hope so' can all be answers to a question such as 'Did Monica catch the train?'. However, most 'attraction' verbs cannot be used in the same way ('Did she catch the train?' 'I want so', 'I wish so'). So, again, this use of 'hope' suggests that it belongs to the epistemic group as well as the 'attraction' group.

In summary, there are persuasive reasons for believing that the verb 'hope' belongs to both 'attraction' and epistemic families, as White et al. (2018) argue. The constructions 'hope to', 'hope that', S-lifting and 'hope so' are among the syntactic markers of this dual membership.

8.3.3 The implications of dual membership

In virtue of this dual citizenship, the verb 'hope' is like both 'want' (in some respects) and 'believe' (in others). It conveys both a preference and a proposition. It is natural to associate its *preferential* side with element [a] of the basic schema, and its *propositional* side with elements [b], [c] and [d] – especially [b]. In some contexts, it will be the preferential side that is more salient; in others, it will be the propositional side. There will be times when a person uses 'hope' to empha-sise her preference for a certain outcome, and when her belief that this outcome is possible will be implied or assumed. There will be other times when she uses 'hope' to convey her belief that the outcome is possible, and to signal that her preference for it can be taken as read.

Which of these applies on any given occasion depends on a number of factors, including (and especially) what is already assumed, by both speaker and audience, about the background situation.

An example of the first type of situation. It is early September 2015, and the assisted dying bill is due to be voted on by MPs later this month. All the signs are that the bill is likely to be rejected by a substantial majority. The subject of the bill comes up in a conversation between me and a new acquaintance, whose views I am unsure of, but who appears to be well informed on political matters. At one point, I ask her whether she thinks the bill will be rejected. 'I hope so', she replies. In this context, what information is she giving me? She is clearly not stating that it's possible the bill will be rejected. We both already know that. What she's doing instead is telling me that she is in favour of rejection. It is her *preference* that the bill is rejected. In this case, then, element [b] is assumed. The salient new information is that she doesn't support the bill. This is element [a].

An example of the second type of situation. An old friend and I are discussing the latest developments in the House of Commons arising out of the UK's decision to leave the European Union. It is January 2019, and the date for departure is 29th March. In this case, it is common background knowledge that we both favoured remaining in the EU, and are both worried about 'crashing out' with no deal. Following a crucial debate, my friend asks: 'Do you think we'll avoid the no-deal option?' If I now reply 'I hope so', what information am I giving him? Unlike the first example, this is a case in which he already knows my *preference*. So I can't be telling him that. What I'm doing instead is saying that I still think it is *possible* that a no-deal scenario can be avoided. In this case, then, element [a] is assumed. The salient information is my belief that a deal of some kind is still a possibility. This is element [b].

Of course, there will also be cases in which neither element [a] nor element [b] is part of the taken-for-granted background, and in which both the 'attraction' and 'epistemic' dimensions of a 'hope' sentence provide new information. For example, the statement 'I hope that I don't fall in love with you' (Waits 1973) is richly informative. It tells the person it's addressed to that Waits does not want to fall in love with her, element [a]; and that he thinks that it's possible he won't, element [b]. At the same time, it tells her that he is aware of factors which might prevent this not-falling-in-love outcome occurring, element [c]; and that his control over these factors is limited, element [d]. Moreover, the fact that he is informing her about elements [c] and [d] – combined with the fact that he bothered to mention any of it in the first place – might suggest to her that there is a distinct possibility that he will fall in love with her anyway.

Although all three of these examples fit the basic schema, the 'hope' statement does a different job in each case. This is because what can be assumed at the outset by speaker and audience varies with the context. Consequently, a different element of the basic schema is salient in each of the examples, with the element in question signalling the 'new' information which is conveyed (or can be inferred) over and above what is already 'given'.[15] The verb's dual membership of the 'attraction' and 'epistemic' families is marked syntactically by the features reviewed above. It is realised functionally by the context-related salience of one or more elements of the basic schema.

This is one reason why the job done by a 'hope' statement is not always the same from one occasion to the next. But it is not the only reason, as we will see in the next two chapters. In particular, 'hope' as a mass noun, and constructions involving negation, can amend the word's function to a striking degree. For example, when the noun is used in phrases such as 'without hope', or when the verb is negated in expressions such as 'cannot hope', element [a] of the basic schema becomes recessive, in the sense that it is confined largely to the 'given' function of the statement, while element [b] becomes dominant, almost always providing the 'new' information. The basic schema remains in place, but different constructions significantly modify the work that can be done by the word.

8.4 The present continuous

The basic schema tabulates four (sometimes five) inferences that can be drawn when it is claimed that 'A hopes for/that X'. This kind of statement incorporates the simple present tense. Here, I want to raise the question as to what difference it makes if the present continuous is used instead: 'I am hoping', 'she is hoping' and so on.[16] Look at some examples:

(21) Flynn is hoping for a pardon before charges are brought against him.
(22) Levesque said he is hoping to announce a woman's tournament soon.
(23) The company is hoping to launch a prototype next year.
(24) The Senate is hoping to complete its work on the bill by 4th July.
(25) Lorna is hoping to qualify for the Olympic Games.
(26) He is hoping that the election will proceed more smoothly than the primary.

One interesting thing about these examples is the sense of imminence. Or, if not imminence, then at least a timetable, an agenda, a goal that is being worked towards. Another is the frequency of the construction 'is hoping *to*' compared to 'is hoping *that*'. In COCA, for example, the former outnumbers the latter by a ratio of about 3:1.[17] The two features together suggest that the present continuous is used especially in situations where there is a sense of limited time, and/or where there is an ongoing process of some kind. The 'is hoping *to*' construction is used, as one might expect, where the individual concerned has some active role in the developments concerned. The Senate is working on the bill; Levesque is organising a woman's tournament; the company is building a prototype.

The implication is that 'is hoping' applies particularly to circumstances which involve current activity of some kind. Where the subject of the sentence is directly involved in this activity, we can infer that one aspect of it is related to elements [c] and [d] of the basic schema. For example, the Senate will be trying to overcome or minimise the factors which might prevent work on the bill being completed by 4th July. Lorna is aiming to record a time that will qualify her for the Olympics. Levesque is busy organising the tournament. All of them are seeking to overcome the factors that might prevent the goal being achieved.

This is consistent with the work done on the present continuous by cognitive linguists (Langacker 2001, De Wit & Brisard 2009). It has traditionally been assumed that the present continuous refers to activity that is concurrent with the statement's being made. 'She's listening to Leonard Cohen' implies that she's listening to him at the moment; 'She listens to Leonard Cohen' implies something habitual. Cognitive linguists see this as an expression of modality. It is not so much the fact that some activity is *ongoing*, as the fact that it is *contingent on the present circumstances*. Consequently, as De Wit and Brisard (2009: 11) observe, 'connotations such as surprise or atypicality feature quite frequently'. The circumstances on which the activity is contingent do not have to be exceptional, but they often are. In examples (21) to (26), the exceptional circumstances are the prospect of charges being brought, the organisation of a tournament, a prototype in development, a new piece of legislation, the Olympic Games, and an election.

But what of hoping-situations in which the person concerned is unable to affect the outcome at all, and is therefore in no position to invest activity in trying to overcome or mitigate the factors that might prevent it? Consider, for example:

(27)   Kate is hoping that Clinton will win.

If Kate is a citizen of the UK, then she has no control over the outcome, not even minimally (not being able to vote). So what kind of 'current activity', contingent on the circumstances of a USA election, can she be involved in? We can contrast this with:

(28)   Kate hopes that Clinton will win.

If the cognitive linguists are right about the modal implications of the present continuous, then (27) has the sense that something *depends* on the outcome. Kate is hoping Clinton wins because the outcome will have some repercussions for her. (28) does not convey this to the same extent. She hopes Clinton wins because she generally favours the Democrats, or dislikes Trump; but nothing of any consequence hangs on it as far as she personally is concerned.

This is a very subtle difference, of course, and there will certainly be contexts in which (27) is intended to convey no more than (28). However, (27) will be particularly apt when the person concerned feels that there are consequences for her personally; and when, as a result, she finds herself wanting a Clinton victory especially strongly, takes a consistent interest in newspaper stories about the election, keeps up to date with the polls and spends a significant proportion of time thinking about the political situation.

In circumstances of this kind, then, 'hoping' is more active. There is nothing the person can do to affect the outcome, so she cannot be active in that sense. Instead, her 'activity' is mental. She thinks about the situation a great deal, acquires relevant information, discusses it with friends and anticipates the likely consequences of one outcome or another. This may seem a lot to hang on the choice of tense; but, as I've already suggested, none of this *follows* from (27). My observations do not amount to an analysis of (27). They are merely indicators of the considerations that might be involved in choosing to say (27) rather than (28). There is no inconsistency about conceding that, on occasion, (27) may be intended to convey no more than (28) does. It is rather a matter of what options and communicative opportunities different constructions offer.

The activity implied by the 'is hoping' construction echoes what I said about the element of attention in Section 8.2.3. In particular, the kind of mental activity implied by statements like (27) corresponds to the element [e] inference outlined there. The idea is that the present continuous suggests this sort of activity more strongly than the simple present. The same applies to the physical activity characteristic of (21) to (26), though perhaps at one remove. The kind of preparations involved in hoping to launch a prototype, or in hoping to qualify for the Olympic games, can hardly be undertaken in the absence of the kind of attention associated with element [e]. Indeed, it is not unlikely that the people concerned have said both to themselves and to others: 'We are hoping to launch a prototype', and 'I am hoping to qualify for the Olympics'. The option of 'unconscious' or 'inexplicit' hoping does not seem to be available here.

First-person uses of 'hoping to' introduce the same sense of imminence, agenda or a goal as third-person uses; and they inherit from the first person, simple present tense the inference to element [e].

(29)   I am hoping to get a greenhouse built this year.
(30)   I am hoping to meet Obama before he leaves Washington.
(31)   I am hoping that things will change after the election.
(32)   I am hoping that effective therapies will eventually be found.

First-person uses of 'hoping that' also support the inference to element [e] and usually, but not always, introduce the theme of contingency or atypicality.

I will return to the present continuous when I discuss 'hoping against hope' in Chapter 11. In certain health and illness situations, there is a sense of imminence, and of limited time. There is an acute sense of contingency, and of what hangs on the outcome. And there is an awareness that the person concerned has little or no control at all over the factors that will determine that outcome – and, perhaps, that no-one else has either.

8.5 Conclusion

Here is a nutshell summary of this chapter. The verb 'hope' gives simultaneous expression to desires and beliefs, either of which can be dominant or recessive. Its 'belief' component involves, most significantly, an assessment of probability. The verb and the count noun both take a grammatical object, which is what individuates the hope concerned.

A background theme of the chapter is that the word 'hope' has several different uses, partly dependent on syntax. Those who talk about 'analysing the concept of hope', or who ask 'What is hope?' (Kwong 2019), tend to overlook this. As I observed in Part I, 'the concept of X' is assumed to be a singular *thing* (whether mental or abstract) which accounts for the different uses of the word 'X'. So whenever you use the word 'hope', you are expressing, or voicing, or articulating, or applying the same *concept*. But, as I also suggested in Part I, this is a misleading picture. The various uses of the word 'hope' have different functions. There is no 'concept of hope' which underlies them all, and no single analysis which accounts for the whole range.

This chapter has focused mainly on uses of 'hope' the verb, with some reference to the count noun. In the next chapter, I turn my attention to uses of the mass noun.

Notes

1 I had originally intended to write only one chapter on 'hope'. However, as we'll see, the pattern of use is so complex that a single chapter would have been insufficient.

2 I borrow 'attraction' from Martin (2014), and 'preferential' from White et al. (2018). The terms are used by these authors to designate this family of verbs, though White et al. use 'preferential' to refer to 'negative preference' verbs as well, for example 'loathe' and 'dislike'.

3 Including 'desire', 'favour', 'aspire', 'dream', 'hanker', 'crave', 'wish', 'lust', 'long', 'yearn', 'covet', 'fancy', 'incline' and 'thirst'. Grammatically, they don't all take the infinitive. 'I'd like to climb Ben Nevis', but 'I fancy climbing Ben Nevis'. 'I wish to speak to the manager', but 'I'm lusting after those chocolates'. As with the verbs discussed in the text, the nuances vary.

4 According to Holmes (1982: 24), people learning English as a second language have often 'found it difficult to master the expression of degrees of certainty and conviction in English. Without a command of such skills speakers tend to sound abrupt, rude or didactic in different situations'. Wierzbicka (2006: 251) makes a similar point: 'Acquiring the means of qualifying one's statements is a matter of great importance for the learner of English'. She adds that the need to master this skill 'can be compared with the need to master honorifics in Japanese'. People for whom English is a first language generally underestimate this aspect of Anglo linguistic culture.

5 For example, 'I long to see her again' suggests a long-standing, unfulfilled desire, while implying that there are factors which prevent the speaker from fulfilling it in the near future, or which have prevented it from being fulfilled until now. On the other hand, it is difficult to imagine a situation in which 'I long to catch the 6:45 train' could be anything other than a piece of ironic humour.

6 I've used 'outcome' here because the use of 'hope' is generally future-orientated. However, it's quite possible to hope about things in the past. Most philosophers use 'desire' or 'wish' instead of 'would like'. I think both these terms muddy the waters. 'Desire' is a useful generic term, but it has distracting connotations. 'Wish' has a different set of functions. In fairy tales, you're granted three wishes, not three hopes; you toss a coin into the wishing well, not the hoping well; you might wish upon a star, but you don't hope upon a star. 'Wish that' (as opposed to 'wish to') is counter-factual. Contrast 'I wish to talk to my father' and 'I wish that I could talk to my father'. The latter acknowledges that, much as I might want to, I won't be able to.

7 I suppose this counts, weakly, as a form of inferentialism, but I don't think I'm going all the way with, for example, Brandom (1998). There are too many things in his ver-

sion that I don't see the need for. See the interesting discussions of Brandom in Turner (2010, 2014).

8 Day actually uses 'p' instead of 'X'. I have changed this for two reasons. First, to prevent confusion with the use of 'p' for probability, which occurs later in the text. Second, to be consistent with my formulation of the basic schema. In this context, 'X' stands for any proposition/statement/clause that can follow 'hopes that'.

9 I don't have the space to examine the contributions to this debate. However, I do discuss Martin's book in Section 11.9.

10 For example, as I noted in Section 8.2.1, Day's (1969) analysis of 'A hopes that X' is: 'A wishes that X, and A thinks that X has some degree of probability, *however small'* (my italics).

11 Again, there are many more verbs in the 'epistemic' family, including: 'think', 'gather', 'presume', 'guess', 'believe', 'find', 'expect', 'take it', 'bet', 'suspect', 'assume' and 'trust'. This rather long list of verbal epistemic phrases is apparently a peculiarity of English. According to Wierzbicka (2006: 206), it is 'probably without parallel in other languages of the world'. For an analysis of the differences between 15 of these epistemic phrases in English, see Wierzbicka's Chapter 7.

12 The pragmatic analysis of these expressions can be traced back to Austin's observations on the use of 'I know' (Austin 1961), Urmson's discussion of what he calls 'parenthetical verbs' (Urmson 1952) and Wittgenstein's discussions of 'mental process' verbs such as 'believe', 'understand', 'fear' and 'think' (Wittgenstein 1963, Baker 2004). The idea is that we should be trying to give up the assumption that 'I know' (for example) describes a state of mind or refers to a 'propositional attitude'. In response to the statement 'Charles has left Fiona!', the replies 'I know', 'I heard', 'Apparently', 'So I understand' and 'Yes, Fiona told me' are functionally the same. They are confirmations (or assurances) that the speaker is aware of the circumstances. In this sort of context, 'I know' and 'I understand' are not intended to be descriptions of one's state of mind, any more than 'Apparently' and 'Yes, Fiona told me' are.

13 'Is that really going to happen?' 'I'm afraid so.' The second speaker is not saying that she is in a state of fear. She is saying, first, that it is likely to happen; second, that she recognises that this will be an unwelcome development. Pragmatically, third, she may also be making an apology. In the same way, 'I hope so' can function, pragmatically, as reassurance.

14 Given its positive valence, 'hope' only works where the situation/event described is a welcome one. 'Colin fell and broke his leg, I understand' is fine. 'Colin fell and broke his leg, I hope' is unexpected. It could be used only in unusual circumstances, or by someone with a sadistic attitude towards Colin.

15 The difference between 'given' and 'new' is a key feature of Halliday's functional grammar. See Chapter 3 of Halliday (2014). In my terms, what is 'given' is what the speaker and/or audience can take as read; while 'new' is that element of the basic schema which is most salient, either in the conveying or in the inferring.

16 The recent linguistics literature prefers the term 'present progressive' (De Wit & Brisard 2009). I have retained 'present continuous' because it is more familiar.

17 Interestingly, this relation is reversed for first person constructions. 'Am hoping that' outnumbers 'am hoping to' by a ratio of 5:2.

References

Anand, P., & Hacquard, V. (2013). Epistemics and attitudes. *Semantics and Pragmatics*, *6*(8), 1–59.

Austin, J. L. (1961). *Philosophical Papers*. Oxford: Clarendon Press.

Baker, G. (2004). *Wittgenstein's Method: Neglected Aspects*. Malden, MA: Blackwell Publishing.

Bovens, L. (1999). The value of hope. *Philosophy and Phenomenological Research, 59*(3), 667–681.

Brandom, R. (1998). *Making It Explicit: Reasoning, Representing and Discursive Commitment*. Cambridge, MA: Harvard University Press.

Clayton, J. M., Hancock, K., Parker, S., Butow, P. N., Walder, S., Carrick, S., … Tattersall, M. H. N. (2008). Sustaining hope when communicating with terminally ill patients and their families: A systematic review. *Psycho-Oncology, 17*, 641–659.

Cutcliffe, J. R., & Herth, K. (2002). The concept of hope in nursing 1: Its origins, background and nature. *British Journal of Nursing, 11*(12), 832–840.

Day, J. P. (1969). Hope. *American Philosophical Quarterly, 6*(2), 89–102.

De Villiers, J. G., & De Villiers, P. A. (2000). Linguistic determination and the understanding of false belief. In P. Mitchell & K. J. Riggs (Eds.), *Children's Reasoning and the Mind* (pp. 191–228). Hove, UK: Psychology Press.

De Wit, A., & Brisard, F. (2009). Expressions of epistemic contingency in the use of the English present. *Papers in the Linguistic Society of Belgium, 4*, http://uahost.uantwe rpen.be/linguist/SBKL/sbkl2009/dew2009.pdf.

Dorcy, K. S. (2010). Hegemony, hermeneutics, and the heuristics of hope. *Advances in Nursing Science, 33*(1), 78–90.

Downie, R. S. (1963). Hope. *Philosophy and Phenomenological Research, 24*(2), 248–251.

Eliott, J. A., & Olver, I. (2002). The discursive properties of "hope": A qualitative analysis of cancer patients' speech. *Qualitative Health Research, 12*, 173–193.

Halliday, M. A. K. (2014). *Halliday's Introduction to Functional Grammar*. 4th ed. New York: Routledge.

Harrigan, K., Hacquard, V., & Lidz, J. (2016). Syntactic bootstrapping in the acquisition of attitude verbs: Think, want and hope. In K.-M. Kim, et al. (Eds.), *Proceedings of the 33rd West Coast Conference on Formal Linguistics*. Somerville, MA: Cascadilla Proceedings Project.

Holmes, J. (1982). Expressing doubt and certainty in English. *RELC Journal, 13*(2), 9–28.

Kiss, T., Pelletier, F. J., Husić, H., & Poppek, J. (2017). Issues of mass and count: Dealing with 'dual life' nouns. In *Proceedings of the 6th Joint Conference on Lexical and Computational Semantics* (pp. 189–198). Vancouver: Association for Computational Linguistics.

Koslicki, K. (1999). The semantics of mass-predicates. *Noûs, 33*(1), 46–91.

Kwong, J. M. C. (2019). What is hope? *European Journal of Philosophy, 27*(1), 243–254.

Langacker, R. W. (2001). The English present tense. *English Language and Linguistics, 5*, 251–273.

Larsen, D. J., & Stege, R. (2010). Hope-focused practices during early psychotherapy sessions: Part II: Explicit approaches. *Journal of Psychotherapy Integration, 20*(3), 293–311.

Martin, A. M. (2014). *How We Hope: A Moral Psychology*. Princeton, NJ: Princeton University Press.

Meirav, A. (2009). The nature of hope. *Ratio, 22*(2), 216–233.

Nierop-van Baalen, C., Grypdonck, M., van Hecke, A., & Verhaeghe, S. (2016). Hope dies last: A qualitative study into the meaning of hope for people with cancer in the palliative phase. *European Journal of Cancer Care, 25*, 570–579.

Pelletier, F. J. (2010). Mass terms: a philosophical introduction. In F. J. Pelletier (Ed.), *Kinds, Things, and Stuff: Mass Terms and Generics* (pp. 161–169). Oxford: Oxford University Press.

Pelletier, F. J. (2012). Lexical nouns are both +MASS and +COUNT, but they are neither +MASS nor +COUNT. In D. Massam (Ed.), *Count and Mass Across Languages* (pp. 9–27). Oxford: Oxford University Press.

Pettit, P. (2004). Hope and its place in mind. *The Annals of the American Academy of Political and Social Science*, *592*(1), 152–165.

Ross, J. R. (1973). Slifting. In M. Gross, M. Halle, & M.-P. Schützenberger (Eds.), *The Formal Analysis of Natural Languages* (pp. 133–169). The Hague: Mouton de Gruyter.

Segal, G., & Textor, M. (2015). Hope as a primitive mental state. *Ratio*, XXVIII, 207–222.

Stalnaker, R. (1984). *Inquiry*. Cambridge, MA: MIT Press.

Turner, S. P. (2010). *Explaining the Normative*. Cambridge, UK: Polity Press.

Turner, S. P. (2014). *Understanding the Tacit*. New York: Routledge.

Urmson, J. O. (1952). Parenthetical verbs. *Mind*, *61*(244), 480–496.

Waits, T. (1973). I hope that I don't fall in love with you. *Closing Time*. Los Angeles, CA: Asylum Records.

White, A. S., Hacquard, V., & Lidz, J. (2018). Semantic information and the syntax of propositiomal attitude verbs. *Cognitive Science*, *42*, 416–456.

Wierzbicka, A. (2006). *English: Meaning and Culture*. Oxford: Oxford University Press.

Wittgenstein, L. (1963). *Philosophical Investigations*. Oxford: Basil Blackwell.

9 'Hope'

The mass noun

The uses of 'hope' associated with the basic schema involve the verb and the count noun, both of which take an individuating object. In this chapter, I look at four ways in which 'hope' can be used as a mass noun. The first is its function as a shell noun (Schmid 2000) or signalling noun (Flowerdew & Forest 2015); the second is its use with ellipsis; the third is its function as a domain noun (Section 5.4); and the fourth is when it occurs as the subject of a sentence. These terms will all be explained as we proceed.

9.1 'Hope' as a shell noun

Shell nouns are a group of abstract nouns which can exercise a particular function.[1] They are not shell nouns 'because of some inherent property', but because they are *used* in a certain way (Schmid 2000: 4). The best way to explain the 'shell noun' idea is to give some examples:

(1) The **problem** was that Sam had basically no idea how airplanes worked.
(2) The Government's **aim** is to make GPs more financially accountable.
(3) It's impossible, given the **fact** that some areas are not contiguous with others.
(4) The **advantage** is that there is a huge audience for this sort of thing.
(5) My faith is rooted in the **belief** that we are all part of the great creative force.
(6) Don't let the **idea** of making these major changes to your life overwhelm you.

In each of these examples, a situation, thought, project, possibility, proposal or piece of information is temporarily *associated with* a single word. In Schmid's terminology, the single word is the 'shell noun', and the idea/project/information is the shell 'content'. So the shell, metaphorically speaking, 'encloses' the content. In the typography of Schmid (2000) and Flowerdew and Forest (2015), the word in bold is the shell noun (or signalling noun), and the underlined phrase is the 'content'.

One significant function of a 'shell noun' construction is that it makes possible anaphoric reference. For example, a sentence which follows (3) might begin:

'This fact explains why…' Here, 'this fact' refers anaphorically to the circumstances in question – that 'some areas are contiguous with others' – without having to repeat that phrase.

These are not unusual words. Schmid (2000) lists 670 of them, and 'hope' is one. 'Hope' as a shell noun can be either count or mass.[2] Some examples of the count noun acting in this way:

(7)   My one **hope** is <u>that I'll find a new job</u>.
(8)   <u>Discovering life on other planets</u> is a realistic **hope**.
(9)   His **hope** <u>for a large-scale overhaul</u> proved to be a vain one.
(10) There's not a **hope** in hell <u>of these targets being achieved</u>.

And some examples using the mass noun:

(11) There is no **hope** <u>of making a perpetual motion machine</u>.
(12) Any remaining **hope** <u>of reviving the cease-fire evaporated</u>.
(13) There is some **hope** in the industry <u>that these restrictions will be lifted</u>.
(14) **Hope** <u>of finding survivors</u> faded.

Discursively, a shell noun *characterises* the idea/information it encloses. It places the idea in a particular attitudinal or narrative context. Consider the following:

(15) The **idea** is <u>that these men will be released from prison</u>.
(16) The **fact** is <u>that these men will be released from prison</u>.
(17) The **risk** is <u>that these men will be released from prison</u>.
(18) The **suspicion** is <u>that these men will be released from prison</u>.
(19) The **reason** is <u>that these men will be released from prison</u>.
(20) The **hope** is <u>that these men will be released from prison</u>.

The choice of a shell noun conveys something about the background situation, and/or the speaker's view of it. It's as if each of these statements is taken from a different story. (15) implies that the men's release from prison is still just a proposal. (16), by contrast, implies that the decision has been taken and it will happen. (17) and (18) imply that the release will not be a good thing: (17) suggests that it could be an unwelcome consequence of some other decision or development, while (18) refers indirectly to people anticipating this possibility, and not liking it. (19) characterises the men's release as an explanation of some event or situation. (20) implies, as we have seen, that the release-outcome would be welcome, and that it is a possibility. Each statement belongs, as it were, to a different narrative, the outline of which we get a sense of from the particular shell noun used.

Notice, too, that the shell 'content' in (20) functions as the object of hope. As I observed in Chapter 8, verb and count-noun hope is never hope-full-stop.[3] In both cases, it must be hope that, hope of, hope to or hope for. We get a glimpse here of how aspects of the word's use fit together. In this one example, the noun 'hope' takes an object (technically, a noun clause), functions as a shell noun, sets up an anaphoric role and characterises its 'content' relative to an implied narrative background... all at the same time. This versatility is, however, typical of the construction.

We can see, too, that the use of 'hope' as a shell noun is consistent with the basic schema, even though 'hope' is a noun in this context rather than a verb. The shell's 'content' corresponds to the desired outcome, element [a]; and the use of 'hope' as the shell itself signals the 'positive valence' of element [a] and the 'open possibility' of element [b]. In (7), for example, finding a new job is the outcome; it is the one the speaker prefers; and she believes that it is possible. We can also infer elements [c] and [d]: there are factors that might prevent the desired outcome occurring, and the speaker's control over these factors is limited. Since she is referring to her own hope, as opposed to somebody else's, we can infer [e] as well: she is aware of all four elements, and is likely to be engaged in relevant activity, both physical (making applications for jobs) and mental (focusing her attention on the project of securing one).

In the next chapter, I'll take a closer look at examples which involve negation, as in (10) and (11). It turns out that the relation between the basic schema and sentences involving negation is of particular interest.

9.2 'Hope' with ellipsis

The object-of-hope is not always made explicit, at least not in the immediate linguistic vicinity. I will suggest that there are two main circumstances in which it is absent. One is where there is an obvious ellipsis, and the object can be retrieved from the context – sometimes from text belonging to the same passage in which 'hope' occurs, but not necessarily in the same sentence or paragraph. The other is where there does not appear to be an ellipsis at all, and the work done by 'hope' shifts dramatically.

I cited two examples of ellipsis in Section 8.2.2. Here is another, drawn from a newspaper article about the return to the UK of Matthew Hedges, a doctoral student at Durham University, following his arrest and imprisonment in the United Arab Emirates.

> The 31-year-old, who has been back in the UK for a week, said he suffered seizures and other health problems and began to lose hope during the long months of captivity, which began when UAE security services swooped at Dubai airport in early May.
>
> (Rawlinson 2018)

At no point in the article is it stated what Hedges was hoping for. This is not a case in which the object of hope can be retrieved from the text in the immediate vicinity of the sentence. Later in the article, we read:

> During his detention, he begged for medication for a pre-existing condition, he said, and was given a cocktail of drugs his doctors have since described as concerning. It was at that stage that he began to lose hope, he said.

Even here, the object-of-hope is not spelled out; but it is not difficult to imagine what the author has in mind: the hope of being released from prison; of being able to return to the UK; of not being tortured; and (possibly) of receiving proper medication for his condition. This is a little vague and, technically, speculative. But it would be surprising if these were not the kinds of thing filling the elliptical gap; and we can be fairly confident that the author of the article assumes that his readers will understand this.

The expression 'to *lose* hope' is a reference to the assessment of probability. Hedges began to believe that the likelihood of his being released – having been jailed for life, having been interrogated for up to 15 hours a day, and having been told that he would be taken to a military base where he would be beaten and tortured – was decreasing. He began to question element [b] of the basic schema. In losing hope, he did not lose his desire to be released, element [a]. What he lost, or what he began to lose, was the belief that this was possible. We will return to this idea in the next chapter.

However, the main point I want to make here is that the uses of 'hope' with ellipsis form a spectrum. At one end of this spectrum are the cases in which the 'missing object' can be retrieved from the immediate vicinity of text, and in which there is no ambiguity about what is hoped for. In a dialogue such as:

(21) A Will Olga be attending the conference?
     B That's the hope.

there is no doubt that 'the hope', as referred to by B, is the hope that Olga will attend the conference. But, as we have just seen in the Matthew Hedges story, there are two ways in which the retrieval of the 'missing object' can be less straightforward. First, the object-of-hope may be referred to in a part of the text that is *more remote* from the occurrence of 'hope' than in (21). Second, it may be referred to *more vaguely* than in (21). This is an 'and/or'. The reference may be more remote, but not vague. Or it may be vague, but in the same vicinity. Or it may be both more remote and more vague. Consider this example:

(22) Moseley Braun's charisma galvanized voters of all backgrounds and inspired new hope in American politics.

The newspaper article from which this sentence comes is a review of a book (Morris 2015) about Carol Moseley Braun's campaign for the US Senate in 1992. Here is the text either side of (22)

> Moseley Braun, a long-time Illinois state politician, leapt onto the national scene as feminist voters exerted political muscle. Many women were enraged by the confirmation of Clarence Thomas to the U.S. Supreme Court despite Anita Hill's damning testimony of his sexual harassment. Some male lawmakers brushed off Hill's claims as inconsequential, inciting women to fight back — at the ballot box ... *[(22) appears here]* ... She upset incumbent

Alan Dixon in the Democratic primary and went on to win the election. Her campaign served as a harbinger for another black rising star from the rough side of Chicago: President Obama.

(Torres 2016)

Morris does not make the 'new hope' explicit. There is no 'hope for...', or 'hope of...' or 'hope that...' So the object-of-hope is left somewhat vague. However, the political context sketched here is enough to give the reader a general sense of what she has in mind. Something along the lines of: a hope (among 'voters of all backgrounds', but perhaps especially among women and African Americans) that it was possible to elect senators who would not just represent them, but understand their struggles; the hope that, as a consequence, they could aspire to a better life. However, there is something of a Rorschach effect here. The fact that the object-of-hope is not specified, but left as a vague gesture against a lightly sketched background, means that readers will project their own ideas and preconceptions into the text.

This is no doubt what I have done myself. Indeed, I hesitated before attempting to spell out what kind of hope Morris was referring to, and it took several edits before I decided on a final version. There seemed to be too many ways of getting it wrong, too many ways of going beyond what the article actually says. However, this seems to be part of the point when 'hope' is used this way. The elliptical gap is so large that the reader has little choice. Either she just skims past, not worrying about what the specifics-of-hope are in this particular case, but with a general sense of 'good things now seeming possible'. Or she tries to articulate the hope less vaguely than the author has done, through an act which is as much self-revelation as interpretation. It is the ellipsis itself which creates this situation.

In the book review, and in the Matthew Hedges story, it does not greatly matter that the object-of-hope is left vague. The sense of 'good things seeming possible' in a certain context – American politics, or a man in prison – is enough to secure an emotional cadence (Velleman 2003) for the reader; and this is all that is required for a book review or newspaper article to work. For texts of this kind, a carefully described filling out of what Hedges thought, or what American voters anticipated, is not necessary. The details, in such a case, are beside the point. In this context, vaguely referring – without any itemising, identifying or describing – more than fits the bill.[4]

So the picture I am suggesting is ellipsis-as-a-spectrum, ranging from examples like (21) at one end, to examples like (22) somewhere in the middle... and beyond that to examples such as:

(23) The birth of a new baby gives us hope for the future.
(24) Something inside told me there might still be hope for us.

In these examples, 'hope' is being used in a very broad context. In (23), the arrival of a baby conjures up... well, possibilities of some sort: the start of a new family, parents investing in new projects, new aspirations, new relationships. All very non-specific in terms of what objects-of-hope are being alluded to, but the reader does have some sense of what the relevant possibilities are, and can distinguish them from obviously irrelevant ones. In (24), 'us' refers to the narrator and a woman who is engaged to somebody else, so the possibilities concern: persuading her not to marry the other guy, perhaps; or the two of them getting together; or establishing a friendship; or sorting out past misunderstandings; and so on. Again, very non-specific, but with a general sense of a distinction between relevant and irrelevant possibilities.

This is the far end of the spectrum, where the elliptical gap is at its greatest. At this point, the array of intelligible possibilities – characteristic of (22) and the Matthew Hedges story – has become a large, amorphous cloud, expanding to the point where one cannot enumerate them. If pressed, one can offer examples of the kinds of thing (23) and (24) might be referring to; but there is an indefinite number of possible objects-of-hope which could, in different circumstances, fill the ellipsis slot. This is exophoric 'hope' at its most vague. Nearly.

9.3 'Hope' as a domain noun

There comes a point when to talk about 'ellipsis' is artificial. So far, I have defined the elliptical gap in terms of a non-explicit object-of-hope, which may be retrievable – at least in broad, cloud-of-possibility terms – from the text in which 'hope' occurs. However, there are uses of 'hope' which appeal, not just to potential hope-objects, but also to a wider domain of things-we-associate-with-hope. Consider, for example, a series of statements taken from an article entitled 'A land of hope again?' (Moïsi 2008):

(25) The United States will have to recover or reinvent the culture of hope.
(26) You seem to have dropped the mantle of hope that once made you unique.
(27) The country has to reinvigorate its capacity to symbolize hope.
(28) Pragmatism is not incompatible with hope.

There is, in these sentences, no indication of a hope for.../ to.../ of.../ that... But what is being referred to here seems to go beyond hope for any particular outcome, or even a range of outcomes. The fact that expressions such as 'culture of hope', 'mantle of hope' and 'symbolise hope' are used, and that hope is compared to pragmatism as if it were a philosophical or political principle, suggests that something far wider than an object-of-hope, or a group of related objects-of-hope, is being invoked.

This use of 'hope' exploits a double generalisation. In the first place, there is a generalisation from the idea of a desired-outcome-believed-to-be-possible to the idea of lots-of-potentially-desirable-outcomes-seeming-possible. This is no longer just an outcome that has *already* been identified as desirable, as with (21); nor is it a limited range of outcomes, which are broadly consistent with the text, as in (22). Rather, it includes outcomes we cannot anticipate, outcomes which we might not even have thought of yet. In a 'culture of hope', or in a country which 'symbolizes hope', the outcomes we might (at some point) come to identify as desirable – whatever they prove to be – will also seem possible. So 'hope' in sentences (25) to (28) stands for: *good things seeming possible in general*. It lassoes actual, conceivable and as-yet-unimagined desired-outcomes together, and refers to them in the vaguest possible way (i.e. without specifying, itemising or describing any of them). I will call this 'outcome generalisation'.

The second generalisation is from objects-of-hope to the various circumstances associated with hope. If 'outcome generalisation' indefinitely extends the range of 'X' in elements [a], [b] and [c] of the basic schema, the second goes beyond the schema altogether, and invokes the conditions and consequences of hoping. Much as 'the world of theatre' refers to actors, buildings, institutions, audiences, tickets, critics, rehearsals, producers, opening nights, impresarios, stage traditions and so on, this use of 'hope' refers to ideals, aspirations, projects, plans, motivation, decision making, information, evaluation, support and encouragement from others, struggles, risk, recovery from setbacks, optimism, psychological states such as pleasure, excitement and uncertainty, a better life… and more. It does so with the same vagueness as 'the world of theatre', lassoing these disparate elements together in a broad gesture, without itemising or describing them. It evokes much of what we know about situations in which there is hope, and especially situations in which hope is fulfilled. In the terminology of Section 5.4, it is a domain noun. This really is 'hope' at its most vague, its most elliptical, a use I will call 'context-generalisation'.

Two further comments on the implications of seeing 'hope' (in these linguistic contexts) as a domain noun. First, in lassoing together such a disparate and indefinite range of elements, this use of 'hope' is not susceptible to definition. The basic schema echoes a philosophical definition for statements of the form 'A hopes for/ that X', discussed in Section 8.2. In these cases, a definite preferred-outcome, X, is specified; so there is no outcome generalisation. Nor is there any context generalisation, since these statements are tied to a particular and identifiable context. But where 'hope' is used as a domain noun, neither of these restrictions applies, since vague reference to an unspecified cluster of elements is the whole point of this usage. So any attempt to define 'hope' as it appears in, say, (26) or (27) is doomed to failure. It would not be able to 'capture' the range of elements in any concise formula, and would have to resort to listing examples of the 'kind of thing' referred to by 'hope' when it is used in this way (this, of course, is what I have done in the previous paragraph). One could describe this use as 'subject to outcome- and context-generalisation'; but that would not help to identify 'instances' of 'hope' – even if the domain noun function were in the business of identifying 'instances', which it isn't.[5]

Second comment. Although I have suggested that the domain noun use of 'hope' is not susceptible to definition, one feature of it encourages the assumption that it is. For in this use, 'hope' appears to be independent of the basic schema. It permits reference to 'hope' without having to specify any particular object-of-hope, and independently of any particular context. ('Permits' is not quite the right word here, given that this is the whole point of using 'hope' as a domain noun.) As a result, it comes to resemble other, non-abstract mass nouns.

Consider 'water' and 'concrete', for example. Like 'hope' they can be used without a determiner, and can be the first word in a sentence. But with 'water' and 'concrete' there is nothing which corresponds to the basic schema. Both words are taken to denote a form of (more or less) undifferentiated *stuff*, rather than something that can be counted (like, say, 'person', or 'fork'). One can refer to a chunk of concrete, or an expanse of water; but these expressions just refer to the way in which some of the stuff in question can be collected into one place or another. In each case, it makes sense to ask what kind of substance we are dealing with. What is it made of? What are its properties? How does it behave in certain conditions? And so on.

Detach 'hope' from the basic schema – which is what happens when it is used as a domain noun – and it can appear to resemble 'concrete' and 'water'. In the absence of an explicit link to outcomes, objects-of-hope and relevant contexts, it can look as if it is another kind of *thing*... a stuff, a substance, a structure, a process, a force or whatever. Not, of course, a physical stuff... but a certain kind of *something*, none the less. This being so, it then becomes tempting to ask questions similar to those asked about concrete and water. What kind of thing is it? What does it consist of? What are its properties? How does it react to certain conditions? In many cases, asking questions of this sort prompts a search for definitions. We read that 'hope is defined as...(something)'. For example: 'a *multidimensional* dynamic life force characterized by a *confident* yet *uncertain* expectation of achieving a future *good*' (Dufault & Martocchio 1985: 380). Like a physical type of force, it can be empirically analysed into dimensions, components, parts, spheres and facets. Like a physical kind of stuff, it can be measured.

If I am right about the domain noun use of 'hope', this all seems substantially off-target. A noun used to refer, in the vaguest terms, to an indefinite, unspecified range of possibilities and contexts is construed as a noun used to denote a... kind of *something*. The temptation to think of nouns and nominalisations as names for certain kinds of things has been with us since Chapter 2, and this is arguably a variation on the theme. However, the next section considers one further use of 'hope' as a mass noun, a use which is distinct from the domain noun function. Perhaps that will serve to vindicate the idea that 'hope' denotes something which can be characterised in the way that writers like Dufault and Martiocchio suppose.

9.4 'Hope' in the subject position

Consider the use of 'hope' in (29) to (32). Unlike the examples in the previous section, these all have 'hope' in the subject position, the first word of the sentence. Moreover, whereas (25) to (28) appear to tell us something about a country, or about pragmatism, these sentences seem to tell us something about *hope*. They ascribe a property to it. 'Hope' is clearly not being used here as a domain noun, and these statements certainly look as if they are referring to *something*, even if it is not a physical object.

(29) Hope always incites change.
(30) Hope is a thin and slippery thing, sorely tested and hard to come by.

(31)   Hope is made of memories.
(32)   Hope dies last.

None of these statements would be classified as a definition of hope (I will be looking at definitions in Chapter 11), but they all characterise it in some way; and it is
easy to slip into *nouns-are-naming-words* mode, and assume that what (29) to (32)
are doing is ascribing a property to a 'mental' object. This is a temptation reinforced
by the fact that, in (29) and (32), hope *does* something; in (30) it is described as a
thing; and in (31) it is *made* of something. This is the language we apply to physical
objects and/or stuff. Concrete sets, ice is a slippery thing, beer is made with hops,
glyphosate causes cancer. So why would we *not* think that the hope-sentences are
doing exactly what they appear to be doing; that is, referring to a certain kind of
object (or state, or phenomenon) and identifying one of its attributes?

I will leave this possibility open for the time being; but it's worth pointing out
that it raises some tricky metaphysical questions about the nature of the object
being described. We know what concrete is, what ice is, what beer is and what
glyphosate is. But there is no consensus about what hope is. It is said to be an
emotion (Lazarus 1999), an 'inner power' (Herth 1990), an 'adaptive mechanism'
(Folkman 2010), a 'theological virtue' (Lebacqz 1985), a 'life force' (Dufault &
Martocchio 1985) and more. Presumably, this emotion/power/virtue/mechanism/
force is present in everybody,[6] so there are further questions about how it got
there, how it works, what other biological or psychological systems it's connected
to, whether there is independent evidence for its existence and so on.[7] Since characterisations of this kind turn up a lot in the health care literature, I will return to
them in Chapter 11.

However, the main point I want to make at this stage is that the metaphysical
problems are unnecessary. We can finesse them. They start with the assumption
that the grammar of statements like (30) and (31) can be taken as a metaphysical
guide.[8] Syntactically, we have a grammatical subject ('Hope') which has a predicate ('is a thin and slippery thing'; 'is made of memories') attached to it. This is
the most familiar construction in English. The metaphysical jump we make is to
infer that this subject-predicate structure *reflects how the world is*. We assume that
what the sentence is doing is picking out some kind of object or phenomenon (corresponding to the grammatical subject), and then identifying a property that it has
(corresponding to the predicate). With sentences referring to physical objects, states
or substances, this assumption creates few problems. 'Tigers have stripes', 'water is
wet', 'diabetes is caused by a lack of insulin' can all be treated in (roughly) this way.

It's less obvious that the 'metaphysical guide' assumption works with sentences like 'Hope is made of memories'. As I have already implied, 'what hope
is made of' is not as straightforward as 'what beer is made of'. But to understand
how the finessing of this type of sentence might go, we need another idea from
linguistics.

Linguists have long had 'an acute awareness of the strong similarity between
plurals and mass nouns' (Chierchia 1998: 54). In fact, some – including Chierchia
himself and Gillon (1992) – have argued that mass nouns are in effect disguised

plurals. The Inherent Plurality Hypothesis, as Chierchia calls it, takes issue with the assumption that a mass noun, such as 'ice', 'courage', 'glyphosate', 'footwear', stands for 'a mereological whole of some kind': a natural kind, a substance, a species, a *type* of thing. It proposes, instead, that mass nouns 'come out of the lexicon with plurality already built in' (Chierchia 1998: 53); and this is the only way in which they differ from count nouns. The implication is that, in terms of what they denote, there is no significant difference between mass nouns and plurals.

The argument implies that there is a spectrum of cases. At one end, the potential equivalence of plurals and mass nouns is not difficult to accept. Chierchia's examples are 'shoes' and 'footwear', 'coins' and 'change', 'clothes' and 'clothing', 'carpets' and 'carpeting'. These are all cases in which there is a count noun term for the individual items. However, the idea can also be applied to mass nouns like 'furniture' and 'cutlery', which do not have corresponding count nouns (although examples can be itemised), but which are clearly plural in the way 'change' and 'footwear' are. From there, you can extend the same line of thought to 'sand' and 'rice', which do not have corresponding count nouns either (though we can refer to 'grains of...' in each case). These can be construed as plural in a similar way; it's just that there is no term, in English, for individual particles of rice or sand, in the way that there is for individual items furniture ('table', 'chair') or cutlery ('knife', 'fork'). From there, we can proceed to 'water', 'concrete' or 'glyphosate'. In these examples, not only are there no corresponding count nouns, and no names for individual instances; we cannot even *see* the individual instances concerned (that is, molecules).

So the spectrum of cases ranges from middle-sized objects, such as coins (for which we have a count noun); through smaller sized objects, such as grains of sand (for which we don't); to invisible objects, such as molecules of water (which we can't even see). With the middle-sized objects, we have plurals ('coins') and sometimes mass nouns ('change', 'cutlery');[9] with smaller objects, we usually just have mass nouns ('sand', 'rice'). Where the smallest particle of a substance is invisible, we only have mass nouns ('water', 'concrete'). The plurality option is available at all points on the spectrum; but in the case of fluids or substances, where no individual objects are visible, plurality is *all* there is. And this plurality is represented by a mass noun.

The discussion so far has considered only physical objects, or stuffs. In fact, most examples used in the linguistics literature are concrete, and the analysis of abstract nouns in count, mass and plural terms has barely begun (Zamparelli 2019). However, it is possible that the idea of mass-nouns-as-plurals can be applied to at least some of them, especially dual-life nouns associated with mental states: 'fear', 'love', 'ambition', 'belief', 'desire', 'thought' – and 'hope'. The idea is certainly plausible for 'subject position' cases, like (29) to (32), which arguably generalise over individual cases of hope and hoping.[10] Indeed, apparently equivalent sentences beginning with a plural subject are not difficult to devise:

(29[a]) Hopes always incite change.
(30[a]) Hopes are thin and slippery things, sorely tested and hard to come by.

(31[a]) Hopes are made of memories.
(32[a]) Hopes die last.[11]

These reformulations reduce the temptation to think that 'hope' is the name of an object/state/power of some sort, and so alleviate worries about what kind of object it is. The metaphysical questions recede. Of course, there *are* still questions about what is conveyed, or inferred, when we speak about individual instances of hope and hoping: when we say that someone hopes, or finds themselves hoping, or admits that there's no hope, or asks whether there is any hope. But we have the basic schema to help with that.

However, I am not dismissing the idea that 'hope' in the subject position does name an object, or a force, or a state, or a mechanism, or a process, or a virtue, or a *something* of a certain type. Instead, I will leave this possibility open for now, given that it turns up a lot in the health care literature. In Chapter 11, we'll come back to it.

9.5 Overview: 'hope' as a mass noun

The nutshell message here is that what we can infer from the use of 'hope' as a mass noun depends on the degree to which the desired outcome is identified. The way in which 'hope' alludes to the object-of-hope varies from explicit and highly specific to implicit and extremely vague. At its most vague, 'hope' becomes a domain noun, referring indirectly to a cloud of possibilities which do not need to be specified. The function of this use is largely rhetorical, as its emotional cadence is: 'good things seeming possible'.

Before turning to the functions of 'hope' in the context of health care, I want to consider some further syntactic variations. These are almost always overlooked, but are extremely instructive. They include negation, interrogatives, 'hope' combined with modals, and 'hope' used with modifiers. In every case, these variations modify the tasks that 'hope' can be used to perform.

Notes

1 Several expressions have been used to refer to this class of nouns: 'carrier nouns', 'general nouns', 'metadiscursive nouns', 'type 3 vocabulary', 'metalanguage nouns', 'unspecific nouns', 'low content nouns' and 'advance labels'. As Flowerdew and Forest (2015: 9) suggest, these terms 'are all attempts to characterise the same word class'.

2 This is an example of the count noun and the mass noun sharing a function. As I suggested in the last chapter, and as we will see later in this one, the mass noun has various other functions which the count noun does not have.

3 To be clear: count noun 'hope' always takes an object. Mass noun 'hope' *can* take an object, but (as the rest of this chapter explains) doesn't always.

4 We've been here before, of course, in Chapters 4 and 5. What I am here calling 'hope with ellipsis' is another form of anaphoric, cataphoric or exophoric reference.

5 The domain noun use of 'hope' is consistent with the view that there is no distinction to be made between linguistic knowledge and non-linguistic knowledge (Peeters 2000). See Chapter 4, Note 4. In this case, the use of 'hope' is explicitly encyclopaedic. It can be described only by listing examples of 'general knowledge about hope'. An audience

encountering this use draws on background knowledge of hope-related situations. In a comparable but more restricted way, an audience encountering a statement of the form 'A hopes that X' draws on its background knowledge of what can standardly be inferred from this type of sentence, and makes an inference of that kind. This is why the basic schema is a schema of inference, not a definition – even though, in this restricted range of cases ('A hopes that X'), it approximates to one.

6 Nobody thinks that hope is some kind of independent object, just hanging in the ether. So if it's an object or a quasi-object, it must be *inside* the person. The metaphysical problems referred to in the text concern this kind of object: something which is a force, a power, a virtue, a mechanism... or one of the many other characterisations. From my point of view, as will be clear from Part I of this book, once you have got to this point you're already in a cul-de-sac. 'Nouns are names of objects; so "hope" must be the name of an (intra-personal) object; so the project is to determine what sort of object it is'. I would argue that 'hope' is not the name of any sort of object or quasi-object; so there are no difficult questions to be answered about what sort of object it is.

7 In conversations, I have sometimes been told that this reference to a 'life force' (for example) is just a metaphor. This is okay, as long as you're prepared to explain what makes it an appropriate metaphor. If I use the metaphor 'blanket of snow', I can explain why 'blanket' works as a metaphorical description of certain kinds of snowy landscape. So the question is whether you can explain why 'life force' works as a metaphorical description of hope. If you do offer an explanation, we can then have a debate about how far it is a persuasive one. Sometimes, though, people want to say 'it's just a metaphor', and leave it at that. When this happens, the phrase is a dodge, a get-out-of-jail-free card. It's being used as a licence to say whatever takes your fancy. More on this theme in Sections 11.4 and 11.6.

8 To use Matthews' (2007) phrase, this is the assumption that the metaphysics can be 'read off' from the syntax. See my preamble to Chapter 3.

9 That there is a degree of arbitrariness in the distinction been mass nouns and plural count nouns is suggested by cross-linguistic considerations. For example, 'hair' in English can (as a count noun) refer to individuals hairs; but it can also be a mass noun (referring to the hair on someone's head). In Italian, the mass noun use of 'hair' would be translated by a plural: 'capelli'. Similarly, 'cutlery' would have, as its Italian equivalent, the plural 'posate'.

10 It should be emphasised that I'm not claiming that the domain noun version of 'hope' is equivalent to a plural. It obviously isn't. This is another illustration of the fact that 'hope' in all its forms – count noun, mass noun, verb – has more than one function.

11 Both versions of this proverb occur in English: 'hope dies last' and 'hopes die last'.

References

Chierchia, G. (1998). Plurality of mass nouns and the notion of "semantic parameter". In S. Rothstein (Ed.), *Events and Grammar* (pp. 53–103). Dordrecht: Kluwer.

Dufault, K., & Martocchio, B. C. (1985). Hope: its spheres and dimensions. *Nursing Clinics of North America, 20*(2), 379–391.

Flowerdew, J., & Forest, R. W. (2015). *Signalling Nouns in English: A Corpus-Based Discourse Approach*. Cambridge, UK: Cambridge University Press.

Folkman, S. (2010). Stress, coping, and hope. *Psycho-Oncology, 19*, 901–908.

Gillon, B. (1992). Towards a common semantics for English count and mass nouns. *Linguistics and Philosophy, 15*, 597–640.

Herth, K. (1990). Fostering hope in terminally ill people. *Journal of Advanced Nursing, 15*, 1250–1259.

Lazarus, R. S. (1999). Hope: an emotion and a vital coping resource. *Social Research*, *66*(2), 653–678.

Lebacqz, K. (1985). The virtuous patient. In E. E. Shelp (Ed.), *Virtue and Medicine* (pp. 275–288). Berlin: Springer.

Matthews, R. J. (2007). *The Measure of Mind: Propositional Attitudes and Their Attribution*. New York: Oxford University Press.

Morris, J. (2015). *Behind the Smile: A Story of Carol Moseley Braun's Historic Senate Campaign*. Chicago, IL: Agate Midway.

Moïsi, D. (2008). The land of hope again? An old dream for a new America. *Foreign Affairs*, *87*(5), 140–146.

Peeters, B. (2000). Setting the scene: Some recent milestones in the lexicon-encyclopedia debate. In B. Peeters (Ed.), *The Lexicon-Encyclopedia Interface* (pp. 1–52). Oxford: Elsevier.

Rawlinson, K. (2018). Matthew Hedges says UAE asked him to spy on Britain. *The Guardian*, 05 December 2018. https://www.theguardian.com/world/2018/dec/2005/matthew-hedges-says-uae-asked-him-to-spy-on-britain.

Schmid, H.-J. (2000). *English Abstract Nouns as Conceptual Shells*. The Hague: Mouton de Gruyter.

Torres, B. (2016). 'Behind the Smile': The rise and fall of Carol Moseley Braun. *The Seattle Times*, 7th February 2016.

Velleman, J. D. (2003). Narrative explanation. *Philosophical Review*, *112*, 1–25.

Zamparelli, R. (2019). *Countability Shifts and Abstract Nouns*. Department of Psychology and Cognitive Science, University of Trento.

10 'Hope'

Negations, modals and modifiers

As I suggested in Chapter 8, philosophical analyses of hope focus on sentences of the form 'A hopes that X' or 'A hopes for X', even if they begin with the question 'What is hope?' (Kwong 2019). Sentences of this kind are positive, indicative, simple present, third-person uses of the verb. This is a highly restricted range. We have already seen, in Chapter 8, that the present continuous tense has a different nuance from the simple present, and that first-person uses are not identical to third-person uses. In the last chapter, we saw that the mass noun has functions which differ from both verb and count noun. In this chapter, I will present further variations – negation, interrogatives, impersonal constructions, the use of ancillary modal verbs, together with adjectival and adverbial modifiers – and argue that by limiting their attention to 'A hopes that X', many authors have overlooked important aspects of what the word 'hope' is employed to do.[1]

In contrast to philosophers, many writers in health care and psychology attempt to define 'hope' in the absence of any grammatical construction. In doing so, they are inevitably focusing on the mass noun, and their definitions begin with 'Hope is a...', which places the noun in the subject position. Equally inevitably, in presenting their definitions, they take themselves to be describing an intra-personal object, state, process or power. 'Hope' is a noun; so it names an object of some kind; so the task is to determine what kind of object it is, and to identify its properties. In the next chapter, we will see how this project unfolds. Here, I simply want to make the point that this approach, like that of the philosophers, focuses on an extremely restricted range of 'hope' uses. Where the philosophers examine only the verb, and limit their interest in *that* to positive, indicative, simple present, third-person uses, health care writers are more interested in the mass noun. This chapter will help to loosen things up a bit.

I will begin with negations of 'hope'. These have many variations. For example:

(1)   She did not hope for much success.
(2)   Texas cannot hope to remain competitive.
(3)   Believe me, I'm not hoping for anything right away.
(4)   Don't get your hopes up.
(5)   We have no hope of winning.
(6)   There's not a hope in hell that he'll be quiet.

(7)   They are hired at low pay, without hope of tenure.
(8)   He was left with a sense of hopelessness.

Three of these involve the verb; of the others, two involve the mass noun, two involve the count noun and one involves 'hopelessness', also used as a mass noun. In the first half of the chapter, I will take a closer look at statements like these, and suggest that 'negations of hope' have several different functions (though all of them can be indexed to the basic schema).

I will start with sentences involving '…no hope…'. There are several different syntactic constructions which include this pairing. The two which occur the most frequently are 'there is no hope' and 'A has no hope'. Less frequently, we find 'A sees no hope' and 'X offers no hope'.

10.1   There is no hope

Examples of 'there is no hope' from COCA:

(9)   There is no hope of a return for Carrasco.
(10)   There is no hope for Senator Clinton to win over the Conservative vote.
(11)   If we stick with the American way of doing things, there is no hope for America.
(12)   With the hiring freeze, there is no hope of hiring a trained toxicologist.
(13)   There is no hope of making a perpetual motion machine.
(14)   You may have to fight when there is no hope of victory.

What precisely is being negated in these examples? Consider sentence (14) with reference to the basic schema. Is it element [a] that is being denied? Is it being suggested that 'you' do not *want* victory? In (12), does the speaker not *wish* to hire a trained toxicologist? In (10), is it being implied that Senator Clinton would not *like* to win over the Conservative vote? In all cases, the answer is presumably 'no'. What is being revoked here is element [b]. In each example, the speaker is denying that the desired outcome is possible. The negating emphasis, as it were, is on the *probability* not the *wanting*.

This emphasis is so marked that, in five of the examples, 'hope' could almost be replaced by 'chance',[2] 'possibility' or 'prospect'. 'You may have to fight when there is no chance of victory'; 'With the hiring freeze, there is no prospect of hiring a trained toxicologist'. (In some cases, a slight adjustment in syntax might be more idiomatic: 'There is no chance of Senator Clinton winning over the Conservative vote'.)

I say 'almost' because there is, of course, a subtle nuance. Although it is element [b] that is being denied, not element [a], the use of 'hope' does imply that the outcome is something to be desired, even if it is not regarded as possible. Obviously, 'you' would *prefer* victory, the speaker *wants* to hire a toxicologist and Senator Clinton *would like* to win over the Conservative vote. This is not implied – to the same extent – by the use of 'chance' (although there is probably a default assumption that people want victory, that the hiring of a toxicologist is desirable and that politicians want to win over voters).

We can dramatise this point by comparing three possible claims:

(15)   There is no hope of X happening.
(16)   There is no danger of X happening.
(17)   There is no chance of X happening.

The explicit claim being made in each of these is that the likelihood of X happening is zero. There is no possibility that X will happen. The difference is what is implied in each case. In (15), it is implied that X would be a good thing. In (16), it is implied that it would be a bad thing. In (17), the matter is left open.

In summary, then, the function of the THERE IS NO HOPE OF construction appears to be: to revoke element [b] of the basic schema, while letting it be inferred that element [a] remains true. What is being denied is the possibility of the outcome, not its desirability.

The question arises, though, as to *whose* belief the revocation of [b] involves. In the basic schema, [a] A would like X as an outcome, and [b] A believes that X is possible. But in a THERE IS NO HOPE sentence, there is no A; that is, there is no subject of the sentence.[3] In (13), for example, there is no reference to anyone who might be doing the hoping, or who might believe that perpetual motion is possible (or not). So the answer to the 'Who is doing the negating?' question can only be: the speaker/writer. In (13), it's the speaker who believes that a perpetual motion machine is impossible. It's the speaker who is revoking the [b] element of the basic schema.

How about (9), though? Who is denying that there is any chance/hope of Carrasco's return? Might it be Carrasco himself? I don't think so. 'There is no hope of a return for Carrasco' is quite compatible with: '... even if Carrasco thinks there is'. In other words, Carrasco himself might still be asserting [b]; but, in a THERE IS NO HOPE sentence, it is the speaker's revocation of [b] which counts. Similarly with (10). It is the speaker who thinks that Senator Clinton has no chance of winning over the Conservative vote; and this is independent of whatever Senator Clinton herself thinks. The same is true of all the examples (9) to (13). The odd one out is (14), in which there is a slight ambiguity, given that the speaker might mean: 'You may have to fight when, in your view, there is no hope of victory'.

So there is an interesting switch here. With positive sentences of the form 'A hopes for X', we can infer something about the *grammatical subject* of the sentence: '*A* believes that X is possible'. However, with sentences of the form 'there is no hope of X', we can infer something about the *speaker*: it is the speaker who believes X is not possible. Belief about the likelihood of X is attributed to the grammatical subject in 'A hopes for X'; but, in 'there is no hope of X', it is the speaker's belief. This is why I said earlier that focusing on positive sentences, in which 'hope' is a verb, leads to authors missing aspects of how 'hope' is used. In particular, they overlook its function when it appears as a noun in negative sentences.

10.2 She has no hope

We can now turn to 'she has no hope' and its variations:

(18)   She has no hope of getting them on the stand.
(19)   Many people living in our inner cities have no hope.
(20)   We have no hope of finding work.
(21)   At this range, he had no hope of surviving.
(22)   When I was sick, I had no hope. I had no inspiration.
(23)   A system that most scientists say has no hope of working.
(24)   Jim has no hope of raising the money.

The construction HAVE NO HOPE is a little less clear-cut than THERE IS NO HOPE. But there are obvious parallels. In five of these examples – the exceptions are (19) and (22) – it is again possible to substitute 'chance' for 'hope' and leave the core sense intact. This is especially true in (23), where the reference (in a 1995 news item) is to the Star Wars missile defence system. In this case, it is not even clear that the scientists in question would regard this system – if it did work – as a good thing. In the other three cases, the use of 'hope' rather than 'chance' implies that the outcome would certainly be welcome; it's just that there is no prospect of it occurring. Surviving, finding work and 'getting them on the stand' are all things one would want to happen in principle; but, as with the THERE IS NO HOPE construction, what is asserted is the zero likelihood of the outcome. The in-principle desirability of that outcome is implicit in the choice of 'hope' as the appropriate term.

Another parallel is that sentences like this are perfectly consistent:

(18$^+$) She has no hope of getting them on the stand, even though she thinks she has.
(24$^+$) Jim has no hope of raising the money, even though he thinks he has.

These are both comparable to: 'there is no hope of a return for Carrasco, even if Carrasco thinks there is'. From that point of view, there is little to choose between 'she has no hope' and 'there is no hope'. In both cases, the evaluation of likelihood switches from the person referred to *in* the sentence to the person who is the *speaker of* the sentence.

In the first instance, then, HAVE NO HOPE, like THERE IS NO HOPE, appears to be revoking element [b] of the basic schema, with the revocation being performed by the speaker.

However, there is a difference between the two 'no hope' constructions. THERE IS NO HOPE is an impersonal form, and makes no direct reference to any individual's state of mind. HAS NO HOPE appears to refer to someone's ('she') state of mind; and it appears to assert that this state of mind does not include hope. There are some exceptions. For example in (23) it is the 'system' that 'has no hope of working'; and the system does not have a state of mind. This is why, in (23), 'hope' is almost synonymous with 'chance'.

Still, suppose that someone insists on the literalness of 'Jim has' in (24), and suggests that something is being said about what Jim wants or believes. Since it is highly unlikely that Jim has no *desire* to raise the money ('A wants X as an outcome' remains true), this suggestion implies that it is Jim, not the speaker, who believes that he has no chance of raising it. On this view, then, sentences like (24) ascribe a belief about the impossibility of X to the grammatical subject.

To my mind, this is a bit of a stretch. For one thing, as I've already noted, the statement 'Jim has no hope of raising the money, even though he thinks he has' is perfectly consistent. For another, there is a form of words that is more plausibly regarded as referring to Jim's state of mind. Ironically, this involves the use of the plural:

(25)   Jim has no hopes of raising the money.

Idiomatically, I think this does imply the ascription of a belief to Jim. It suggests more than 'Jim has no hope of raising the money', and the substitution of 'chances' for 'hopes' does not work. It is surprising, perhaps, that the plural of 'hope' (in a negation sentence) can refer to the subject's state of mind, even when the singular 'hope' does not. But that is how it seems to be. Compare:

(26)   She has no hopes of singing with the angels.
(27)   He had no hopes of obtaining a commission.

The implication here is that 'She' and 'He' both recognise that their preferred outcome is not possible; so saying that they have 'no hopes' can be legitimately taken as a reference to their states of mind, and specifically the absence of hope. By default, I think it is also implied that the speaker agrees with their assessment: the outcome *isn't* possible. On the other hand, in an interesting reversal, these two sentences are both consistent:

(28)   She has no hopes of singing with the angels... but she will!
(29)   He had no hopes of obtaining a commission, even though his chances were good.

In these examples, the speaker clearly disagrees with the subject's assessment. So perhaps we can say that the use of the plural introduces an ambiguity. A belief is ascribed to the grammatical subject, but it is unclear what the speaker's view is. The default assumption might be that the speaker agrees with the assessment; but it is also possible for the speaker to 'correct' the subject, and suggest that her/his belief is wrong. Either way, 'She has no hopes of...' is different from 'She has no hope of...' The latter is, I would argue, the equivalent of 'There is no hope of...' In effect, it is a syntactic variation.

Of course, I can't prove it. Like most of the claims in this book, there are no conclusive arguments to be had. The only available strategy is to examine various constructions, provide objects of comparison and study the ways in which one use of 'hope' differs from another.

10.3 Cannot hope

I originally assumed that I'd have a section on DOES NOT HOPE, but I was sty-
mied by the discovery that there is not a single instance of 'does not hope' in
COCA.[4] There are numerous occurrences of '...not hope...', but nearly 75% of
them involve modal auxiliary verbs: 'cannot hope' and 'could not hope'. In this
section, therefore, I will consider 'cannot hope' and 'could hope'. (So we are
now returning to 'hope' as a verb, after Sections 10.1 and 10.2, both of which
concerned the noun.)

Modal verbs include verbs such as 'can', 'could', 'may', 'might', 'must',
'shall', 'should' and 'would'. They refer to questions of likelihood, possibility,
permission, capacity, obligation and so on. They are morphologically unusual in
that they do not have an infinitive form ('to must'?), and they are not inflected ('I
should, you should, she should': not 'she shoulds').[5]

Some 'cannot hope' examples:

(30)   If they play like this, the Panthers cannot hope to win anything.
(31)   Falling fertility rates mean that our culture cannot hope to sustain itself.
(32)   The position paper cannot hope to answer all the specifics.
(33)   Hillary cannot hope to be so lucky.
(34)   We cannot hope to rely on Morgase: she is in Caemlyn.
(35)   China cannot hope to match total OECD military expenditures any time
       soon.

Two things are striking about these examples (and most of the occurrences in
COCA). First, it is almost always 'cannot hope *to*', very rarely 'cannot hope
that' or 'cannot hope for'. Second, the grammatical subject of these sentences
is normally a collective, a group, an abstraction or a general reference to 'we',
or 'you' (in the sense of 'one'). In this respect, (33) is rather unusual. It is one
of only a handful of examples in which the subject is an individual person. The
other subjects in (30) to (35) are: a football team, a culture, a document, 'we' and
a nation state.

(32) is interesting for different reasons. A position paper doesn't have states
of mind, so this example can only be saying that it is impossible for the paper to
address every issue. Once again, then, we have a preliminary indication that the
main function of 'not hope' sentences is to revoke [b] in the basic schema. There
is no hope – it is just not possible – that the position paper can answer all the
specifics. Roughly the same can be said of (31). 'Our culture' is not an inanimate
object like the position paper, but it does not include any direct reference to people, whether individually or as a group. It is equivalent to 'Falling fertility rates
mean that there is no chance/prospect/likelihood of our culture sustaining itself'.
As with previous examples, the use of 'hope' implies that it would be better if the
culture *could* sustain itself. But the function of the sentence is to claim that the
likelihood of its doing so is zero.

The remaining sentences are of a similar kind. In each case, it is claimed that
the likelihood of a certain outcome is zero, while the use of 'hope' implies that

this outcome would, in principle, be the preferred one. In two cases – (31) and (32) – the preference is that of the speaker. In (35) it is attributed to the grammatical subject: the Chinese may wish to match total OECD expenditure, but the speaker does not necessarily share this preference. In (30) the outcome is presumably desired by the Panthers; however, the speaker may (or may not) have the same desire. In (33), the in-principle preference is attributed to Hillary, but (again) may or may not be shared by the speaker. In (34), the preferred possibility – relying on Morgase – is presumably that of the 'we' group; but it is unclear whether the speaker herself shares it.

'Could not hope' sentences are comparable to 'cannot hope', but in the past tense:

(36)   She was told she could not hope to beat Heseltine in the second ballot.
(37)   The review could not hope to be exhaustive.
(38)   These were forces he could not hope to control.
(39)   The army could not hope to progress more than a few miles before dusk.
(40)   Britain and France could not hope to beat Germany without Russia.

Collective and abstract subjects are common again, as in (37), (39) and (40); however, the proportion of personal subjects, as with (36) and (38), is higher here. As before, 'hope' alludes to what would be the desired outcome; but what is asserted is that there is no chance of that outcome being attained.

10.4 Without hope

'Hope' appears in this construction as a mass noun, sometimes with ellipsis and sometimes with a fully specified object. In these examples, (41) and (42) are elliptical, while (43) and (44) identify the *specific* hope which the people concerned are 'without'.

(41)   New Orleans is a city without hope.
(42)   Without hope, the present becomes unbearable.
(43)   Life imprisonment without hope of parole is a just punishment.
(44)   They are hired at low pay without hope of tenure.

In (41) and (42) the elliptical gap is so great that 'hope' effectively becomes a domain noun, referring vaguely to a loose assortment of aspirations, possibilities and resources – or lack of them. In (43) and (44), one could substitute 'any prospect' (or even 'any chance') for 'hope' without compromising the sense. In both cases, the most salient feature of the basic schema is element [b]. It is the *possibility* of parole and tenure that is being denied. However, the use of 'hope', rather than 'prospect' or 'chance', signals the speaker's recognition that parole/ tenure would be welcomed by the prisoners/lecturing staff.

So even a construction like WITHOUT HOPE does not have just one function. The claims made in (43) and (44) are different from those made in (41) and (42). In the non-elliptical cases ('hope of...'), a statement about zero probability is being made. In the elliptical cases, what is lacking ('without') is not merely 'possibility' (in any case, the possible outcome is not specified). Rather, what is lacking is an ill-defined, non-itemised domain of possibilities, states of mind, decisions, beliefs, options, values, resources and so on. If the phrase 'without hope' can have two such markedly different uses, then the prospects of being able to define 'hope' (or hope) *tout court*, independently of context or construction, are negligible.

10.5 'Hopeless' and 'hopelessness'

Let's begin with 'hopeless', and the obvious point that this generally does *not* mean 'lacking hope'. It's true that it is sometimes used this way when the predicate 'is hopeless' is applied to people; but, almost always, 'he is hopeless' is a way of suggesting that he is incompetent – even if, like 'you're hopeless', it can be intended affectionately. This is not just a semantic oddity, since element [b] of the basic schema is lurking in the background. 'He's hopeless', when it is a synonym for 'he's incompetent' (relative to a certain context), tells us that the probability of his performing adequately (in that context) is, if not zero, then very low. It is close to: 'There's little hope of him succeeding at this'. It is, however, interestingly different from 'He's useless', which also ascribes incompetence, but does so in a more generalised and derogatory manner. 'He's useless' suggests that, for *all* tasks of this kind, he is incapable of performing adequately. It is dismissive. 'He's hopeless' *can* imply the same thing, but more often refers to a specific task, or a particular kind of task. It is more localised, and potentially less derogatory.

COCA suggests that it is not *people* who are usually described as hopeless, but situations, tasks, causes, cases and so on. This is true when 'hopeless' is a predicative adjective ('the situation is hopeless'), but more especially when it is an attributive adjective ('a hopeless situation'). For example:

(45)   Legally, he's in a hopeless position.
(46)   Getting rid of these insects is a hopeless task.
(47)   To him, the situation looked hopeless.
(48)   Trying to teach them science is a hopeless endeavour.

When 'hopeless' is an attributive adjective, the nouns it most frequently qualifies are: 'situation', 'case', 'romantic', 'task', 'cause'. Of these, only 'romantic' refers to a person; and 'a hopeless romantic' is *not* 'a romantic who lacks hope'. Rather, s/he is someone who has no chance of being anything other than romantic. So, once again, the revocation of element [b] is the key to understanding why an 'incurable romantic' can also be described as a 'hopeless romantic'.

As for the other nouns: expressions such as 'hopeless position', 'hopeless cause' and 'hopeless task' all refer to circumstances in which a desired outcome cannot be achieved. In (45) to (48), it is being claimed that there is zero probability of winning the court case, getting rid of the insects or teaching science. The negation of 'hope' implied by the suffix '-less' (just like the other negations we have considered) is a revocation of element [b] in the basic schema.

10.5.1 'Hopelessness'

Turning from the adjective to the noun, we should note first that the uses of 'hopelessness' range along a spectrum from non-elliptical to elliptical, just as with 'hope' (Sections 9.2 and 9.3). Some examples of the non-elliptical end of the spectrum:

(49) Churchill laments the hopelessness of this assault on the enemy.
(50) We must acknowledge the hopelessness of eradicating sin.
(51) I learned the hopelessness of hunting eland in their own country.
(52) He talked about the hopelessness of a long-distance relationship.

Each of these examples specifies the situation, task, cause or project which is regarded as hopeless, in the sense described in the last section: the *impossibility* of achieving the outcome (a successful assault, the eradication of sin, hunting eland, a settled long-distance relationship). In all cases, element [b] of the basic schema is revoked, whether by the speaker or by the subject of the sentence.

In the middle of the spectrum are anaphoric uses, in which a term such as 'situation', 'predicament' or 'task' is used anaphorically to refer to a set of circumstances previously described in the text:

(53) We're the first to admit the hopelessness of the task.
(54) The true hopelessness of my sister's situation dawned on me.
(55) Billy saw the hopelessness of his predicament.
(56) He refused to concede the hopelessness of his cause.

In each case, the specific task, situation, cause or predicament can be retrieved from earlier in the text.

By way of contrast, maximum ellipsis – the far end of the spectrum – turns 'hopelessness' into a domain noun, just as it does with 'hope'. At this point, too, 'hopelessness' is unambiguously a mass noun, not a count noun. In these examples, the definite article disappears.

(57) I can see hopelessness in your father's eyes.
(58) She sensed hopelessness behind his frightened face.
(59) Hopelessness threatened to overwhelm him.
(60) I had such a feeling of hopelessness.

These examples go beyond (49) to (56) in an interesting way. In the earlier examples, hopelessness is attributed to a *set of circumstances*. It is the hopelessness of the task, the cause, the situation – or, less elliptically, an assault on the enemy or the eradication of sin. In (57) to (60), however, hopelessness is attributed to a

person. It has become something that can be seen in someone's eyes, or someone's face. The individual concerned can experience feelings of hopelessness,
or hopelessness can overwhelm him. Why does this transition from situation to
person come about?

There are two possibilities. The first is that the outcome referred to in element
[a] of the basic schema has a pronounced significance for the person concerned.
For example, comments such as (57) to (60) would be, at the very least, exaggerated (possibly for comic effect) in a situation where the individual concerned was
contemplating an inevitable loss in a game of tiddly winks. In matters of life and
death, on the other hand, or in situations where the individual cannot escape some
terrible predicament, they would not be. In such cases, 'hopelessness' is used to
refer (vaguely) to the emotions occasioned by an unavoidably appalling outcome.
Hence, 'the sense of hopelessness', 'feelings of hopelessness' or just (as an example of metonymy) 'hopelessness'.

The second possibility involves an outcome generalisation of the kind described
in Section 9.3. In (49) to (56), 'hopelessness' applies to particular situations –
one-offs, as it were – and implies a revocation of element [b] with respect to the
situation concerned. An outcome generalisation, however, suggests that not just
one situation, task or cause is hopeless, but many (and, it might seem, all). When
every desirable outcome appears impossible, 'hopelessness' can be used to refer
(vaguely) to this state *as a whole*,and to the emotions precipitated by it. This is an
alternative reading of examples (57) to (60).

Notice that, as with outcome generalisation in the case of 'hope', the outcome
generalisation implied by this use of 'hopelessness' includes outcomes which the
individual cannot anticipate, or has not thought of yet. Whereas 'hope' used with
an outcome generalisation stands, roughly, for *good things seeming possible in
general*, 'hopelessness' used in the same way refers to *nothing good seeming
possible at all*.

Hopelessness of this generalised kind may be associated with one type of clinical depression, described as 'hopelessness depression' by Abramson et al. (1989:
359).[6] These authors suggest that:

> A proximal sufficient cause of the symptoms of hopelessness depression is
> an expectation that highly desired outcomes will not occur or that highly
> aversive outcomes will occur coupled with an expectation that no response in
> one's repertoire will change the likelihood of occurrence of these outcomes
> … We use the phrase *generalized hopelessness* when people exhibit the neg-
> ative-outcome/helplessness expectancy about many areas of life. In contrast,
> *circumscribed pessimism* occurs when people exhibit the negative-outcome/
> helplessness expectancy about only a limited domain (emphasis in original).

It should be noted that Abramson et al. are here offering a causal account of *one
form* of depression, not proposing hopelessness as a cause, predictor or symptom
of depression *in general*. However, it is not definitively established that 'generalised hopelessness' inevitably leads to this form of depression; and the 'outcome

generalisation' reading of (57) to (60) does not *require* the inference that the individuals concerned are depressed.[7] It is hardly in dispute that hopelessness of an extreme, generalised kind can dispose to at least one type of clinical depression; but we should not imagine that the two are always or necessarily associated.

'Hopelessness' can, like 'hope', imply a context generalisation as well as an outcome generalisation. In this usage, the word extends beyond outcomes, and lassoes together the conditions and consequences of hopeless situations conceived as pervasive. These conditions and consequences might include the failure of ideals, aspirations, projects and plans; the culture to which this wholesale failure may give rise; and the various psychological states associated with it: pessimism, lack of motivation, addiction, rejection of relationships and community. Again, these disparate elements are referred to only in a broad gesture, and none of them are identified or described.

(61) The themes of homelessness, hopelessness, lack of work, lack of education.
(62) Hopelessness and lack of opportunity breeds this type of desperation.
(63) She had escaped a life of poverty, abuse and hopelessness.
(64) The hopelessness of the poor, the marginalisation of the oppressed.

In these examples, the combination of outcome and context generalisation is associated with a shift of emphasis from the psychological to the sociological. 'Hopelessness' as a domain noun has become the mirror image of 'hope' as a domain noun. Unlike 'hope', however, 'hopelessness' the domain noun typically appears in lists, as in (61) to (64). It is as if 'hope' is a symbol of inspiration in its own right, whereas 'hopelessness' requires the support of other privations to achieve the desired rhetorical effect.

As with 'hope' – and largely for the same reasons – 'hopelessness' as a domain noun is not susceptible to definition. However, the fact that it is a noun, and therefore the 'name' of something, encourages the search for one, just as it encourages the devising of scales to measure it. It is hardly surprising, then, that attempts to formulate both scales and definitions can run into problems. For example, 'hopelessness' and 'pessimism' are often used interchangeably (Minkoff et al. 1973, Beck et al. 1974, Greene 1989);[8] while the Beck Hopelessness Scale has a history of analyses showing inconsistent factorial structures, as well as factors which are difficult/impossible to interpret (Steed 2001, Iliceto & Fino 2015), particularly with cancer patients (Spangenberg et al. 2016).

10.6 False hope

If element [b] of the basic schema is true, but the belief that X-is-possible is mistaken, or very probably mistaken, then we are inclined to speak of 'false hope'. Examples:

(65) Does the Clinton camp have a shot, or is it false hope?
(66) The afterlife is just another tale designed to offer false hope.
(67) It's better knowing than wondering: false hope's the worst kind there is.

(68)   We do not want to give our patients false hope.

In all these cases, 'false hope' is a reference to someone believing that a desirable outcome is possible when objectively it is not. For example, in (66) the belief that survival of death is possible is said to be false. In (68), health professionals refrain from encouraging patients to believe that recovery is possible when it isn't.

This appears straightforward enough, but there are some wrinkles, particularly in the context of health care. For example, who is to determine that X is *not* ('objectively') possible, and on what basis? How does this square with what was said, in Section 8.2.4, about the probability of X never being zero? Does the possibility of 'hoping against hope' (Martin 2014) suggest that 'false hope' is a misnomer? What importance should we give to the idea that, according to some authors, false beliefs can have beneficial consequences (Taylor 1989, Flanagan & Graham 2017)? One cannot deal satisfactorily with how 'hope' is used in health care without addressing these questions, and I'll return to them in Chapter 11.

10.7 Other 'there' constructions

In this section, I want to consider three constructions that are not negations, but which do not involve direct reference to any A, as in 'A hopes for X'. One is THERE IS HOPE, the apparent opposite of THERE IS NO HOPE. The second is the interrogative: IS THERE HOPE? The third is a variant: IS THERE ANY HOPE? The first of these is quite common in COCA, the second and third much less so. However, given that the questions 'Is there hope?' and 'Is there any hope?' are often mentioned in the health care literature, it's worth having a brief look.

Some examples of 'there is hope':

(69)   There is hope in the travel industry that these restrictions will be lifted.
(70)   There is hope of finding a cure for glaucoma, say scientists.
(71)   There is hope that war can be avoided.
(72)   But now there is hope for people with tinnitus.
(73)   There is hope beyond the grave because of Jesus Christ.
(74)   Maybe there is hope for us, Selar.
(75)   There is hope.

Most of these refer, vaguely, to groups: people in the travel industry, people with tinnitus and so on. No individuals are identified, and it is not implied that the 'hope' claim is true of *every* member of the group concerned. Rather, we can infer that, for *some* people in the relevant group, it *is* true: there are members of that group for whom 'A hopes that X' applies. For example, (69) can be read as: 'There are people in the travel industry who hope that the restrictions will be lifted'. The implication is that this hope is fairly widespread, if not universal. At any rate, given that (69) is a partial generalisation of 'A hopes that X', the basic schema will apply. For every case in which 'A hopes that X', [a] A would like the restrictions to be lifted, and [b] A believes there is a chance, perhaps a good chance, that they will be. The same kind of thing can be said about (70).

Other examples partially generalise 'A hopes that X' in the same way; but more of what is said depends on context, with either A or X (or both) not being specified. In (71), the group is not identified, but the hoped-for outcome (that war can be avoided) is. In (72), the group, people with tinnitus, is specified, but the outcome is not. In context, of course, it will be clear what the 'hope' consists of: the alleviation of symptoms, perhaps. In (73), the group is not specified, but by implication it is every human being; the outcome is only hinted at. In (74) the group is identified as 'us', but the outcome cannot be determined. In (75), neither group nor outcome is specified, although both may be clear in context.

Some examples of 'Is there hope?' and 'Is there any hope?'

(76)   Is there hope that North Carolina can turn President Obama's way?
(77)   Is there any hope that the world can really change for the better?
(78)   Is there any hope of this becoming a more customer-friendly service?
(79)   Is there hope for people who are HIV positive?
(80)   Is there any hope for me?
(81)   Is there any hope for me? Do I have comic talent?
(82)   Is there (any) hope?

With the interrogative, we have a similar pattern, *mutatis mutandis*. Sometimes both A (group) and X (outcome) are specified. Sometimes one or both are not. In (79), for example, A is identified, but X is context-dependent, though it is not difficult to imagine the kind of X the speaker has in mind. In (78), it is the other way round. In (80), the A is 'me', but X could be almost anything. In (81), the X is implied by the second sentence; so that 'Is there any hope for me?' is equivalent to something like: 'Is there any chance that I will make it as a stand-up comedian?' In examples (76) to (78), 'hope' can be replaced by 'chance', 'a chance', or 'prospect', leaving the desirability of the outcome implicit. In (82), everything is context-dependent. What is hoped for, and who is hoping, are left open. (This is another expression that turns up in the health care literature, and I will mention it again in Chapter 11.)

'Hope' in this interrogative construction makes no reference to a state of mind. If hope were an inner something – a power, a force, a mechanism, an emotion – then no-one would have any reason for asking whether they hoped that X, or hoped for Y. Presumably, it would be enough to introspect, to turn one's attention 'inwards', in order to detect the existence of this force, or determine whether the mechanism has been activated. In some cases, a speaker might want to ask herself whether she really does *want* the outcome concerned; and perhaps she will look 'inside' for an answer. But this possibility does not seem plausible in (76) to (82). In any case, if (77), say, is construed as 'Do I hope that the world can really change for the better?', it is not clear what the point is of asking it – unless it is a rhetorical gesture: 'Do I hope that the world can really change for the better? Yes, I certainly do!' In these interrogatives, then, as in negations, 'hope' is a way of referring to the *chance* that a positively valenced outcome will occur.

10.8 Other modal constructions

I want to return briefly to the modal expressions with 'hope', comparing positive assertions ('can hope', 'could hope') with negative assertions ('cannot hope', 'could not hope'), as discussed in Section 10.3. The constructions CAN HOPE and COULD HOPE are both common.

Examples of 'can hope':

(83)   A November return is the earliest he can hope for.
(84)   The best we can hope for now is the best of the worst outcomes.
(85)   The only thing we can hope for is to have a colour-blind government policy.
(86)   The chances of it happening are not great, but it may be all you can hope for.
(87)   One can hope that a future translation will find a happy medium.
(88)   Paul can hope to earn more in future than he does now.

The most frequent use of this expression is to identify a 'limit' outcome, as with (83) to (86): the best you can hope for, the earliest you can hope for, the only thing you can hope for and so on. Something like a preference/probability vector is involved here. Of all the outcomes you might want (in a certain context), this is either the most likely, or the only possible one (85, 86). Alternatively, of the outcomes that are possible, this is the best, or the earliest, or some other preference-superlative (83, 84).

These examples, then, represent an interesting difference, between the best-of-the-possible and the only-one-possible-of-the-desirable; that is, 'the best he can hope for' and 'the only thing he can hope for'. In both cases, however, 'hope' refers to the possibility element, [b], not the preference element, [a]:

Of the things you can hope for (= that are possible), this is the best.
Of the things you would like, this is the only one you can hope for (= only one possible).

This is another illustration of how different uses of the same word – including apparently identical uses ('can hope') – are capable of performing subtly different functions. In both (84) and (85), for example, 'hope' is used to identify what-is-possible; but, even so, the work the two sentences do is not exactly the same.

This is also true of (87) and (88). One might imagine that examples like this are simply the opposite of 'cannot hope'; and, in a sense, they are. But 'one can hope' isn't the same as 'one hopes'; and 'he can hope' is not the same as 'he hopes'. For example, (88) does not make the claim that, as a matter of fact, Paul *does* hope that he will earn more in future. He may not think it possible; he may not have thought about it. Still, if he *were* to hope that he would earn more in future than he does now, that hope would be warranted. The speaker, then, asserts [b] on Paul's behalf, hypothetically. A's belief that X is possible *would* be justified, even if A has not yet entertained the idea. So, in this kind of construction, 'can hope' signals that the speaker believes X is possible, and suggests that A is entitled to the same belief.

Examples of 'could hope':

(89) She has all the qualifications you could hope for.
(90) It was the best present I could hope for.
(91) He was as safe here as he could hope to be anywhere.
(92) Only a ground invasion could hope to accomplish that.
(93) It was something that other states in the region could hope to exploit.

The first four have 'limit' functions again. In (89), list *all* the qualifications you could hope for – that is, the ones you would like the candidate to have, and which are *possible* in the circumstances – and those qualifications, all of them, are the ones she's actually got. In (90), if I had listed all the *possible* presents (afford-able, available and so on) I might have received, the best of those was the one I did receive.

However, (93) is slightly different; it's like (88), but in the past tense. If (the leaders of) other states were hoping to exploit the situation, they would have been entitled to do so because, according to the speaker, exploiting the situation would have been possible. Once again, it is the possibility of the outcome that is asserted – hence justifying the hope – with the use of 'hope' also implying that this was an opportunity the other states would presumably have welcomed.

10.9 Degrees of hope

Finally in this chapter, I will turn to three other modifiers of 'hope'. One of them is related to 'no hope', and is akin to negation: 'little hope'. The other two are rough opposites of 'little hope', in the sense that they suggest greater possibility rather than less: 'a lot of hope' and 'real hope'. All three are modifiers which refer to what we might call the 'degree' of hope.[9]

'Little hope' functions in the same way as 'no hope': the only difference is that the speaker assesses the probability of the outcome as being very low rather than zero. As with 'no hope', the two most common syntactic environments are 'there is...' and 'has...':

(94) Most prisoners had little hope of ever getting out.
(95) There is little hope of the reforms being implemented.
(96) They faced an overpowering enemy with little hope of success.
(97) I have little hope that this case will be investigated properly.

'A lot of hope' is heavily dependent on the wider context, as the following exam-ples indicate:

(98) Following Trump's election, as a businessman I have a lot of hope.
(99) Blockchain technology offers a lot of hope.

(100) I have a lot of hope for Baltimore.
(101) There was a lot of hope for Bill Clinton.

In none of these cases is the object-of-hope specified, and one has to read the paragraph from which each example comes to understand, roughly, what is being said (this is another example of ellipsis). In (98), the businessman's hope concerns the prospect of deregulation. In (99), the hope is that blockchain will increase efficiency and reduce costs in the financial sector. With (100), the source is very unclear, but the comment appears to have something to do with employment conditions. (101) is not dissimilar, as it is unclear what specific type of hope the author is referring to. The sense is of a general hope that 'things will improve'. With (100) and (101), then, we have ellipsis again, but this time a more 'distant' form of it, as the immediate context does not identify any particular object.

In all four examples, 'a lot of hope' signals the speaker's belief that there is a relatively high probability that the desired outcome (whatever it is) will happen. It is, in this sense, the opposite of 'little hope', as one would expect.

Examples of 'real hope' (adjective + noun) and 'really hope' (adverb + verb):

(102) We really hope that people come and support us.
(103) I really hope that you'll come and work for us.
(104) There is real hope for a safe haven when Assad falls.
(105) It offered real hope to people suffering from type 2 diabetes.
(106) There was real hope for the future.

Like 'a lot of hope', 'real hope' is used to assert that the likelihood of the outcome is relatively high (its desirability is presupposed by the positive valence). The object of hope is specified in (104), but ellipsis occurs again in (105) and (106).

'Really hope' is nearly always used in the first person ('really hopes' is rare). This construction is very different from the others we have considered, since the 'really' does *not* refer to probability. These are not claims about the *likelihood* of a particular outcome. Rather, they are intensifiers of the 'wanting' element of the basic schema. They emphasise element [a], not element [b]. So, for example, (102) is the equivalent of 'We would really like people to come and support us'; and (103) is equivalent to 'I would really like you to come and work for us'. In these cases, it is *assumed* that the outcome is possible. What is *asserted*, in using 'hope', is that it is also desirable.

There is an interesting reversal here. In the 'real hope' examples, what is asserted is the relatively high probability that an outcome will occur; what is implied is that the outcome is desirable. In the 'really hope' sentences, in contrast, what is asserted concerns the strength of the desire for a given outcome; what is implied is that there is at least a possibility that this outcome will occur. That 'real hope' and 'really hope' should have these reverse functions is unexpected. It is confirmation of the fact that, in examining usage, we have to be careful about the details, and recognise that shifts in what is conveyed can occur even between constructions that look very similar.

10.10 Summary of Chapters 8–10

Before turning to the use of 'hope' in health care, I think it would be useful to provide a brief summary of the last three chapters.

The basic schema (Section 8.2) indicates what can generally be inferred from statements of the form 'A hopes that X'. According to the schema, 'hope' has an object, referring to a preferred outcome; and this object is what distinguishes one hope from another. However, 'hope' is an epistemic verb as well as a verb of attraction, its primary function in this respect being to report on assessments of probability. The present continuous is used when an activity is contingent on present circumstances, and there is a sense of imminence. In this construction, 'am/is hoping' may refer to activity designed to minimise the effects of the factors referred to in elements [c] and [d] of the basic schema. Alternatively, it may refer to forms of 'mental' activity if the person concerned has no control, rather than limited control, over the factors in question.

The basic schema and its variations apply to 'hope' when it acts as a verb or count noun. 'Hope' as a mass noun extends through a spectrum in which the object-of-hope is articulated with varying degrees of specificity. When 'hope' is used as a shell noun, the degree of specificity is high. Ellipsis occurs when specificity is low and, in the extreme case, 'hope' becomes a domain noun referring, vaguely, to 'good things seeming possible' without itemising or describing what is thereby referred to. In the subject position, 'hope' permits generalisation over instances of hope (though I haven't ruled out the possibility that it may also be used to describe the object, state, power or force which 'hope' names, or to introduce a definition).

Negations of 'hope' revoke element [b] of the basic schema, the belief that the preferred outcome is possible. In these constructions, 'hope' is frequently an alternative to 'chance', 'risk' or 'danger', an alternative which signals that the preferred outcome has a positive valence. In negations, interrogatives, modal constructions and 'there is hope' sentences, the most salient element of the schema is [b], given that these constructions all make claims about probability. They acknowledge the positive valence of the outcome, but they make no reference to anyone's state of mind. An exception is 'hopelessness', but even then only certain uses of it (those which refer to a state in which nothing good seems possible).

Notes

1 There are, of course, some exceptions. For example, van Hooft (2014: 11) mentions the construction 'He doesn't have a hope'. However, he gives it only a few lines because there is a 'meaning we are more interested in'.

2 The exception, of course, is: 'If we stick with the American way of doing things, there is no hope for America'. (Even here, the substitution of 'chance' would still be intelligible, and would approximate to the sense of the original.) The question is whether 'hope' in 'there is no hope for America' has the function of a domain noun or whether, in context, it is exploiting ellipsis. If the latter, the next question would be: 'Specifically, hope of/for what?'

3 Grammatically, 'There' (in sentences beginning 'There is…') *can* be classified as the 'subject' of the sentence; but its role is that of a 'dummy'. Its function is to satisfy English's structural requirement for an initial subject in indicative sentences. See (Quirk et al. 1985: 1402–6).

4 There are, however, four cases of '…did not hope…' It is interesting, and unexpected, that there are virtually no examples of this construction, and the few that do exist are in the past tense.

5 For more technical detail on modal auxiliaries, in the context of corpus linguistics, see Coates (1983). Chapter 5 deals with 'can' and 'could'. Coates also analyses the effects of negation for different types of modal.

6 The Abramson et al. paper has well over 4,000 citations, so has decent claims to being a landmark work. The hopelessness theory of depression retains its currency, with recent reviews (Liu et al. 2015) and research activity (Giollabhui et al. 2018).

7 What does appear to be established, though, is that hopelessness is a predictor of suicidal ideation, independently of any association with depression. Indeed, it predicts suicide better than a summed score from an inventory assessing multiple depressive symptoms. See the review by Fried and Nesse (2015). This again suggests that, if hopelessness *is* associated with depression, it is a very specific form of the latter; and that it is ill-advised to regard hopelessness as a 'symptom' of depression-in-a-global-sense.

8 'Negative expectancies' is another expression that is taken to be synonymous with 'hopelessness'. But these, and 'pessimism', are distinct. I have negative expectancies about my ability to play the flute, but 'hopelessness' doesn't come into it. Similarly, I'm pessimistic about my team's chances of winning the FA Cup; but to talk of hopelessness in this context is ridiculous. There is a widespread assumption that 'hope' and 'hopelessness' are 'opposites'. At best, this is a massive over-simplification.

9 I will discuss the question of how degrees of hope can be measured in Section 11.5.

References

Abramson, L. Y., Metalsky, G. I., & Alloy, L. B. (1989). Hopelessness depression: A theory-based subtype of depression. *Psychological Review*, *96*(2), 358–372.

Beck, A. T., Weissman, A., Lester, D., & Trexler, L. (1974). The measurement of pessimism: The Hopelessness Scale. *Journal of Consulting and Clinical Psychology*, *42*, 861–865.

Coates, J. (1983). *The Semantics of the Modal Auxiliaries*. Abingdon, UK: Routledge.

Flanagan, O., & Graham, G. (2017). Truth and sanity: Positive illusions, spiritual delusions, and metaphysical hallucinations. In J. Poland & S. Tekin (Eds.), *Extraordinary Science and Psychiatry: Responses to the Crisis in Mental Health Research* (pp. 293–314). Cambridge, MA: MIT Press.

Fried, E. I., & Nesse, R. M. (2015). Depression sum-scores don't add up: Why analyzing specific depression symptoms is essential. *BMC Medicine*, *13*(72), 1–11.

Giollabhui, N., Hamilton, J. L., Nielsen, J., Connolly, S. L., Stange, J. P., Varga, S., … Alloy, L. B. (2018). Negative cognitive style interacts with negative life events to predict first onset of a major depressive episode in adolescence via hopelessness. *Journal of Abnormal Psychology*, *127*(1), 1–11.

Greene, S. M. (1989). The relationship between depression and hopelessness: Implications for current theories of depression. *British Journal of Psychiatry*, *154*, 650–659.

Iliceto, P., & Fino, E. (2015). Beck Hopelessness Scale (BHS): a second-order confirmatory factor analysis. *European Journal of Psychological Assessment*, *31*(1), 31–37.

Kwong, J. M. C. (2019). What is hope? *European Journal of Philosophy*, *27*(1), 243–254.

Liu, R. T., Kleiman, E. M., Nestor, B. A., & Cheek, S. M. (2015). The hopelessness theory of depression: A quarter century review. *Clinical Psychology, 22*(4), 345–365.

Martin, A. M. (2014). *How We Hope: A Moral Psychology*. Princeton, NJ: Princeton University Press.

Minkoff, K., Bergman, E., Beck, A. T., & Beck, R. (1973). Hopelessness, depression, and attempted suicide. *American Journal of Psychiatry, 130*(4), 455–459.

Quirk, R., Greenbaum, S., Leech, G., & Svartvik, J. (1985). *A Comprehensive Grammar of the English Language*. London: Longman.

Spangenberg, L., Zenger, M., Garcia-Torres, F., Mueller, V., Reck, M., Mehnert, A., & Vehling, S. (2016). Dimensionality, stability, and validity of the Beck Hopelessness Scale in cancer patients receiving curative and palliative treament. *Journal of Pain and Symptom Management, 51*(3), 615–622.

Steed, L. (2001). Further validity and reliability evidence for Beck Hopelessness Scale scores in a nonclinical sample. *Educational and Psychological Measurement, 61*(2), 303–316.

Taylor, S. E. (1989). *Positive Illusions: Creative Self-Deception and the Healthy Mind*. New York: Basic Books.

van Hooft, S. (2014). *Hope*. Abingdon, UK: Routledge.

11 'Hope' in health care

In the last three chapters I've explored the variegated usage pattern of 'hope' as a verb, count noun and mass noun, drawing attention to the wide range of functions the word has, and linking these functions to the different constructions it appears in. At the outset, I suggested that, by focusing narrowly on 'hope' as a mass noun, the academic literature in nursing (but also in psychology) has overlooked a significant portion of this pattern. In this chapter, I will provide some evidence for this claim, taking a more detailed look at discussions of hope in nursing and, to a lesser extent, in psychology and philosophy.

First, however, I will give a very brief summary of where the chapter is going, and head off one possible misunderstanding.

11.1 The appropriation of 'hope'

As the last three chapters show, 'hope' has an extensive range of uses, dependent on the constructions and contexts it occurs in. The word performs different tasks in these different constructions. Sometimes it refers to an inner state of the person; often it doesn't. Sometimes it expresses the speaker's preference; at other times not. Sometimes it indexes the speaker/writer's assessment of the probability of a particular outcome, making no reference to anybody's state of mind; but there are also exceptions. And so on. I have pictured 'the concept of hope' as a loose, highly permeable boundary round these variegated uses. That expression refers to them (vaguely) without identifying or describing any of them.

There are two important aspects of what nursing (and health care generally) has done in its discussions of hope. First, it has overlooked many – in fact most – of these uses. Second, it has appropriated the word 'hope' for new tasks, and one kind of task in particular. In health care, 'hope' has functions it does not have in ordinary usage. In some instances, ordinary usage effectively disallows or repudiates these new functions.

The soundbite version of the previous paragraph is: 'hope' in health care does not always 'mean' what it 'means' in other contexts. This does not, however, imply that its use in health care is wrong. This is the possible misunderstanding I referred to above: I am *not* saying that because health care usage is at odds with established use it is therefore somehow mistaken.[1] It is a familiar thing for technical disciplines to appropriate familiar words, ignore many of their ordinary uses, and give them new functions. In physics, 'work' and 'force' are technical terms, only distantly related to how they are used in ordinary discourse. The same can be said of 'bit' and 'bug' in computer science, or 'cell', 'reaction' and 'limb' in biology, chemistry and astronomy, respectively. In a similar way, 'hope' is (often) a technical term in health care.

There is no problem, then, about familiar terms being appropriated for new tasks. However, there might be a problem if you create a technical term without realising that this is what you've done. That, I think, is often the situation in nursing. Many of the writers who have helped to attach 'hope' to these new functions do not recognise their achievement for what it is. They think they have 'analysed' or 'defined' hope as it is ordinarily understood (while making its boundaries sharper, perhaps). Sometimes, this lack of awareness has no practical consequences; but sometimes it has unfortunate methodological or clinical implications.[2]

Figure 11.1 is a rough visual representation of the view I have sketched in this section. Theories of hope, in both health care and psychology, are based on a narrowly selective range of uses of the word 'hope', disregarding the others. At the same time, they draw on different – but still anticipatory – concepts such as optimism or ambition in order to fit 'hope' for its new function(s). This is particularly noticeable, as we shall see, in instruments used to measure 'hope' (which, on this analysis, measure something else). I will return to this point in Sections 11.7 and 11.8.

In the rest of this chapter, I will try to justify what I've said in this summary, citing the work of several authors who have contributed to the literature on hope.

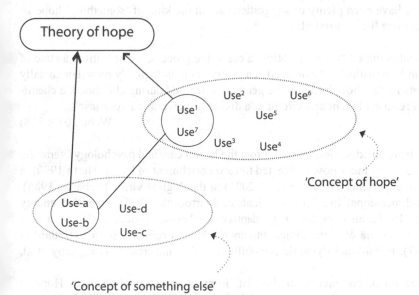

Figure 11.1 Theories of hope and uses of 'hope'.

I will also identify the health-related functions which 'hope' has acquired, and suggest an explanation of why this word, rather than any alternative, has been appropriated for these functions.

11.2 Hope as something

In the health literature, 'hope' is generally assumed to be the name of something. That I am sceptical about this assumption will be evident from the discussion in Part I, and from the approach adopted in Chapters 8–10. However, I am not alone in this scepticism. Eliott (2005) attributes to Menninger (1959) the introduction of the idea that hope is a 'thing' that can be objectively studied, that it is a measurable 'entity' inside people. She adds: 'Menninger convincingly employed the language of medical discourse to market hope to the medical community. Inherent in this medicalisation of hope is the objectification of hope' (11).

Menninger seems to have envisaged hope as a psychological equivalent of a homeostatic substance like blood sugar, something which must be kept within a narrow range of values, neither too much nor too little, and which can be increased or decreased exogenously. Indeed, this regulation of hope is said to be a task of health professionals, administering the psychological equivalent of glucose or insulin in order to maintain the correct levels.

I will return to the project of fostering and maintaining hope in Section 11.10. In this section, I want to focus on the picture of hope which underlies that project. The picture, which appears to be ingrained in the literature, suggests that hope is a psychological or spiritual *something* which 'resides', or perhaps manifests itself, in the individual. I'm trying to avoid premature ontological commitments here; but there have been plenty of suggestions about the kind of 'something' hope is. Consider one list of possibilities:

> What is hope? Is it an emotion, a cognitive process, a disposition, a state of mind, an instinct, a basic need, a mystery? Is it biologically rooted or socially constructed, hotwired into the genome or learned during childhood, a chemical reaction in a neural circuit or a divine gift awaiting a response?
>
> (Webb 2010: 328)

This is from an education journal. From the health care and psychology literature, we can add: an inner power directed toward enrichment of being (Herth 1990), a dynamic experience (Benzein et al. 2001), a theological virtue (Lebacqz 1985), a multidimensional life force (Dufault & Martocchio 1985), cognitive energy (Snyder 1995), an evolutionarily adaptive mechanism (Folkman 2010), a way of *being* (Kylmä & Vehviläinen-Julkunen 1997), a robust resource (Ballard et al. 1997), transitional dynamic possibilities within uncertainty (Duggleby et al. 2010).

Three quick comments on this list. First, it is extremely varied. Hope is described as an emotion, a need, a life force, possibilities, a virtue and so on. Second, several of the descriptions fall quite a long way short of being crystal clear (cognitive energy, life force, transitional dynamic possibilities?). Third, it's a little surprising, given that hope is allegedly a 'universal human phenomenon' (Leung et al. 2009) and 'central to life' (Miller 2007) that it is so difficult to pin down. The normal case is that, in situations where we are confident about making statements of this kind, we know what the entity/state/process in question is, and how it works. Glucose, for example, is definitely a 'universal human phenomenon', and 'central to life'. But the reason we're able to make such claims is that we know precisely what glucose is, we understand its biochemistry, and we've learned why the maintenance of certain glucose levels in the blood is essential to the life of any human being. So being in a position to make similar claims about hope – universal human phenomenon, central to life – while having no clear idea about what it is, can be regarded as an unusual state of affairs.

Still, if you start with the assumption that hope is a *something* when in fact it isn't, you'll find it difficult to say what sort of something it is.[3]

Reader: So you're saying hope isn't anything? It doesn't exist? Isn't that ridiculous?

Me: Well, we've had this a number of times before. Nouns that are useful to the point of being indispensable, but not because they *name* anything.

Reader: But if hope isn't a something, how can we talk about it? If there's no such thing, how can we refer to it, think about it, or recognise examples of it? How we can we experience it? Or are you saying that's just an illusion?

Me: Obviously, I'm not denying that it's often true to say that people hope for things. What I'm denying is that this implies they 'possess', or have some other relation with, a 'something' called 'hope'.

Reader: But if we experience hope, there must be *something* we are experiencing.

Me: That's the root of the problem. We assume that the metaphysics can be read off from the syntax. She's drinking coffee, so there must be something (called 'coffee') she's drinking. That works. She's experiencing hope, so there must be something (called 'hope') she's experiencing. That doesn't.

11.3 Hope as something inner

I said that the suggestions about hope's nature are very diverse. However, there do appear to be certain underlying assumptions common to all or most of them. Here is a bullet point summary of what I take five of these assumptions to be:

- Hope is just one kind of thing.
- Hope is something that can be characterised universally.
- Hope is inside, or manifested in, a person.
- Hope is something mental, or possibly spiritual.
- 'Hope' is the name of this inner something.

One kind of thing. As I suggested in Section 2.2, what is analysed is *the* concept of hope; and when a description is offered, or a definition is formulated, it consists of a predicate attached to 'hope' in the subject position of a sentence: 'Hope is a multidimensional dynamic life force'. 'Hope is a theological virtue'. 'Hope is a positive goal-related motivational state'. It is, inevitably, something singular being described. There is no sense that hope, or the *uses* of 'hope', might be plural, variegated, heterogeneous.

Universality. The predicate which does the describing applies to that singular thing in its entirety. It is possible to make generalisations about hope, statements which are always true of the something we are referring to. Nobody suggests that 'hope is a theological virtue *for some people*'; or that 'hope is central to life *part of the time*'; or that 'hope is a multidimensional life force *in certain circumstances*'. 'Hope' statements are typically made without qualification, rather like: 'Water is a transparent, tasteless liquid, a compound of hydrogen and oxygen, freezing at 0°C and boiling at 100°C'.

In the person. Irrespective of the specific predicates attached to hope, it is (in some sense) a state of the person. A disposition, a state of mind, an instinct, a need, an experience, cognitive energy, a virtue. Even when something more mysterious is suggested – a divine gift, an inner power – it is always implied that this whatever-it-is manifests itself *in* the individual.

Mental or spiritual. Explicitly or implicitly, hope is construed as 'inner', in the sense of being a mental state/process/power/resource, or perhaps a spiritual one. In whatever way it is described, hope is always something of which the person is conscious. There may be such a thing as '*un*conscious hope' (Fromm 1968), but it is rarely discussed in the nursing literature.

'Hope' as a name. I have not come across any author in the health care literature who states, explicitly, that 'hope' is the name of this inner something, but neither have I come across any author who suggests it isn't. It is assumed in virtually every discussion. The very fact that defining or characterising claims typically begin 'Hope is…' implies that the writer takes herself to be describing something denoted by the word 'hope'. She does not think that her task is to propose alternatives to the view that 'hope' names something. Rather, she assumes that she is trying to find the correct description of the thing named.

What these assumptions add up to can be described as a *referentialist* view of 'hope' and, beyond that, a referentialist view of mental terms generally. This is a view which is ubiquitous not just in health care, but in philosophy and the study of language acquisition. 'Theory of mind researchers typically assume that mental verbs are referring to internal states' (Montgomery 2017: 242). On this view, '*hope* is simply referring to an experience'. More generally, Childs (2014: 106) has suggested that language acquisition studies 'are grounded in a referential view of language, which assumes that mental state terms develop as names referring to private entities'. She adds that the referential view 'is dominant in the field of social cognition'. It is a variation on the *noun-name-object* picture which has been with us since Chapter 3.[4] 'Cake' is the name of something in the tin. 'Hope' is the name of something in the mind.[5]

According to referentialism, says Ter Hark (2000),'the primary role of psychological words is to stand for or refer to things, properties and processes'. It is, he adds, one of the main targets of Wittgenstein's philosophy of psychology (196). Wittgenstein (1963) rejects the idea that words such as 'remember', 'understanding', 'think', 'pain', 'belief' and 'hope' *denote* inner objects, inner processes. The 'naming diagram' (Section 3.1), a picture-of-language which works for physical-object and physical-activity words leads us astray when we insist on trying to make psychological words conform to the same model.

In the case of 'hope', Chapters 8–10 have already provided numerous examples of the word *not* denoting an inner object/state, although sometimes it can certainly be interpreted that way:

(1) I hope to climb Ben Nevis.
(2) As darkness fell, hope faded.
(3) New Orleans is a city without hope.

(1) and (2) can be construed according to the 'inner something' paradigm. (1) refers to my state of mind. (2) refers, indirectly, to the states of mind of unnamed individuals, who are all hoping to find survivors of some disaster. Stretching it a bit, (3) can be construed in the same way, referring even more indirectly to the inhabitants of New Orleans, implying that 'hope' is not currently a feature of their 'inner' states.

However, the 'inner something' model seems to break down with examples like this:

(4) It's your only hope.
(5) There's not a hope in hell he'll be quiet.
(6) The review could not hope to be exhaustive.
(7) Mike hasn't a hope of winning.
(8) Is there any hope?
(9) It's a hopeless task you've given Trevor.
(10) David's hopeless.

It's difficult to see how 'hope' can be denoting an inner something in (4). The 'it' refers to some device, option or strategy which, the speaker claims, is the only way 'you' can achieve a good outcome or avoid a bad one. 'Hope' in this sentence is virtually synonymous with 'chance'. Indeed, 'It's your only chance' could be substituted without any loss of meaning, given that (in this context) the project of salvaging the situation is already implied.

Of course, a different story can always be told. 'Hope', it might be said, *does* denote an inner state, since the person addressed *hopes* to achieve a good outcome. It is the sentence's syntax which, misleadingly, implies that 'hope' is equivalent to 'chance'. A reformulation of the sentence would correct this: 'It's the only chance you have of attaining what you hope for'. As always, there is no way of refuting this view. I have no conclusive argument against it. However, the question I would ask is: what warrant is there for this claim? What justifies it other than the prior conviction that 'hope' *must* denote an inner something?

Can the person taking this line offer any evidence which is independent of that conviction?

The 'inner something' story gets progressively more difficult to tell with the remaining examples. In (7), for example, it is clearly *not* being said that Mike lacks a certain inner state; that he is not nurturing the hope of winning. In fact, the statement may be true even if Mike passionately wants to win, and thinks he can. Rather, the claim is being made that (in the speaker's opinion) he has no *chance* of winning, whatever his own thoughts on the matter might be. In this case, it's not even clear how the alternative, 'inner something' story would go. Whose inner state is being referred to? Obviously not Mike's, if he is hoping to win. And obviously not the speaker's, since (7) is not the same as 'I hope Mike doesn't win'.

Similarly, (8) is not asking whether someone is in a certain state of mind. It is certainly not the same as 'Do you have any hope?' It is closer to 'Is there any chance?' In both cases, the context will determine what outcome is in question; and in both cases the sense is: is there any possibility of that outcome being achieved? Likewise, in (9), neither Trevor nor the task is 'lacking in hope'. Tasks cannot possess 'inner states'; so neither can they fail to possess them. Trevor, meanwhile, may not yet be aware that his task is hopeless; he might not even be aware, at this stage, that he has been given a task at all. (10), of course, does not imply that David is lacking in hope. It implies, rather, that he is lacking in competence.

Ordinary usage, then, is not consistent with the assumption that 'hope' *always* denotes an inner state. It is more consistent with the idea that the function of 'hope' varies with the construction, and the context, it occurs in.[6]

11.4 Interlude: ordinary use and Wittgenstein

The 'inner something' account, then, is consistent with some uses of the word 'hope', but ignores others. For example, it ignores uses in which 'hope' is combined with negating words such as 'not' and 'no'. In these constructions, 'hope' is not used to say whether somebody is (or is not) in a particular inner state, but to convey the *speaker's* belief that the likelihood of a specific, positively valenced outcome is very low. The 'inner state' view is based on a narrowly selective range of uses: those which, like examples (1) to (3), allude (or can be taken to allude) to someone's psychological state.

So am I claiming that, because the 'inner something' idea does not reflect ordinary use, it is mistaken? Not at all. That would be to regard ordinary usage as the ultimate benchmark, the criterion by which we legislate what it is permitted to say. It would be to take Wittgenstein's observation about 'meaning as use' (Section 7.5) as a general theory of language, and effectively to ban any and all uses that conflict with 'ordinary use'. It would be to believe that selective use, poetic use, stipulative definitions or new technical terms are automatically wrong. Wittgenstein is *not* an 'ordinary language philosopher', if by that we mean someone who condemns non-ordinary usage simply because it conflicts with ordinary usage (Kuusela 2013, Read 2014). He is perfectly willing to countenance non-ordinary uses, whether they are advanced on scientific or philosophical grounds.

But there are conditions. Wittgenstein is not so permissive that he will accept *any* novel or selective use. Notice the final word of the last paragraph. There have to be grounds: there has to be some justification for the new technical term or the new coinage. Without this condition, we could invent any old gewgaw, any old seductive phrase, that sounds impressive. In the case of 'hope', for example, it would not be too difficult to produce a whole series of vacuous expressions and announce that hope is *that*. It's a spiritual energy field, an instantiation of the Law of Attraction, an ontological wave function, a connection with the Absolute Thou. There will always be somebody who finds the phrase, whatever it is, appealing. A resonant phrase is added to the list, and a new picture gets hung in the Gallery of Hope for people to feel uplifted by. However, *by themselves*, these phrases are not adding to the *knowledge* of anything.

I can call the expressions in the previous paragraph 'vacuous' because I devised them myself. But how can we distinguish between 'connection with the Absolute Thou', on the one hand, and expressions such as 'inner power directed toward enrichment of being', on the other? Why is the latter an acceptable new use, while 'connection-with-the-Absolute-Thou' isn't? Answer: it's only acceptable if there is a coherent explanation, amounting to an explicit justification, of the use of words like 'inner', 'power', 'directed' and 'being' in this context.

Witherspoon (2000: 345) presents us with a Wittgensteinian perspective on questions like this:

> When Wittgenstein is confronted with an utterance that has no clearly discernible place in a language-game ... he invites the speaker to explain how she is using her words, to connect them with other elements of the language-game in a way that displays their meaningfulness. Only if the speaker is unable to do this in a coherent way does Wittgenstein conclude that the utterance is nonsense.

Read (2014), commenting on Wittgenstein's discussion of Freud, echoes Witherspoon:

> Freud uses words in ways that conflict with their original usage *without fully admitting (or realizing) that he is doing so*, and this for Wittgenstein is a sign that what we have in Freud is a mythology ... [However,] the problem with Freud is *not* – and this is crucial – the extended use *itself*; it is that the extended use is not in fact scientifically justified.
>
> (67: italics original)

This, as Read says, is crucial. Using a certain expression in a new, or narrowly selective, way is not in itself a problem. It only becomes a problem if no justification for the new/selective use is offered; and *not* offering a justification is obviously more likely if the person concerned does not even realise that she is using words 'in ways that conflict with their original usage'.[7]

11.5 'Hope' without an object

There is a sixth feature of 'hope' (as used in the health and psychology literatures) in addition to the five described in Section 11.3. It routinely occurs without an object. Section 8.2.2 suggested that in ordinary language, the verb 'hope' (in common with the count noun) always takes an object. In fact, the object of hope – what is hoped for – is what *individuates* particular hopes. 'I hope to be knighted, and you hope that the President is not re-elected'. Remove the objects from this sentence, and all we're left with is: 'I hope, and you hope', which tells us nothing.

At least since Menninger, hope has often been discussed in the health and psychology literatures without any reference to an object at all. It is, of course, legitimate to use 'hope' on its own to identify a concept: 'Hope: a construct central to nursing' (Miller 2007), or 'Stress, coping, and hope' (Folkman 2010). This is typical of the use of plurals and mass nouns to introduce a topic: 'Unicorns: the myth', 'Phlogiston: an 18th century theory'. However, that is not what I'm referring to here. To see what I'm driving at, think instead about the project of *measuring* hope. What are the implications of this?

The most obvious implication is that hope is something which admits of degrees. The basic schema accommodates this idea in two ways.

[a] People can want the same thing, but to different extents. You might *really* want a certain outcome, whereas I would welcome it, but I'm not as exercised about it as you are.

[b] The probability we assign to the outcome varies. You assign it a somewhat higher degree of probability than I do. You are 'more hopeful', we might say, than I am (though 'hopeful' here is extremely close to 'optimistic').

One can imagine measuring either of these elements, using a simple rating system. For example, you might rate your desire for an end to the monarchy as 9 on a scale of 1–10, while I might rate my desire for the same thing as 7. In much the same way, you might rate the probability of an end to the monarchy actually occurring at 30%, while I rate it at a mere 10%. The idea of measuring hope is, in this respect, quite legitimate. Notice, however, that what is being measured here is the extent of your/my desire for a *specific outcome* – the end of the monarchy – or the probability that each of us assigns to that specific outcome. It is not, so to speak, our hoping-for-things *tout court*.

In contrast, the scales that measure hope are silent about what it is, specifically, that's hoped for. Hope is construed as a singular thing which you can have less or more of, and which is not directed towards any particular outcome. You can, in the terms adopted by Snyder et al. (2018), be a 'high hoper' or a 'low hoper', full stop. The level of 'hope' you have is not with respect to this or that outcome.[8]

It is a trait (or state) that can be identified and measured independently, without reference to any particular object.

This would be a rather odd way of talking in the case of other attraction verbs (see Sections 8.2 and 8.3). Consider 'like', for example. 'Like' obviously takes an object in the same way 'hope' does. We have to like *something* (this is another grammatical remark: Section 6.4). I like coffee, and you like tea. Remove the objects, and we have: 'I like, and you like'. It would be odd if someone proposed to measure 'liking' as a trait or disposition without any reference to *what* is liked. Would Snyder suggest that one person is a 'high liker' and that another person is a 'low liker'? Similarly for verbs such as 'want', 'prefer', 'fancy' and so on. We don't distinguish between 'high fanciers' and 'low fanciers', or 'low preferers' and 'high preferers', without any reference to *what it is* they fancy or prefer.

In the most highly cited paper on hope in the nursing literature, Dufault and Martocchio (1985) distinguish between particularised and generalised hope. It is a distinction between hope with an object, and hope without.[9] 'Particularized hope is concerned with ... a hope object', whereas generalised hope 'is a sense of some future but indeterminate developments ... It is expressed to others in such statements as "I don't hope for anything in particular, I just hope. Things have worked out before"'. It casts 'a positive glow on life'. This account might seem to justify, in the concept of generalised hope, the assumption that hope is an inner state that can exist without an object.

However, by removing the object from particularised hope, and by making no reference at all to ellipsis, Dufault and Martocchio merely confirm that generalised hope is not 'hope' at all, but something closer to 'optimism', a term used to denote a general inclination to expect things to 'work out'.[10] Optimism 'casts a positive glow on life'. It is not 'generalized *hope*', but rather a 'generalized positive *expectation*' (I'll come back to the distinction between 'hope' and 'expectation' in Section 11.6.2). In saying this, I am not implying that 'optimism' has no significance in health care. Actually, I think it has. Instead, what I am suggesting is that it is not the same as 'hope'. And *that* will be important if one of nursing's 'fostering hope' projects is really the project of 'fostering optimism'.

11.6 Dufault and Martocchio

This is my cue to say more about Dufault and Martocchio's (1985) influential paper. The most frequently quoted passage is the point at which they suggest that hope is:

> a *multidimensional* dynamic life force characterized by a *confident* yet *uncertain* expectation of achieving a future good which, to the hoping person, is *realistically* possible and personally significant.
>
> (380: italics original)

From the perspective of the ordinary use of 'hope', this description includes a number of oddities, none of which is discussed by the authors. I'll focus on two claims: (a) hope is a dynamic life force; (b) hope is a form of expectation. This will lead to a discussion of (c) the relation between 'hope' and a number of other anticipatory words.

11.6.1 Dynamic life force

Dufault and Martocchio never explain what they mean by 'dynamic life force'. In the context of the paper, 'dynamic' seems to mean that, for any given individual, hope does not always occur at the same level of intensity, nor is it always hope for the same thing. This is straightforward enough, so here I will restrict my comments to 'life force'.

It is difficult to generalise about the 'ordinary' use of 'life force'. COCA has 326 occurrences, but they are extremely varied. The following examples reflect only a rough, and certainly incomplete, typology.

(11)   George Clooney is a life force for the film industry.
(12)   She was brimming with life force, generosity, humour and talent.
(13)   The life force, qi, flows through channels, or meridians.
(14)   There is something else, a life force or a spirit, that survives the body.
(15)   Statistically, more people now believe in God as a life force.
(16)   *Giardia lamblia* is a quasi-dominant life force that can survive for months.
(17)   Shaw's belief in a life force is opposed to Darwin's natural selection.

So we have 'life force' as: a person, exuberance, a bodily substance, the soul or spirit, God, the extreme hardiness of an organism and a mechanism at work in nature (maybe). All of these – and a few other categories – are multiply represented in COCA.

Granted that 'life force' is used in this wide variety of ways, one problem with Dufault and Martocchio's paper is that it makes no attempt to show how their own use of the expression connects with *any* of the established uses. This is precisely Witherspoon's point (Section 11.4): Wittgenstein 'invites the speaker to explain how she is using her words, to connect them with other elements of the language-game in a way that displays their meaningfulness'. This is something which Dufault and Martocchio fail to do. Their use of 'life force' in the paper is unanchored. We have no idea what kind of thing they are referring to.

11.6.2 Hope and expectation

'Hope' is an anticipatory word: it is usually, although not always, employed when talking about future events (or possible events). There are, of course, many other words that are anticipatory in roughly the same sense. One in particular, 'expectation', is often mentioned in discussions of hope. For example, it plays a significant role in Dufault and Martocchio's characterisation of hope: 'a confident yet uncertain *expectation* of achieving a future good'. Many other authors associate hope and expectation in the same way: Benzein and Saveman (1998), Cutcliffe and Herth (2002), Parker-Oliver (2002), Miller (2007).[11]

   Despite Dufault and Martocchio's characterisation, in ordinary usage 'hope' and 'expectation' are often explicitly distinguished. Consider the following examples:

(18)   I hope it will win, but I don't expect it to.
(19)   She did it more in hope than expectation.
(20)   He hopes I'll help him? Or he's expecting me to?
(21)   Expect the worst, but hope for the best.
(22)   Julie's hoping for a baby. Kate's already expecting.

Crudely, 'hope' and 'expectation' are at different points on the assessment of probability scale. If you expect something to happen, you assume it has a very high probability of occurring. If you only hope it will happen, your assessment of its probability is (usually) significantly lower. There's also a difference with respect to what is implied about preference. 'Hope' has a positive valence. You hope for outcomes you would welcome.[12] 'Expect' has no valence. You can expect outcomes you would *not* welcome.

   In summary, the circumstances in which we use 'hope' are generally different from the circumstances in which we use 'expect'. The two words are both antici-patory, but they imply different things about both likelihood and valence. So to suggest that hope is a form of expectation, or that it is 'characterised' by it, does conflict with established usage.[13]

11.6.3 Other anticipatory words

As I noted above, there are many anticipatory words. In addition to 'hope' and 'expect', verbs include 'aspire', 'predict', 'speculate', 'promise' and 'anticipate' itself. Nouns include 'ambition', 'optimism', 'resolve', 'aspiration', 'intention' and 'threat'. Most of these words can also generate adjectives, usually through the use of a suffix ('hopeful', 'expectant', 'speculative').

   I have already suggested that Dufault and Martocchio (1985) characterise hope as a form of expectation, even though ordinary usage recognises a clear distinc-tion between them. I now want to suggest that their characterisation of hope also fails to discriminate between 'hope' and several other anticipatory terms.

   Read the characterisation again, this time omitting the reference to 'the hoping person':

   a *multidimensional* dynamic life force characterized by a *confident* yet *uncer-tain* expectation of achieving a future good which is *realistically* possible and personally significant.

This description could apply equally well to 'ambition', 'intention', 'aspiration', 'optimism', 'resolve'. Take 'ambition', for example. *Ambitious* people have a confident expectation of achieving a future good that is significant to them, and which they regard as eminently possible. The uncertainty lies in the fact that it is not absolutely *certain* that they will attain that future good. Similarly, a person who *intends* to do something has a confident expectation of achieving a future good which is realistically possible, and of personal significance. In this case, the uncertainty lies in the recognition that it is not always possible to fulfil one's intentions, so the future good may not in fact be achieved, even though it is currently the individual's intention to achieve it.[14]

'Optimism' is a particularly interesting example. Optimistic people have a confident expectation that a future good will be achieved, a good which is possible and personally meaningful. Perennial optimists adopt this outlook on a regular basis. Once again, the uncertainty lies in the fact that the outcome is not guaranteed. As with 'expect', ordinary usage makes a clear distinction between hope and optimism:

(23) I hope she'll agree, but I'm not optimistic.

However, there is a tendency in the hope literature to conflate the two, as I will suggest in Section 11.8 (there are also critics of this tendency). The question is not so much whether this assimilation is right or wrong, although it does constitute a departure, at odds with ordinary use. The more important question is what the consequences of making the assimilation are.

One consequence I will mention briefly now. There are several measures of hope. One of them is the Herth Hope Index, which is one of the three most commonly used (Eliott 2012). According to Herth (1992), the Herth Hope Scale (HHS) 'is based on Dufault & Martocchio's model of hope' (40); and the Herth Hope Index (HHI) is a shorter version of the HHS. In this section, I've suggested that Dufault and Martocchio's characterisation of hope does not clearly distinguish between 'hope' and a number of other anticipatory words. If that's correct, then there is a possibility that HHS and HHI inherit this ambiguity. In other words, it is possible that these scales measure, not hope, but a hope-optimism-confidence mash-up. This is one of the possible methodological consequences to which I referred earlier; but I will defer further discussion of this possibility until Section 11.8.

In summary, Dufault and Martocchio's account of hope is based on a narrowly selective range of uses of 'hope'. However, it also incorporates the pattern of usage associated with different terms, in particular 'expectation'. This suggests a picture like that in Figure 11.1. Dufault and Martocchio's characterisation *both* ignores many established uses of 'hope', *and* reflects the use of at least one significantly different anticipatory term. This again may have implications for any measures of hope which, like those devised by Herth, are based on Dufault and Martocchio's account.

11.7 Snyder

Snyder's hope theory 'has been the most commonly studied approach to hope within psychology since the early 1990s', and is 'certainly the most influential model of hope in psychology' (Snyder et al. 2018: 14/15). The theory is not often cited in the health care literature (exceptions include Penz 2008, Leung et al. 2009, Berendes et al. 2010), but it is discussed here because of its wider significance.

11.7.1 Hope theory

Hope theory emerged from work on goal attainment. Snyder et al. (2018) report that the 'breakthrough' came when they asked 'people to talk about their goal directed thoughts' (27). Interviewees 'repeatedly mentioned the pathways to reach their goals and the motivation to use those pathways'. Consequently, Snyder and his team homed in on 'two components of goal-directed thought – pathways and agency'. An individual's 'pathways thinking' is the process of 'generating workable routes' towards her goals. It is characterised by 'affirming internal messages that are similar to the appellation "I'll find a way to get this done!"' (28). 'Agency thinking' is the motivational component of the theory, and refers to 'self-referential' thoughts about moving along a particular pathway, and the determination to continue doing so. 'We have found that high-hope people embrace such self-talk agentic phrases as "I can do this" and "I am not going to be stopped"' (Snyder et al. 2018: 28).

Both 'pathways thinking' and 'agency thinking' are necessary for what Snyder calls 'hopeful thinking'; and this leads to an account of hope which suggests that it is:

> a positive motivational state that is based on an interactively derived sense of successful (1) agency (goal directed energy) and (2) pathways (planning to meet goals).
>
> (Snyder et al. 1991: 287)

Research indicates that the application of 'hopeful thinking' leads to improved outcomes: for example, higher academic achievement, and greater success in athletics. In health care,

> people with high versus low hope ... appear to remain appropriately energized and focused on what they need to do in order to recuperate. This is in stark contrast to the counter-productive self-focus and self-pity ... that can overtake people with low hope.
>
> (Snyder et al. 2018: 34)

It is interesting to note that the 'breakthrough' to hope theory was a series of interviews in which people were asked to talk about goal-directed thought, rather than (for example) hope. Certainly, the idea of 'pathways to energetically pursued goals' dominates the theory and the measurement scales derived from it. Goal directedness, however, represents a very narrow range of uses of the word 'hope', as will be clear from a comparison of hope theory and the discussion in Chapters 8–10. It does not begin to account for the majority of functions associated with 'hope' constructions.

11.7.2 Ambition, optimism, tenacity, determination

As suggested above, Dufault and Martocchio's characterisation of hope is consistent with the use of other anticipatory terms, such as 'ambition' and 'optimism'. The same is true of Snyder's. Indeed, there is a degree of overlap with Dufault & Martocchio, since 'ambition' is also a term which refers to a positive motivational state based on an 'interactively derived sense of successful agency (goal directed energy) and pathways (planning to meet goals)'.

However, where Dufault and Martocchio emphasise the *expectation* of achieving a future *good*, Snyder and his colleagues emphasise the *cognitive process* that leads to the achievement of *personal goals*. These are alternative takes on the 'anticipatory' theme, and the difference between them is marked, given that the 'determination to attain an aim' is much more specific than the 'expectation of something good'. 'Expectation' does not necessarily imply that you are working towards anything. 'Personal goals' represent an aimed-for target in a way that 'future good' does not.

Look again at the 'self-talk agentic phrases' that Snyder et al. (2018) associate with hope: 'I can do this'. 'I'll find a way to get this done!' 'I am not going to be stopped'. High-hope people are 'energised' and focused. Low-hope people are inclined to self-pity. There is, at the very least, a sense of confidence and determination in the 'agentic' pronouncements (accompanied by the rather judgmental dismissal of 'low hopers'). Show these statements to people who don't know their provenance, and ask what sort of person would make them, and you tend to get 'focused', 'confident', 'determined' and 'purposeful' by way of answers. What you don't tend to get is 'hopeful'.

Critics of hope theory in psychology have made the same kind of point, suggesting that Snyder's theory is a better fit for tenacity, optimism or perseverance than it is for hope (see, for example, Aspinwall and Leaf 2002, Tennen et al. 2002, Callina et al. 2015). The philosopher Adrienne Martin (2014) has said: 'Perhaps there are reasons to call this set of attitudes "hope" in a technical way, but it is clearly not the same attitude I have been discussing' (86). My own view is that Snyder's construct can be diagrammed as in Figure 11.1. It is derived from a (very) narrowly selective range of 'hope' uses, and it has distinct overtones of other concepts such as ambition, confidence, determination, purposefulness, tenacity and optimism. This, of course, is not surprising given the origins of hope theory in research on goal-directed thinking. Whatever label is attached to this construct – and I will suggest in Section 11.8 that it does have value – it cannot realistically be interpreted as 'the concept of hope', not if this expression refers to the wide range of uses sketched in Chapters 8–10.

11.7.3 Morse and Penz

I will close this section by mentioning two nurse authors. One of them gives an account of hope that has some similarity to Snyder's. The other is one of the few writers in the nursing literature to discuss hope theory explicitly.

Morse (2017) reports on two studies (Laskiwski & Morse 1993, Morse & Doberneck 1995), along with a television film, which led to the identification of a set of 'attributes' of hope. Like Snyder's theory, this is a very goal-oriented account. The first attribute is: 'the envisioning of alternatives and the setting of goals'. The fifth is: 'the continuous evaluation for signs that reinforce the selected goals'. In between, we have 'a realistic assessment of personal resources and of external conditions and resources', which is Morse's equivalent of pathways thinking. Finally, there is: 'a determination to endure': 'the maintenance of hope requires focused energy to get through the situation and to reach the goal' (Morse & Doberneck 1995: 278). This is more stoic than Snyder's 'I'm not going to be stopped'; but it does make the same reference to determination, and the expression 'focused energy' is akin to the 'energised and focused' attitude that Snyder attributes to 'high hopers'.

As with Snyder, this 'goal' emphasis is unsurprising in view of the account's origins. The first study was of patients with spinal cord injury, together with family members and rehabilitation staff. The television film was about a young couple and their child, lost in a blizzard in the Rockies. Both scenarios require goal-setting and planning. The rehabilitation of patients with spinal cord injury is a classic example of a clinical context in which goal-setting is regarded as essential (for example, Byrnes et al. 2012). Morse's account of the couple lost in the Rockies constantly emphasises goals and planning, while insisting that this is an 'exemplar of hope'. In the sense that it reflects *one type of situation* in which we might use the word 'hope', this may be true. But there are countless 'hope' situations that do not involve goals and/or planning, whether of the spinal cord injury kind or the lost-in-a-blizzard kind. The craving for generality has encouraged Morse to assume that her two 'exemplar' situations apply to all instances of 'hope'.

Penz's (2008) paper comments on both Morse and Snyder, arguing that their theories are (in my terms) narrowly selective. Hope theory, she says, has 'a narrow emphasis on examining self-motivation and mental events' (410). Noting that Snyder's account is focused on setting and achieving goals, she points out that in studies of hope from the perspective of palliative care professionals 'there was little evidence to substantiate the importance of goal-setting and other cognitive processes'. Her main claim is that 'the assumptions of a cognitive psychological and anthropological approach may not be congruent with the philosophical foundation that defines the nursing discipline in the broad sense and that defines aspects of palliative nursing practice' (ibid.).

In general terms, this is about right, though I don't think it has anything to do with hope-from-this-or-that-perspective. The goal-focused accounts of Snyder and Morse are narrow, not because they do not take account of palliative nursing, but because they ignore a very large proportion of the uses that the word 'hope' is put to – in *any* disciplinary, professional or non-professional context. Of course, the lop-sidedness of hope theory is going to show up in some contexts more than others; and palliative care is certainly going to be one of those contexts, an observation that can be illustrated by looking again at some of the 'agentic' statements Snyder refers to: 'I can do this', 'I'll find a way to get this done!', 'I am not going

to be stopped'. It is difficult to believe that hope among palliative care nurses –
and even less so among their patients – is ever expressed in this way.

11.8 A note on scales

I should say a little more about scales designed to measure hope. According to
Eliott (2012), there were (as of 2011) over 25 English-language scales in the
health care literature designed to measure hope or hopelessness. Since they all
measure a generic state or trait, detached from any specific object-of-hope, they
cannot be measures of 'hope' in the ordinary sense. This does *not* mean they are of
no value; but it does mean that what they are measuring is something else.

There are two scales associated with hope theory, the Trait Hope Scale and
the State Hope Scale. On both, people who rate as 'high hopers' agree that they:

1 Are good at solving any problems they face.
2 Can think of several different ways to solve these problems.
3 Have plenty of ideas about how to get what they want.
4 Set themselves goals.
5 Put a lot of energy into achieving these goals.
6 Regard themselves as pretty successful.

The first three reflect the 'pathways thinking' dimension of hope theory, while the
second three reflect the 'agency thinking' dimension. 'High hopers' say that they
set themselves goals; they can devise ways to achieve them; they pursue them
energetically and successfully; and they are capable of solving problems. There
is a mix here of confidence, optimism, imagination, single-mindedness, ambition,
tenacity and self-satisfaction. But if this set of characteristics reflects 'hope', it
does so in a narrowly selective sense, and it draws heavily on additional concepts,
in the way suggested by the conceptual architecture in Figure 11.1.

Here are some representative items from the Herth Hope Scale (there are 30
items in all):[15]

1   I am looking forward to the future.
3   I have deep inner strength.
4   I have plans for the future.
5   I have inner positive energy.
8   I have a faith that gives me comfort.
11 I feel time heals.
19 I see the positive in most situations.
20 I have goals for the next 3–6 months.

There are some similarities with the 'hope theory' scales, especially in items 4, 19
and 20. But the Herth scale feels far less self-assertive than Snyder's scales, and it
alludes to an 'inner resource' (3, 5, 8) in a way that they do not. It is less difficult
to see 'hope' in these items than in the Snyder There are some similarities with the

'hope theory' scales, especially in items 4, 19 and 20. But the Herth scale feels far less self-assertive than Snyder's scales, and it alludes to an 'inner resource' (3, 5, 8) in a way that they do not. It is less difficult to see 'hope' in these items than in the Snyder equivalents; but it is still a narrowly selective 'hope', relative to Chapters 8–10; and the main impression it conveys – in line with the Dufault and Martocchio characterisation – is one of *confident expectation that all will be well in the end* (1, 3, 5, 8, 11, 19). This hovers somewhere between optimism and faith, and is highly non-specific.

The HHS closely resembles the Life Orientation Test (Scheier & Carver 1985), a well-known optimism measure. The LOT includes items like: 'I always look on the bright side of things'; 'I'm a believer in the idea that "every cloud has a silver lining"'; 'In uncertain times, I usually expect the best' (225). Scheier & Carver's scale also fits the sense of a confident expectation that all will be well in the end, although it differs from Herth's scale in having no undercurrent of 'inner resource'. This is further evidence that the HHS fails to distinguish between 'hope' and 'optimism'.

I should emphasise that nothing I've said is inconsistent with the claim that the Herth and Snyder scales measure *something*, even if there is no single abstract noun (in English) which gives a name to what this something is. Both scales have a reasonably high degree of reliability (Herth 1991, Scioli et al. 2011, Rose & Sieben 2018); and the State and Trait Hope Scales appear to be correlated with athletic success, academic achievement and the ability to cope with some illness/injury conditions (Snyder et al. 2018). The question is whether, for either scale, the what-is-measured can legitimately be described as 'hope'.

11.9 Hoping against hope

Before returning to the project of fostering and maintaining hope in health care, I want to look at some ideas of Adrienne Martin (2014), a philosopher with an interest in bioethics. While based in the NIH Clinical Centre in Maryland, Martin spent two years following a cancer researcher undertaking phase I trials, and attending palliative care team meetings. She became particularly interested in hope, and in how both patients and professionals talked about it. My reason for discussing her work, aside from its intrinsic interest, is that she focuses on a certain form of hope which she describes as 'hope in the fullest sense'.[16] She regards this form of hope as especially relevant to end-of-life care.

Martin starts with the 'orthodox definition' of hope, illustrated by Day (1969) and Downie (1963). Day, for example, defines hope like this:[17]

> 'A hopes that X' is true, if and only if two conditions hold: 'A wishes [desires] that X' and 'A thinks that X has some degree of probability, however small'.[18]

Martin has no problem with the project of defining hope, and would assent to the idea that a successful definition would account for all relevant cases. However, like a number of other philosophers (Bovens 1999, Pettit 2004, Meirav 2009), she thinks the orthodox definition is inadequate. Like these authors, she also believes that what is required to define hope properly is a third condition, to bridge the gap between the orthodox definition and some particularly salient, or paradigmatic, cases of hope.

For Martin, the salient cases are examples of 'hoping against hope'; and her main argument is that the orthodox definition 'cannot accommodate the fact that two people with the same powerful desires can, faced with the same slim odds, seemingly differ in their hopes' (2014: 14). In one example she refers to Alan and Bess, both of whom have advanced (probably terminal) cancer, and both of whom are enrolled in an early-phase trial of an experimental drug. Both understand that there is a less than 1 percent chance that they will receive any medical benefit; and 'they have equally strong desires to find a "miracle cure".' The difference between them is explained as follows:

> If asked, Alan will say he does indeed hope the experimental drug will turn out to be, for him at least, a miracle cure. But he will also emphasize how poor a chance 1 percent is, and he rarely appeals to his hope as a justification for his decisions, moods, or feelings. Bess, instead, while noting that it is almost certain she will not be cured by the experimental drug, says the bare possibility is what keeps her going, and often appeals to her hope as a justification for her decisions, moods, and feelings. One percent is enough, she says. She hopes to be the 1 percent, and that is her main reason for enrolling in the trial. Both people hope for a cure, but Bess is the person we would describe as 'hoping against hope'; there is some sense in which her hope is higher or greater or stronger than Alan's.
>
> (Martin 2014: 15)

Alan and Bess, Martin says, don't differ in their desires, or in the probability they assign to a cure, but their hopes do differ. So 'it seems that the orthodox definition must leave something out'.

This strikes me as an odd inference. Here's an analogy. Chambers defines 'run' like this: 'to proceed by lifting one foot before replacing the other; to go swiftly, at more than walking pace; to hasten; to proceed quickly'. But this definition takes no account of the fact that some people can run faster than others; so it must leave something out. That's a strange argument. Defining what running is, and how people run, has to incorporate the fact that some people are better at it than others? Would Martin argue like this, then? 'Bess and Alan are both lifting one foot before replacing the other, and they are both proceeding at more than walking pace. But Bess is running faster than Alan. So the definition must leave something out'. It seems unlikely.

Setting aside Martin's reasons for thinking that the orthodox definition is inadequate, it is clear that she places great emphasis on hoping against hope, which she regards as a paradigmatic case of 'hope in its fullest sense' (2014: 17). So what, precisely, does it involve? The basic idea is that people who hope against hope treat the *possibility* of the desired outcome as a 'licence' to engage in certain feelings and activities. Even when that possibility is vanishingly small, they judge that there is sufficient reason to engage in these feelings and activities. They stand ready to justify dedicating certain kinds of attention and thought to the outcome, as well as hedged reliance on the outcome in their plans; moreover, they stand ready to appeal to the outcome's probability as part of their justification for these activities. (24)

Which leads to the next question: *which* feelings, activities and plans?

Here are some of the things Martin refers to in the Bess example. Active, narrative fantasising about the desired outcome occurring. Imagining good news from the most recent test or scan. Having positive emotions as a result of these fantasies, and regarding it as justifiable to *feel good* on that basis (Martin's italics). Hopeful anticipation. Prayer, or 'pleading with the universe'. Formulating plans contingent on living well past her expected lifespan, amounting to '*reliance* on a hoped-for outcome' (Martin's italics). In licencing these activities, the person hoping against hope goes 'all in'. This is not just a matter of odd thoughts on the margins, indulged in occasionally. Rather, she invests – and takes herself to be justified in investing – 'a great deal of mental, emotional and physical activity focused on the outcome' (Martin 2014, Chapters 2 and 3, *passim*).

I'm not convinced that Martin has got this right. In particular the 'feeling good', and the 'making plans on the basis of the hoped-for outcome occurring', do not fit many of the examples of 'hoping against hope' in COCA. A few examples:

(24)   Nadia searched desperately for her mother, hoping against hope to find her alive.

(25)   The townspeople were all hoping against hope that Jason hadn't drowned.

(26)   Emily was distraught when I told her, hoping against hope that I'd made it up.

It's possible that there is some fantasising here, and quite possibly prayer or pleading with the universe. But it's difficult to see the 'feeling good' part of Martin's analysis, and equally difficult to imagine that Nadia, Emily or the townspeople were making plans contingent on the hoped-for outcome occurring. We have, in these examples, great anxiety and fear; and the thought is more likely to be: 'Let's get past this, and then we can perhaps think about making plans'. 'Feeling a positive sense of anticipation' (2014: 69) does not come into it.

Incidentally, anxiety is not just a feature of hoping against hope. I think what Martin calls 'prosaic' hope is often accompanied by worry, or even fear (which is *not* to say that fear and anxiety are 'components' of hope). To use one of her examples: if I hope that my friend caught the last train, I worry (a bit) that she might not have done. Many cases of hoping against hope ramp this 'worry' up to fear of an intense kind, as with examples (24) to (26). But I don't think this necessarily applies to all cases in which the term 'hoping against hope' might be used (I'm trying resist the craving for generality). For example, I'm prepared to take Martin's account of Bess's 'hopeful anticipation' at face value, even if I wonder at what point this kind of outlook shades into 'being in denial'.

Still, my purpose here is not to quarrel with Martin's analysis, but to introduce an account of hope which recognises that 'hope' always has an object; which does not appeal to inner powers or life forces; which does not talk about 'generalised' hope, or hope as a trait; and which does not conflate 'hope' with other anticipatory terms. Martin also passes Wittgenstein's litmus test (see Section 11.4): she explains her use of 'hope' in detail, and connects it to established usage (even if I don't think she's right on all points). It is a pity that nurses are not more familiar with her work.

11.10 Fostering and maintaining hope

Finally, we can return to the project of fostering and maintaining hope. What exactly are its aims, and how should it go about achieving them?[19] There is, as we shall see, no one-size-fits-all answer to this question, so I'll organise my comments on it from a number of perspectives, drawing on the discussion in Chapters 8–10.

11.10.1 Hope with an object

Let's start with the basic schema. Here's a reminder:
   If it is true that 'A hopes that/to/for X', then we can generally infer that:

[a]   A would like X as an outcome.
[b]   A believes that X is possible, but not certain.
[c]   A understands that various factors might prevent X.
[d]   A believes that her control over these factors is limited.

With this schema in mind, how might we interpret the idea of 'fostering hope'? In principle, there appear to be several possibilities.
   First, we might encourage A to hope for more things; that is, to have *more* hopes: as if it were a matter of wanting T, U, W, V and Y as well as X. However, I am not aware of any evidence – nor does any writer claim – that the more hopes a patient has, the better off they are. The project of fostering hope is presumably not a matter of counting.
   Second, we might suggest that A should want X more strongly. For some conditions, this appears to be a significant factor. Rehabilitation programmes in a wide range of populations, from children with motor deficits (Meyns et al. 2017) to older cardiac patients (Mikkelsen et al. 2019), are enhanced if the patient is strongly motivated. However, this is not necessarily generalisable to other conditions. It isn't obvious that it applies to palliative care, for example. It is not as if stronger 'wanting' increases the likelihood of either survival or a peaceful death; nor is it clear why palliative nurses should encourage patients to want things such as pain relief more strongly than they already do.
   Third, some patients achieve more in rehabilitation if they recognise that their control over the 'limiting' factors, element [d], may be greater than they assume

(for example, in home exercise programmes: Picha & Howell 2018). This possibility may be more generalisable, given that it could apply to many kinds of rehabilitation process.

Fourth, it might be suggested that patients should be more optimistic, assigning a higher probability to the possibility of X occurring, element [b]. I have already noted that optimism is sometimes associated with beneficial outcomes (Sections 11.7, 11.8). However, this does not appear to be universally true, since the effects of optimism may be illness-specific. For example, optimism has a stronger impact on people with multiple sclerosis than it does on people with Parkinson's Disease (De Ridder et al. 2000). Moreover, it may be important to distinguish between at least two different forms of optimism: naïve optimism, based on the assumption that one is not at risk of illness, and functional optimism, based on the recognition that one is, in fact, vulnerable. Functional optimism is more likely to motivate preventive health behaviour, and the adoption of a healthy lifestyle. It is also more closely associated with health benefits (Schwarzer 1994).

There are, however, limits to promoting optimism. For any condition, it would be unethical, presumably, to suggest that the patient should attach a higher probability to the chance of recovery than is objectively warranted. This is particularly clear in cases of terminal cancer. Even where patients are 'hoping against hope', they are not necessarily (according to Martin) assigning an unrealistically high probability to the chance of cure or remission; rather, they are taking a vanishingly small possibility as a licence to engage in certain feelings, thoughts and activities. In any case, it is not the remit of health care professionals to encourage 'false hope' under the guise of fostering it, although it has been argued that there are cases in which this may be permissible (Begley & Blackwood 2000). Nor is it clear that health professionals are in the business of encouraging, or for that matter discouraging, patients to 'hope against hope', if this is the purely personal decision it appears to be.

The question is further complicated by 'positive illusions' (Taylor 1989, Taylor 2011). There is evidence to suggest that, for certain conditions (including AIDS and breast cancer), if a patient has unrealistically optimistic – but not wildly exaggerated – beliefs about her condition, then she is likely to survive longer (compared to patients whose beliefs are more accurate). Further, the progression of symptoms is likely to be slower, and her psychological adjustment will be better. Does the 'fostering hope' project permit encouraging beliefs of this sort, or at least not discouraging them? This is the kind of question that those who argue in favour of 'fostering hope' should be able to answer.

Fifth, 'fostering hope' could imply encouraging the patient or carer to want Y rather than X in element [a]; that is, to change *what* is hoped for. Examples of this often involve advanced cancer patients being encouraged to 'invest' their hope in a peaceful death, or the love of their family, rather than in a 'cure'. But this amounts to telling people what they should want. For example, some palliative care specialists take it upon themselves to tell patients and/or their carers what they should hope for.

> I suggested that, at various times of illness, there are different things to hope for. At some point, cure may not be realistic, but one can hope for comfort, serenity, to be with certain people, or perhaps to be alone. There can be so much to hope for, based on an individual's life experiences and preferences.
>
> (Lester 2011)

This is an example of regarding hope as a generic 'resource', which can be attached to anything. When a cure is not possible, it is apparently best to attach it to something more attainable. You have 'hope' – it is a resource – and you should invest it more sensibly. However, the man in Lester's story wants his wife to live, he has understandable reasons for wanting that, and he is trying to believe that it is still possible. That is what he implies when he uses the word 'hope'. He is not referring to a transferable quantity of something that would be better directed towards something else. To imply that he is, and to suggest that he ought to spend this resource more wisely by transferring it to a different possibility, could be seen as rather patronising.

This fifth possibility represents a shift from understanding hope as intrinsically hope-with-an-object – in Lester's example, the man's hope that his wife will survive the illness – to understanding it as hope-full-stop, a generic 'resource' transferable from one thing to another. It marks the transition from 'hope' the verb (and count noun) to 'hope' the mass noun, construed as the name of a species of 'inner thing', a state, process or power which has been separated from any connection to a specific outcome, and which correspondingly lacks the 'aboutness' of the basic schema. Lester's narrative reflects the inclination, in health care discourse, to think of hope, not as a particular-something individuated by its object, but as a general-something which can be identified without reference to any object at all.

11.10.2 Hope without an object

If the 'hope' in 'fostering hope' refers to what hope scales measure (Section 11.8), then what is being fostered is closer to equanimity, tenacity, goal-orientation or optimism – faith that things will turn out for the best – depending on which scale is employed. 'High hopers', to use Snyder's expression, will have more optimism, faith, equanimity or tenacity than 'low hopers', without any reference to specific hope-objects. However, the same skewing of 'hope', its transposition into a different concept, can also be observed in qualitative studies carried out by those wedded to mass-noun assumptions.

To illustrate what I mean, I would like to look at one very influential qualitative study (which also used the HHI). Buckley and Herth (2004) replicate Herth (1990), a study with 600 citations in Google Scholar. It arrives at more or less identical findings. The study involved interviews with 16 terminally ill patients receiving hospice care (four of them were also interviewed for a second time). The researchers were particularly interested in things that 'fostered or hindered hope' and, on the basis of the interviews, they identified seven 'hope-fostering categories': love of family and friends, spirituality/having faith, setting goals and maintaining independence, positive relationships with professional carers, humour, personal characteristics, uplifting memories.

The authors' description of these categories does not always make the connection with 'hope' clear. For example, under 'Setting goals', one patient says: 'These days I do small things. Now I'm determined to keep on dressing myself each day'. Under 'Relationships with professional carers', another patient says: 'If I'm low, I tell her [CNS], and we talk. It helps'. According to the authors,

> the striking aspect of this category was how much the 'little things' matter. For example, patients cited the importance of carers 'bothering' to find out what name they preferred to be called by, being courteous and willing to answer questions.

Under 'Humour', a patient says: 'Mixing in the right company, which makes you cheerful, that helps. Their cheerfulness keeps you going'. Under 'Personal characteristics', the authors report that: 'Being positive and determined to maintain optimism in the face of deterioration was the theme of these comments. One said: "I'm the sort of person who always keeps going no matter what"' (37/38).

None of these examples is directly related to 'hope' – at least, not by the patients – and certainly not to any specific hope-with-an-object. Yet these patients are all talking about, very roughly, the same kind of thing. If you want to call that thing 'hope', there's nothing wrong with that, as long as you acknowledge that it's not how we ordinarily use the word. What I see in these extracts, and which I think is cued by what the patients actually say, is a sort of double appreciation: of 'small things', and of anything which helps to 'keep your spirits up'.

'Morale' may be another way of referring to what's going on here.[20] But we don't need to have a single word – 'hope', 'morale', 'cheerfulness', whatever – to identify what these patients find valuable. This is another trap that the *noun-name-object* picture sets for us: the assumption that there must be a concept, a name, a single-word label, associated with whatever it is that emerges from these extracts, or any other 'phenomenon' we think we can identify. A single-word name is a convenience, of course, as it permits succinct reference. But there isn't always a convenient label of that kind. And if we choose 'hope' to do the job, there is a risk of confusing that-which-is-valued by this group of patients – in whatever way we describe it – with the jobs that 'hope' takes on in ordinary discourse.

Here is another illustration (Belchamber et al. 2013). In this study, eight people who attended a day care centre for palliative rehabilitation were interviewed about the effects of the programme. According to the authors, the 'key benefits of rehabilitation' reported by the patients were psychological support and hope (137). So 'hope' was apparently an outcome. The findings are reported under several headings, all of which take the form of: 'Regaining hope through … X'. Specifically, 'hope' is regained by 'sharing' (group work), 'caring' (attentive staff) and 'control' (of symptoms).

The paper has 12 extracts from interview transcripts. Not one of them mentions 'hope'. What these patients do mention is the health-related benefits of attending the programme. They talk about diversion, relaxation, the enjoyment of group activity and the relief of physical symptoms. The programme is good for their morale. It helps them to cope with their illness. It keeps their spirits up.

It appears that 'hope', the mass noun, used without reference to any specific object, is a codeword. It is used by health care professionals to refer succinctly to the kinds of benefits described in Belchamber et al., or the things-valued by the patients in Buckley and Herth. And that's fine, as long as 'hope' in *this* sense is not confused with the verb and count-noun 'hopes' discussed in Section 11.10.1. In this sense, 'hope' in health care has become a technical term.

11.10.3 The opposite of hope

'Hope is the opposite of despair', says Schneider (1980), and she is not alone in construing 'hope' and 'despair'/'hopelessness' as antonyms. For example, Aylott (1998: 231) observes that hopelessness is 'often thought to be at the opposite end of the hope continuum'; Cutcliffe and Herth (2002: 834) refer to 'despair, the opposite to hope'; Lipscomb (2007: 336) talks of 'hope and its converse hopelessness or despair'. Other writers who state, or take for granted, that hope and despair/hopelessness are related in this way include Wiles et al. (2008), Folkman (2010), Duggleby et al. (2012), Herrestad et al. (2014).

Schneider takes herself to be offering a definition; and I propose that we construe 'Hope is the opposite of despair' as precisely that, but as a *stipulative* definition, introducing another technical term. In other words, Schneider stipulates that she will use 'hope' to refer to whatever is the opposite of despair.

It might be argued that 'Hope is the opposite of despair' is a statement of fact, rather than a stipulative definition. However, there are no theoretical or empirical grounds for thinking that hope and despair *are* opposites. The best that Cutcliffe and Herth (2002) can do, for example, is to point out that the dictionary definition of 'despair' is 'to be without hope'. In contrast, Dufault and Martocchio (1985) suggest that 'hope and hopelessness are not the opposite ends of one continuum nor is hopelessness the absence of hope' (389); while Hernandez and Overholser (2020: 28–9) observe that none of the studies they examined 'addressed whether hope and hopelessness are polar opposites or separate constructs, so that conclusions of low hopelessness cannot be readily generalised to high hope'. The assumption that hope and despair are opposites appears to be just that: an assumption. It is probably based on the morphological sequence < 'hope'/'hopeless'/'hopelessness' >, and the belief that 'hopelessness' and 'despair' are synonyms.

Given Schneider's definition, 'fostering hope' is a way of saying: 'minimising the likelihood of despair'. As with 'appreciating small things', 'keeping your spirits up' and the range of health benefits described by Belchamber et al., there can be no objection to using 'hope' in this way – as shorthand, as a codeword – subject to a couple of provisos. First, this use should not be confused with the ordinary uses of 'hope' discussed in Chapters 8–10. Second, we must avoid confusing these codewords with each other: 'hope' as what the scales measure; 'hope' as the opposite of despair; 'hope' as optimism; 'hope' as appreciating the small things; 'hope' as enjoying the company of others; 'hope' as relief from pain. The point is: there is more than one 'technical term' 'here'. The scope for getting them muddled is quite considerable.

11.10.4 Fostering hope: summary

'Fostering hope' might refer to any of a wide range of options: suggesting that the patient changes the object of hope; encouraging her to adopt modestly unrealistic beliefs about her condition; persuading her that she has more control over 'limiting' factors than she imagines; encouraging her to adopt a generally optimistic outlook; keeping her spirits up; promoting a sense that things will work out in the end; trying to prevent a descent into despair; setting goals and helping the patient to achieve them; and several more. The extent to which any of these projects is viable is illness-specific, instrument-specific and dependent on what state of affairs 'hope' is used as a codeword for. It is not my aim to determine which of them is ethical, or clinically worthwhile. I recommend only that we are careful to discriminate between them.

11.11 Conclusion: why 'hope'?

In many respects, 'hope' is a common or garden word. The vast majority of occurrences in COCA are consistent with the basic schema and the numerous-but-everyday variations created by negation, ellipsis and the different grammatical constructions reviewed in Chapters 8–10. Yet, in other respects, 'hope' has a resonance that these ordinary uses would not, by themselves, predict. In this chapter, I have suggested that the word has become something like a technical term in health care, although even in that capacity its functions vary depending on the starting points of the authors concerned. It is used by some writers in preference to 'optimism', 'goal-directedness', 'tenacity', 'the opposite of despair', 'keeping one's spirits up' the 'appreciation of small things', and other expressions which, arguably, would better express what they are talking about. The obvious question is: why? The answer, I think, lies partly in the greater syntactic and morphological flexibility of 'hope', but mainly in the resonance which 'hope' has and these other expressions do not.

What is the source of this resonance? Its origins lie in hope's association with the divine. In Greek myth it is the deceptive gift of the gods. In the Judeo-Christian tradition, it is again bestowed by God, carrying with it the promise of a redemptive future, through either the Messiah or the Second Coming. God will ultimately 'put things right' (Eliott 2005), not just for the individual but for the world as a whole. With the Enlightenment, both the hope and the promise become more secular; but the appeal of redemption does not fade. In secularity, it is not God who will ultimately put things right, but science, or philosophy, or revolution, or Rorty's 'solidarity'. In the 21st century, the religious and the secular currents co-exist, and they are sometimes brought into alignment (Lerner

2015). Hope, as an idea, still has a hold on the narrative imagination; and the hold is not yet broken.

Perhaps it's for this reason, then, that health professionals and academics use 'hope' in preference to less resonant terms. In disciplines whose remit is recovery and rehabilitation, the word has associations that amplify the significance of what can be achieved. Even in palliative care it seems to carry a promise of some kind. As Averill and Sundararajan (2005) suggest, 'hope is both a rhetorical device and a creative emotional experience … [it] is the art of self-persuasion' (127). In my terms, this is elliptical 'hope'; the 'hope' of exophoric reference; and 'creative emotional experience' is one of the main functions this use of 'hope' has. An understanding of 'hope' (mass noun) as rhetoric, rather than as the name of an 'inner something', would be a useful contribution, I think, to the discussion of hope in the health care literature.

Notes

1 I did, however, say something like this in Paley (2014).
2 Not all nurse authors fail to recognise the difference between ordinary uses of 'hope' and their own accounts of hope. Some, for example, are influenced by Gabriel Marcel, who distinguishes between ordinary hope and 'genuine' hope, the latter being a spiritual or quasi-religious resource: 'Hope consists in asserting that there is at the heart of being, beyond all data, beyond all inventories and calculations, a mysterious principle which is in connivance with me' (Marcel 1995: 28). This is clearly not how 'hope' is ordinarily used.
3 For the same reason, it will be equally difficult to achieve a consensus about what its 'attributes' or 'components' are. Eliott and Olver (2002) list the 'elements' of hope as specified by various authors. The list includes: confidence, spiritual beliefs, authentic caring, anticipation, relational thought process, risk, peace, temporality and future, determination to endure, light-heartedness, satisfaction with self, nursing actions and treatment, interconnectedness, uplifting memories, energy, goal-directed determination, planning of ways to meet goals. As Eliott and Olver observe, there 'appears to be no single feature all authors identify as intrinsic' (174). Again, this is puzzling if hope is a universal human phenomenon.
4 Childs (2014) points out that language acquisition researchers routinely use coding schemes, such as that developed by Bartsch and Wellman (1995), which distinguish between *genuine* uses of mental state terms and those that are merely *conversational*. The catch-22 here is that only those uses which can be interpreted as references to 'internal states' are counted as 'genuine'. This criterion is not based on any empirical evidence. It simply reflects the underlying assumption of the researchers: denoting inner states is what these terms do, so any other use can be discounted. Language acquisition researchers who do not share this assumption include Tomasello (2003), Carpendale and Lewis (2004) and Nelson (2009). All three draw explicitly on Wittgenstein.
5 Canfield (2004) is an illuminating essay on Wittgenstein's 'fight against the very idea' of the 'inner' (145). We habitually construe the distinction between physical objects and mental states as a distinction between the 'outer' and the 'inner', the latter pictured as a 'private space' which somehow resides inside us. It is this picture that Wittgenstein thinks we should let go of. *There is no 'inner'*. It's an idea most of us find very counterintuitive. Wittgenstein 'transforms mind-resident entities into aspects of behaviour or behaviour-in-a-context' (153).

6 Some authors have a neat way of getting round the fact that ordinary usage is inconsistent with their preferred account. They make a distinction between a 'higher-grade' form of hope – *true* hope, *genuine* hope, *real* hope, hope in the *fullest sense* – and a 'lower-grade' form, which is less interesting. Ordinary usage is 'lower-grade', so its lack of fit with *genuine* hope isn't relevant. Several writers make this kind of distinction, though in different ways. Marcel (1995), Pettit (2004) and Martin (2014) are examples.

7 Hymers (2017: 11) makes a similar point. Wittgenstein encourages us to be explicit about new ways of speaking, 'so that we do not confuse our new way of speaking with our old'.

8 This is one reason why Snyder's critics have suggested that his theory is better understood not as a theory of hope but as a theory of tenacity or optimism. Both are traits, or dispositions, that can be generalised over particular projects and circumstances. The object-of-a-hope is what individuates it, but tenacity and optimism can be identified and measured without reference to any specific object at all. See Section 11.7.2.

9 The distinction between 'particularized' and 'generalized' hope can be read as another example of what Wittgenstein calls a 'grammatical remark' (Section 6.4). It is a reference to the difference between verb and count noun on the one hand ('particularized'), and mass noun on the other ('generalized'). Of course, Dufault and Martocchio don't understand it this way.

10 As Callina et al. (2018) note, 'several authors have used "optimism" and "hope" interchangeably'. Others insist that they are distinct (Rand 2015, Bury et al. 2019).

11 These are examples from the nursing literature. However, the association of hope with expectation in the psychology literature goes back at least as far as Stotland (1969). It is now so well established that Snyder et al. (2018: 12) can observe: 'Scholars widely agree that hope involves positive expectations for the future'. Widely, but not universally: see Note 13 below.

12 The statement 'You hope for outcomes you would welcome' is another grammatical remark (Section 6.4).

13 This is not a new point. The difference between 'hope' and 'expectation' has been recognised in the health care literature – for example, by Janzen et al. (2006) and Leung et al. (2009). Psychologists who take a similar view include Montgomery et al. (2003), and Miceli and Castelfranchi (2010).

14 Some readers might object that, although ambition or optimism could be described as a 'life force', intention can't plausibly be described in the same way. The objection has no traction. Given that Dufault and Martocchio haven't explained what they think a 'life force' is (Section 11.6.1), we are in no position to say that (for example) 'optimism' is a life force, but 'intention' isn't.

15 The Herth scales are copyrighted. Permission to use them, or quote from them, must be sought from Dr Herth at Minnesota State University.

16 This is a version of 'higher-grade hope', referred to in Note 6.

17 As in Section 8.2.1, I am changing 'p' (in Day's original definition) to 'X'. See Chapter 8, Note 8.

18 So, in philosophy, the analysis is based on 'A hopes that X'. But why that use in particular? Why not: 'A has no hope of X-ing'? Or 'Is there any hope of Y?' Or 'A managed to do Z, I hope'? Why not any of the other uses I've considered in Chapters 8–10? Why is the analysis of hope confined to the narrow defile of 'A hopes that X'? Isn't this use – verb, positive, indicative, third person, present, followed by a noun clause – just an arbitrary point in the whole complex pattern? Why is *that* the benchmark for the entire analysis? Even if you're happy to focus on the present indicative, why the third person? COCA indicates that first person singular (simple present) uses of 'hope' are vastly more common than third person uses. So why do philosophers not analyse 'I hope that X' or 'I hope to Y'? If you're inclined to think it doesn't matter because the pattern of use will be the same – how do you know?

19 A further question is: what evidence is there to support the claim that fostering hope has good health-related outcomes? I don't have the space to deal adequately with this question, but it will become clear that, again, there is no blanket answer. However, see Lipscomb (2007) for comments on some familiar assumptions in the nursing literature.
20 Compare Kleinman's (1988) description of the process of 'kindling hope' as 'remoralization'.

References

Aspinwall, L. G., & Leaf, S. L. (2002). In search of the unique aspects of hope: Pinning our hopes on positive emotions, future-oriented thinking, hard times, and other people. *Psychological Inquiry, 13*(4), 276–321.

Averill, J. R., & Sundararajan, L. (2005). Hope as rhetoric: Cultural narratives of wishing and coping. In J. Eliott (Ed.), *Interdisciplinary Perspectives on Hope* (pp. 127–159). New York: Nova Science Publishers.

Aylott, S. (1998). When hope becomes hopelessness. *European Journal of Oncology Nursing, 2*(4), 231–234.

Ballard, A., Green, T., McCaa, A., & Logsdon, M. C. (1997). A comparison of the level of hope in patients with newly diagnosed and recurrent cancer. *Oncology Nursing Forum, 24*, 899–904.

Bartsch, K., & Wellman, H. M. (1995). *Children Talk about the Mind.* Oxford: Oxford University Press.

Begley, A., & Blackwood, B. (2000). Truth-telling versus hope: A dilemma in practice. *International Journal of Nursing Practice, 6*, 26–31.

Belchamber, C., Gousy, M., & Ellis-Hill, C. (2013). Fostering hope through palliative rehabilitation. *European Journal of Palliative care, 20*(3), 136–139.

Benzein, E., Norberg, A., & Saveman, B.-I. (2001). The meaning of the lived experience of hope in patients with cancer in palliative home care. *Palliative Medicine, 15*(2), 117–126.

Benzein, E., & Saveman, B.-i. (1998). One step towards the understanding of hope: a concept analysis. *International Journal of Nursing Studies, 35*(6), 322–329.

Berendes, D., Keefe, F. J., Somers, T. J., Kothadia, S. M., & Porter, L. S. (2010). Hope in the context of lung cancer: Relationships of hope to symptoms and psychological distress. *Journal of Pain and Symptom Management, 40*(2), 174–182.

Bovens, L. (1999). The value of hope. *Philosophy and Phenomenological Research, 59*(3), 667–681.

Buckley, J., & Herth, K. (2004). Fostering hope in terminally ill patients. *Nursing Standard, 19*(10), 33–41.

Bury, S. M., Wenzel, M., & Woodyatt, L. (2019). Confusing hope and optimism when prospects are good: A matter of language pragmatics or conceptual equivalence? *Motivation and Emotion, 43*, 483–492.

Byrnes, M., Beilby, J., Ray, P., McLennan, R., Ker, J., & Schug, S. (2012). Patient-focused goal planning process and outcome after spinal cord injury rehabilitation: quantitative and qualitative audit. *Clinical Rehabilitation, 26*(12), 1141–1149.

Callina, K. S., Mueller, M. K., Buckingham, M. H., & Gutierrez, A. S. (2015). Building hope for positive development: research, practice and policy. In E. P. Bowers, G. J. Geldhof, S. K. Johnson, L. J. Hilliard, R. M. Hershberg, J. V. Lerner, & R. M. Lerner (Eds.), *Promoting Positive Youth Development: Lessons Learned from the 4-H Study* (pp. 71–94). New York: Springer.

Callina, K. S., Snow, N., & Murray, E. D. (2018). The history of philosophical and psychological perspectives on hope: towards defining hope for the science of positive human development. In M. W. Gallagher & S. J. Lopez (Eds.), *The Oxford Handbook of Hope* (pp. 9–25). Oxford: Oxford University Press.

Canfield, J. V. (2004). Pretence and the inner. In D. Moyal-Sharrock (Ed.), *The Third Wittgenstein* (pp. 145–158). Abingdon, UK: Routledge.

Carpendale, J. I. M., & Lewis, C. (2004). Constructing an understanding of the mind: The development of children's social understanding within social interaction. *Behavioral and Brain Sciences, 27*, 79–96.

Childs, C. (2014). From reading minds to social interaction: respecifying theory of mind. *Human Studies, 37*, 103–122.

Cutcliffe, J. R., & Herth, K. (2002). The concept of hope in nursing 1: its origins background and nature. *British Journal of Nursing, 11*(12), 832–840.

Day, J. P. (1969). Hope. *American Philosophical Quarterly, 6*(2), 89–102.

De Ridder, D., Schreurs, K., & Bensing, J. (2000). The relative benefits of being optimistic: Optimism as a coping resource in multiple sclerosis and Parkinson's disease. *British Journal of Health Psychology, 5*, 141–155.

Downie, R. S. (1963). Hope. *Philosophy and Phenomenological Research, 24*(2), 248–251.

Dufault, K., & Martocchio, B. C. (1985). Hope: its spheres and dimensions. *Nursing Clinics of North America, 20*(2), 379–391.

Duggleby, W., Hicks, D., Nekolaichuk, C., Holtslander, L., Williams, A., Chambers, T., & Eby, J. (2012). Hope, older adults, and chronic illness: a metasynthesis of qualitative research. *Journal of Advanced Nursing, 68*(6), 1211–1223.

Duggleby, W., Holtslander, L., Kylma, J., Duncan, V., Hammond, C., & Williams, A. (2010). Metasynthesis of the hope experience of family caregivers of persons with chronic illness. *Qualitative Health Research, 20*(2), 148–158.

Eliott, J. A. (2005). What have we done with hope? A brief history. In J. A. Eliott (Ed.), *Interdisciplinary Perspectives on Hope* (pp. 3–45). New York: Nova Science Publishers.

Eliott, J. A. (2012). Hope. In M. Cobb, C. M. Puchalski, & B. Rumbold (Eds.), *Oxford Textbook of Spirituality in Healthcare* (pp. 119–126). Oxford: Oxford University Press.

Eliott, J. A., & Olver, I. (2002). The discursive properties of "hope": A qualitative analysis of cancer patients' speech. *Qualitative Health Research, 12*, 173–193.

Folkman, S. (2010). Stress, coping, and hope. *Psycho-Oncology, 19*, 901–908.

Fromm, E. (1968). *The Revolution of Hope: Toward a Humanized Technology*. New York: Harper and Row.

Hernandez, S. C., & Overholser, J. C. (2020). A systematic review of interventions for hope/hopelessness in older adults. *Clinical Gerontologist*. doi: 10.1080/07317115.07 312019.01711281.

Herrestad, H., Biong, S., McCormack, B., & Borg, M. (2014). A pragmatist approach to the hope discourse in health care research. *Nursing Philosophy, 15*(3), 211–220.

Herth, K. (1990). Fostering hope in terminally ill people. *Journal of Advanced Nursing, 15*, 1250–1259.

Herth, K. (1991). Develpment and refinement of an instrument to measure hope. *Scholarly Inquiry for Nursing Practice, 5*(1), 39–51.

Herth, K. (1992). Abbreviated instrument to measure hope: Development and psychiatric evaluation. *Journal of Advanced Nursing, 17*(10), 1251–1259.

Hymers, M. (2017). *Wittgenstein on Sensation and Perception*. New York: Routledge.

Janzen, J. A., Silvius, J., Jacobs, S., Slaughter, S., Dalziel, W., & Drummond, N. (2006). What is a health expectation? Developing a pragmatic conceptual model from psychological theory. *Health Expectations, 9*, 37–48.

Kleinman, A. (1988). *The Illness Narratives: Suffering, Healing and the Human Condition.* New York: Basic Books.

Kuusela, O. (2013). Wittgenstein's method of conceptual investigation and concept formation in psychology. In T. P. Racine & K. L. Slaney (Eds.), *A Wittgensteinian Perspective on the Use of Conceptual Analysis in Psychology* (pp. 51–71). Basingstoke, UK: Palgrave Macmillan.

Kylmä, J., & Vehviläinen-Julkunen, K. (1997). Hope in nursing reseearch: a meta-analysis of the ontological and epistemological foundations of research on hope. *Journal of Advanced Nursing, 25*(2), 364–371.

Laskiwski, S., & Morse, J. M. (1993). The spinal cord injured patient: The modification of hope and expressions of despair. *Canadian Journal of Rehabilitation, 6*(3), 143–153.

Lebacqz, K. (1985). The virtuous patient. In E. E. Shelp (Ed.), *Virtue and Medicine* (pp. 275–288). Berlin: Springer.

Lerner, A. (2015). *Redemptive Hope: From the Age of Enlightenment to the Age of Obama.* New York: Fordham University press.

Lester, P. A. (2011). What to hope for? *Journal of Palliative Medicine, 14*(6), 786–787.

Leung, K. K., Silvius, J. L., Pimlott, N., Dalziel, W., & Drummond, N. (2009). Why health expectations and hopes are different: the development of a conceptual model. *Health Expectations, 12*, 347–360.

Lipscomb, M. (2007). Maintaining patient hopefulness: a critique. *Nursing Inquiry, 14*(4), 335–342.

Marcel, G. (1995). *The Philosophy of Existentialism.* New York: Citadel.

Martin, A. M. (2014). *How We Hope: A Moral Psychology.* Princeton, NJ: Princeton University Press.

Meirav, A. (2009). The nature of hope. *Ratio, 22*(2), 216–233.

Menninger, K. (1959). The academic lecture: Hope. *The American Journal of Psychiatry, 116*, 481–491.

Meyns, P., de Mettelinge, T. R., van der Spank, J., Couseens, M., & Van Waelvelde, H. (2017). Motivation in pediatric motor rehabilitation: A systematic search of the literature using the self-determination theory as a conceptual framework. *Developmental Neurorehabilitation, 21*(6), 371–390.

Miceli, M., & Castelfranchi, C. (2010). Hope: The power of wish and possibility. *Theory and Psychology, 20*(2), 251–276.

Mikkelsen, N., Dall, C., Holdgaard, A., Frederiksen, M., Rasmusen, H., & Prescott, E. (2019). Motivation for physical activity predicts effect of cardiac rehabilitation in an elderly cardiac population. *European Heart Journal, 40*(Supplement 1). doi: 10.1093/eurheartj/ehz1747.0242.

Miller, J. F. (2007). Hope: a construct central to nursing. *Nursing Forum, 42*(1), 12–19.

Montgomery, D. E. (2017). The meaning of *hope*: Developmental origins in early childhood. *Human Development, 60*, 239–261.

Montgomery, G. H., David, D., DiLorenzo, T., & Erblich, J. (2003). Is hoping the same as expecting? Discrimination between hopes and response expectancies for nonvolitional outcomes. *Personal and Individual Differences, 35*(2), 399–409.

Morse, J. M. (2017). *Analyzing and Conceptualizing the Theoretical Foundations of Nursing.* New York: Springer.

Morse, J. M., & Doberneck, B. (1995). Delineating the concept of hope. *Image: Journal of Nursing Scholarship, 27*, 277–285.

Nelson, K. (2009). Wittgenstein and contemporary theories of word learning. *New Ideas in Psychology, 27*, 275–287.

Paley, J. (2014). Hope, positive illusions and palliative rehabilitation. *Progress in Palliative Care, 22*, 358–362.

Parker-Oliver, D. (2002). Redefining hope for the terminally ill. *American Journal of Hospice & Palliative Care, 19*(2), 115–120.

Penz, K. (2008). Theories of hope: are they relevant for palliative care nurses and their practice? *International Journal of Palliative Nursing, 14*(8), 408–412.

Pettit, P. (2004). Hope and its place in mind. *The Annals of the American Academy of Political and Social Science, 592*(1), 152–165.

Picha, K. J., & Howell, D. M. (2018). A model to increase rehabilitation adherence to home exercise programmes in patients with varying levels of self-efficacy. *Musculoskeletal Care, 16*(1), 233–237.

Rand, K. L. (2015). Hope, self-efficacy, and optimism: conceptual and empirical differences. In E. P. Bowers, G. J. Geldhof, S. K. Johnson, L. J. Hilliard, R. M. Hershberg, J. V. Lerner, & R. M. Lerner (Eds.), *Promoting Positive Youth Development: Lessons Learned From the 4-H Study* (pp. 45–58). New York: Springer.

Read, R. (2014). Ordinary/everyday language. In K. D. Jolley (Ed.), *Wittgenstein: Key Concepts* (pp. 63–80). Abingdon, UK: Routledge.

Rose, S., & Sieben, N. (2018). Hope measurement. In M. W. Gallagher & S. J. Lopez (Eds.), *The Oxford Handbook of Hope* (pp. 83–93). Oxford: Oxford University Press.

Scheier, M. F., & Carver, C. S. (1985). Optimism, coping, and health: Assessment and implications of generalized outcome expectancies. *Health Psychology, 55*, 169–210.

Schneider, J. S. (1980). Hopelessness and helplessness. *Journal of Psychiatric Nursing and Mental Health Services, 18*(3), 12–21.

Schwarzer, R. (1994). Optimism, vulnerability, and self-beliefs as health-related cognitions: A systematic overview. *Psychology and Health, 9*, 161–180.

Scioli, A., Ricci, M., Nyugen, T., & Scioli, E. R. (2011). Hope: Its nature and measurement. *Psychology of Religion and Spirituality, 3*(2), 78–97.

Snyder, C. R. (1995). Conceptualizing, measuring, and nurturing hope. *Journal of Counselling and Development, 73*, 379–391.

Snyder, C. R., Irving, L., & Anderson, J. R. (1991). Hope and health: measuring the will and the ways. In C. R. Snyder & D. R. Forsyth (Eds.), *Handbook of Social and Clinical Psychology: The Health Perspective* (pp. 285–305). Elmsford, NY: Pergamon.

Snyder, C. R., Rand, K. L., & Sigmon, D. R. (2018). Hope theory: a member of the positive psychology family. In M. W. Gallagher & S. J. Lopez (Eds.), *The Oxford Handbook of Hope* (pp. 27–43). Oxford: Oxford University Press.

Stotland, E. (1969). *The Psychology of Hope: An Integration of Experimental, Clinical, and Social Approaches*. San Francisco, CA: Jossey-Bass.

Taylor, S. E. (1989). *Positive Illusions: Creative Self-Deception and the Healthy Mind*. New York: Basic Books.

Taylor, S. E. (2011). Positive illusions: how ordinary people become extraordinary. In M. A. Gernsbacher, R. W. Pew, L. M. Hough, & J. R. Pomerantz (Eds.), *Psychology and the Real World: Essays Illustrating Fundamental Contributions to Society* (pp. 224–228). New York: Worth Publishers.

Tennen, H., Affleck, G., & Tennen, R. (2002). Clipped feathers: The theory and measurement of hope. *Psychological Inquiry, 13*(4), 311–317.

Ter Hark, M. (2000). Uncertainty, vagueness and psychological indeterminacy. *Synthese, 124*(2), 193–220.

Tomasello, M. (2003). *Constructing a Language: A Usage-Based Theory of Language Acquisition*. Cambridge, MA: Harvard University Press.

Webb, D. (2010). Paulo Freire and 'the need for a kind of education in hope'. *Cambridge Journal of Education*, *40*(4), 327–339.

Wiles, R., Cott, C., & Gibson, B. E. (2008). Hope, expectations and recovery from illness: a narrative synthesis of qualitative research. *Journal of Advanced Nursing*, *64*(6), 564–573.

Witherspoon, E. (2000). Conceptions of nonsense in Carnap and Wittgenstein. In A. Crary & R. Read (Eds.), *The New Wittgenstein* (pp. 315–350). London: Routledge.

Wittgenstein, L. (1963). *Philosophical Investigations*. Oxford: Basil Blackwell.

12 'Moral distress'

The last four chapters have explored the pattern of use associated with an ordinary word. 'Hope' occurs frequently in everyday conversation (where it performs a range of different tasks), but it has also been appropriated by health care writers, and given jobs other than the ones it has in colloquial discourse. In this chapter, I turn to a different kind of expression, one which was coined in the recent past, and which does not occur in everyday conversation. 'Moral' and 'distress' are, of course, familiar terms when they are considered individually; but the expression 'moral distress' was coined as recently as 1984.[1] It was taken up enthusiastically by the academic nursing community, and has subsequently become a topic in the health care literature more generally.

With 'moral distress', then, there is no pattern of ordinary use we can explore. What there is instead is a trajectory of academic discourse extending (so far) over 35 years; and the most noticeable feature of that discourse is the fact that it is a history of 'definitions'. In this chapter, I propose to trace that history, and (first) exhibit the logical schema these definitions conform to, and (second) make a proposal about what it is they achieve. This achievement, I will suggest, is not to determine what moral distress essentially *is*, but to bolster a narrative concerning nursing's identity.

12.1 Jameton's distinction

'Moral distress arises when one knows the right thing to do, but institutional constraints make it nearly impossible to pursue the right course of action' (Jameton 1984: 6). It is noticeable that, in this original formulation – but also in his later work – Jameton does not use the word 'define'. Instead, he describes himself as 'characterizing' moral distress. It's equally noticeable that he says very little about emotional responses to the kind of situation he outlines, and makes no attempt to unpack the 'distress' part of the expression in terms of 'negative feeling states' and 'pain'. He is not concerned with the 'necessary and sufficient conditions' of moral distress (unlike, say, Morley et al. 2019); nor does he emphasise the suffering that moral distress can cause (unlike Corley 2002, and most subsequent authors).

His primary aim is to distinguish between three kinds of morally difficult situation. The paragraph which introduces moral distress begins like this: 'Moral and ethical problems in the hospital can be sorted into three different types' (Jameton 1984: 6). The types in question are: moral uncertainty, moral dilemmas and moral distress.

It is clear from this sentence, and from the rest of his discussion, that he regards these as three types of *problem*. He does not think that one of them (moral distress) is an emotional response. If he did think that, he would have made a very strange distinction – between, on the one hand, two types of problem, and, on the other, a psychological state. He would not be comparing like with like. Saying:

Moral and ethical problems in the hospital can be sorted into three different types: moral uncertainty, moral dilemmas, and moral distress.

would be rather like saying:

Stage performances can be sorted into three different types: drama, opera and applause.

or:

Books can be sorted into three different types: fiction, non-fiction and reading.

This is clearly not what he had in mind. Instead, he describes three different kinds of *situation*. In the first, there is a sense that something is wrong, but it is not clear what moral principles, if any, should be applied, or whether any particular principle has been violated. This is moral uncertainty. In the second, there is a conflict between two moral principles, each of which is compelling; but in the given situation, acting in accordance with one would mean violating the other. This is a moral dilemma. In the third, it is clear what moral principle should be applied, and equally clear that it is being violated; but institutional constraints make it almost impossible to pursue the right course of action. This is moral distress.

In his subsequent writing, Jameton focused on the difference between moral dilemma and moral distress. During the 1970s, he says (2013), philosophers in bioethics based their teaching on 'ethical dilemmas'. They used 'case studies that stimulated exploring direct conflicts among basic theoretical principles' (298). This approach was not a good match, Jameton suggests, for the experience of nurses, who were more concerned with the fact that their moral principles were being violated, and the difficulty most of them had in expressing their views, given the distribution of power in hospitals. So instead of analysing moral dilemmas in terms of philosophical theories, Jameton encouraged the discussion of situations in which the nurse's moral judgment clashed with institutional and professional structures.

In his 2013 paper, then, Jameton is making a distinction between two different kinds of moral conflict:

- First, how do we (anyone) resolve a conflict between opposing, but equally compelling, moral principles? This type of conflict is a moral dilemma.

- Second, how do we (nurses) resolve conflicts between what the nurse thinks is right and what institutional structures and protocols permit? This type of conflict is moral distress.

There is a case for saying that the expression 'moral distress' was not well chosen, and that it has led to many articles in the nursing literature disappearing down a definitional rabbit hole. I will say more about that later. For now, I would like to be clear about two things. First, Jameton is not defining anything. He is merely distinguishing between two types of moral problem, two types of moral conflict. Second, the word 'distress' in 'moral distress' does not refer to any particular emotion, or to emotional responses in general. Both these points need further elaboration in the light of possible objections.

First point. Jameton is drawing attention to the differences between two types of moral conflict. Now, it might be assumed that, in order to do this, he has to be able to *define* one or both types of conflict. But in fact this is not the case. Drawing attention to the difference between things does not necessarily require definition. In order to distinguish between apples and oranges, for example, I don't need to define either 'apple' or 'orange'. I can just point out that they look different and taste different. I don't need to specify the necessary and sufficient conditions of being an apple, or the necessary and sufficient conditions of being an orange, in order to say: 'Look, I think we can distinguish between apples and oranges'.[2] It's the same with Jameton. He draws attention to two types of moral problem. He does not define either; nor does he attempt to specify their necessary and sufficient conditions.

Second point. The word 'distress' in 'moral distress' does not refer to any particular emotion, or to any psychological state. Jameton is obviously aware that nurses confronted with conflicts between what they believe is right and constraints that prevent them from acting on that belief might experience frustration, anger, disgust, despair and so on. But this is not, for him, the central point. It is tempting to think that:

- 'moral distress' is like 'emotional distress'.

In which case, we are likely to imagine that some kind of feeling – anger, anguish, pain – is an intrinsic part of what Jameton is referring to. It isn't. An alternative comparison would be:

- 'moral distress' is like 'financial distress'.

In this expression, very difficult circumstances are being referred to, but there is nothing which refers to someone experiencing 'painful feelings' or 'psychological disequilibrium'. No doubt people in 'financial distress' do *have* 'painful feelings'. But the expression itself does not refer to those feelings. In a similar way, people who have a 'broken leg' no doubt experience pain. But the expression does not refer to *that*. It merely refers to the fact that the leg is broken.

Other 'distress' expressions that do not have feelings or sensations 'built into' them include: 'economic distress', 'pecuniary distress', 'respiratory distress', 'agricultural distress', 'ship in distress' and 'damsel in distress'. In all these examples, 'distress' has the sense of 'calamity; misfortune; peril; difficulty' (to quote *Chambers*). As with financial distress, the conditions in question presumably do have emotional consequences. But these consequences are not themselves referred to in the expression, any more than pain is referred to in the phrase 'broken leg'. We should not imagine that the emotional *consequences* of the situation referred to in the expression 'damsel in distress' – the damsel's fear, for example – are part of what the expression is *referring* to. Similarly, the consequences of an unexpected defeat may well be disappointment. But disappointment is not part of what the phrase 'unexpected defeat' actually means.

In summary, Jameton is interested in a particular type of moral conflict, one which is different from the traditional 'dilemmas' in which abstract ethical principles clash. His concerns are ethical and practical: 'How can we *resolve situations* of moral distress?' They are not conceptual or linguistic: 'How do we *define* moral distress or "moral distress"?'

12.2 Wilkinson's definition

So Jameton draws attention to a distinction between 'moral dilemmas' and 'moral distress'. At this stage (1984), he does not define either, and does not claim to. However, the nursing literature has a particular attraction to definitions. Three years after Jameton's book was published, a definition was attributed to him by Wilkinson (1987); and, since then, definitions have appeared at regular intervals. Morley et al. (2019) found 20 'key definitions' in the 34 articles they included in a narrative synthesis. They ended their own paper by proposing another one.

I would argue that Wilkinson, not Jameton, is the inventor of the current concept of moral distress. Her 1987 paper makes three key moves. First, it defines moral distress as '*psychological disequilibrium and negative feeling state* experienced when a person makes a moral decision but does not follow through by performing the moral behavior indicated by that decision'. In other words, it defines moral distress as a psychological state, not as a sort of problem/situation. Second, it omits from this definition any reference to *constraints* (although Wilkinson does refer to constraint elsewhere in the article). Third, it refers to 'moral distress *as defined by Jameton*', implying that his 'characterisation' was in fact a definition, or intended as a definition (italics mine). Let's see why these three moves are so important.

First move. Wilkinson's definition puts psychological states centre stage. For Jameton, 'moral distress' is a type of ethically difficult *situation*. For Wilkinson it is a *state of mind*, a subjective experience. This state of mind may be caused by 'situational constraints', but 'psychological disequilibrium and negative feeling state' is what moral distress *is*. There are other modifications, of course; but it is this shift – from moral distress as a type of situation, to moral distress as a state of mind – that marks Wilkinson, not Jameton, as the person who is largely responsible for the current concept of moral distress.

The significance of the shift is as follows. If moral distress is a state of mind, involving 'negative feeling states', then it becomes possible to suggest that these states might be caused by situations other than the one described by Jameton. Crudely, if moral distress is a psychological reaction, we can ask what other situations cause it. On Jameton's account, this question makes no sense because, for him, moral distress is a certain type of *situation*. But if moral distress is 'psychological disequilibrium' or a 'negative feeling state', then the question will be asked: 'Don't other situations cause the same, or very similar, states of mind? Don't people experience disequilibrium and negative feelings in response to other kinds of moral predicament as well?'

Subsequent contributions take up this question. Indeed, the history of moral distress definitions is, in part, the history of writers identifying further sets of (morally inflected) circumstances that precipitate distress, and arguing that the concept should apply to them too. This is why some authors, especially in recent years, complain that Jameton's definition – or perhaps any definition that precedes their own – is 'too narrow' (Fourie 2015, Campbell et al. 2016, Morley et al. 2019).

Second move. Wilkinson's definition leaves out Jameton's reference to institutional constraints. Moral distress is a psychological reaction that occurs when somebody does not 'follow through' on a moral decision she has made. The definition does not specify any particular circumstances that might explain why this 'following through' does not take place. Jameton gave us 'moral judgment plus constraint'. Wilkinson gives us 'moral decision plus not acting on it'. The effect of this change is to set a precedent. It erects a sign marked: 'Queue here if you have any suggestions to make about why nurses sometimes don't act on their moral decisions'.

It is true that Wilkinson does talk about constraints in the rest of the article; but it is interesting that her definition does not include any mention of them. I'm not entirely sure what accounts for this omission, and the author herself makes no attempt to explain it. However, the precedent set by the non-constraint definition was one which, as we'll see in a moment, subsequent authors were quick to follow, especially following an influential essay by Webster and Bayliss (2000).

The first move and the second move are linked. Defining moral distress as a state of mind means that we can ask what other situations might cause it. Omitting constraints from the definition says: 'those other situations don't have to be constraints'. This gives the green light to anyone who wants to include non-constraining circumstances in the list of possible causes. Later writers have accepted this invitation. For example, Campbell et al. (2016: 6) suggest that

> it is possible for one to feel morally compromised or tainted even in cases where one is not constrained and one successfully performs what one judges to be the morally best action … Yet their actions, in conjunction with factors beyond their control, turn out to have morally undesirable consequences. This can lead to feelings of distress.

This illustrates the way in which, following Wilkinson's definition, it is possible to propose no-constraint circumstances as causes of the 'negative-feeling state'.

Third move. Wilkinson's paper attributes a definition to Jameton. She does not claim that his 'definition' resembles her own; but her first page quotes Jameton, and the quotation is immediately followed by her own definition. The association has proved too strong to resist, and several subsequent authors attribute Wilkinson's definition to Jameton. Perhaps the most significant example is Corley (1995), who suggests that:

> Jameton defined moral distress as painful feelings and/or psychological dis-equilibrium caused by a situation in which (1) one believes one knows the ethically ideal action to take and (2) that one cannot carry out that action because of (3) institutionalized obstacles.

This is basically a mash-up of Jameton's characterisation and Wilkinson's definition. The claim, in essentials, is repeated in Corley et al. (2001) and Corley et al. (2005). Other authors assume that Jameton *did* intend to define moral distress, but they do not necessarily attribute Wilkinson's definition to him.

The significance of the third move is as follows. In attributing a definition to Jameton, and in suggesting one of her own, Wilkinson is creating a precedent. She is, in effect, pointing to a certain kind of project: that of defining moral distress. It is a project which the nursing literature has taken up enthusiastically, in a manner to be sketched in the next section, pursuing a trajectory which culminates, as we shall see, in the three papers by Fourie (2015), Campbell et al. (2016) and Morley et al. (2019).

In other respects, however, the third move is no more than a footnote to the main business, which is: (a) defining moral distress as a psychological state; in doing so (b) making it possible to identify situations other than the one described by Jameton as causes of moral distress, including (c) situations that involve no constraint at all. While not exactly setting an agenda, Wilkinson's definition is an invitation to extend – even greatly extend – the range of situations that can be said to cause moral distress, and to diversify and/or intensify the range of psychological states that can be classified in this way.

12.3 The definitional schema

In effect, Wilkinson (1987) created what I will call a 'definitional schema' for moral distress. It consists of two definitional slots: the 'state of mind' slot, and the 'precipitating circumstances' slot. The schema can be pictured like this:

Moral distress is < *state of mind* > caused by < *precipitating circumstances* >.

The nursing literature after 1987 is based on this schema – or so I will argue – with subsequent authors making various proposals about what should go in the two slots. I will also suggest that, in each slot, there has been a discernible trend over time. In the 'precipitating circumstances' slot, the trend has been to extend – and, recently, vastly extend – the range of situations said to cause moral distress. In the 'state of mind' slot, a similar trend is visible, together with an 'intensifying' trend, by which writers propose increasingly 'intense' descriptions of the relevant state of mind.

In the initial stages of the latter trend, for example, 'negative feeling state' is superseded by 'painful feelings' (Corley 1995), which then gives way to 'suffering' (Corley 2002) and 'anguish' (Hanna 2004). To these psychological states, many subsequent authors add physical states. For example, Nathaniel's (2006: 421) definition begins: 'Moral distress is pain affecting the mind, the *body*, or relationships that results from a patient care situation in which...' (see, in addition, Lützén et al. 2003, Kopala & Burkhart 2005). A decade later, McCarthy and Gastmans (2015: 135) were able to observe that there is a 'general consensus ... that the term "moral distress" refers to the psychological-emotional-*physiological* suffering that nurses may experience when, constrained by circumstances, they participate in perceived wrongdoing by action or omission' (italics in this paragraph mine).

Another twist on the state-of-mind slot is the addition of moral harm to psychological harm (Liaschenko 1995). Moral harm is the 'loss of integrity in practice'. In introducing this idea, Liaschenko sets the stage for future developments portraying moral distress as intrinsically harmful, and prepares the ground for identifying moral distress with compromised integrity. A paper by Peter and Liaschenko (2004) continues this theme by depicting inadequate resources and terrible working conditions – examples, in Jameton's terms, of 'institutional constraints' – as an 'assault' on the nurse's 'moral integrity and values', with the risk that her moral values, moral integrity and moral identity will be thoroughly compromised. These two articles have been very influential and, as a consequence, the state-of-mind slot has become a state-of-the-person slot, incorporating both psychological and emotional suffering, physical health risks and seriously compromised moral integrity (Hamric 2014).

Meanwhile, the list of specific psychological states said to be implicated in moral distress has grown ever longer: anger, guilt, resentment, shame, embarrassment, depression, dread, anxiety, sadness, grief, frustration, disappointment, self-doubt, self-blame, reduced self-worth, psychological disequilibrium, psychological disorientation, powerlessness, hopelessness, interior aversion, feelings of being violated and so on. Almost any 'negative feeling state' (in Wilkinson's terms) is a candidate for inclusion.

If we turn now to the 'precipitating circumstances' slot, we find an expansion in the range of situations that may cause these 'feeling states' (and/or compromised moral integrity). Webster and Bayliss (2000), for example, recommend broadening the definition of moral distress in such a way that it includes, not only institutional constraints, but 'an error in judgment' or a 'personal failing' (these are often referred to now as 'internal constraints'). Hanna (2004) goes even further, suggesting that moral distress can be caused by 'facing a moral dilemma' and 'moral uncertainty', situations explicitly excluded by Jameton. The definition proposed by Kälvemark et al. (2004) is very similar: distress, according to this definition, can be caused by moral uncertainty and moral dilemma; 'constraints' are no longer a necessary feature of the precipitating circumstances.

More recent articles take the project of extending the range of 'precipitating circumstances' to its logical conclusion. Fourie (2015) argues that moral dilemma and moral distress are not mutually exclusive, so we should adopt a broader understanding of moral distress, according to which 'moral constraint is not a necessary condition'. Moral distress should therefore be defined as a 'psychological response to morally challenging situations'. Campbell et al. (2016) argue that there appears to be no principled reason why a definition of moral distress should exclude cases of moral uncertainty, 'mild distress', 'delayed distress', moral dilemma, 'bad moral luck' or 'distress by association'. On this basis, they propose that it should be defined as 'one or more negative self-directed emotions or attitudes that arise in response to one's perceived involvement in a situation that one perceives to be morally undesirable'. Morley et al. (2019: 660) also suggest that 'narrow conceptions' of moral distress should be superseded, as 'it seems obvious that any distress causally associated with a moral event … is ipso facto, MD'. Accordingly, they suggest that 'the combination of (1) the experience of a moral event, (2) the experience of "psychological distress" and (3) a direct causal relation between (1) and (2) together are necessary and sufficient conditions for moral distress'.

These three definitions are structurally almost identical:

- Psychological response to a morally challenging situation (Fourie).
- Negative emotions/attitudes in response to a morally undesirable situation (Campbell et al.).
- Psychological distress caused by experience of a moral event (Morley et al.).

Or, in a composite nutshell:

- (Negative) state of mind caused by (morally inflected) situation.

This is a classic of the craving for generality. All three definitions are designed to cover everything that has been inserted into Wilkinson's schema. Each author admits that 'further details are necessary', but each claims to have 'contributed to definitional and conceptual clarity' (Morley et al. 2019). I see it a bit differently. The definitions cover every precipitating circumstance and every state of mind; but for that very reason they cease to be of any use. The craving for generality results in something so distended that it can serve no useful purpose. Below, I will explain more fully why.

Before proceeding, however, I want to be clear. In claiming that the two slots in Wilkinson's schema have been constantly expanded, I am not arguing that the literature has 'got Jameton wrong', or that any of the contributors to that literature is in error. Nor am I arguing that this or that definition is preferable to all the others. I'm simply observing that the concept has developed in a particular way. Its evolution turns on the assumption that 'moral distress' names a certain kind of *experience*, which can be brought about by various situations; and the project has become one of identifying situations that give rise to it (to be placed, as it were, in Wilkinson's suggestions box). But what is the significance of all this?

12.4 An open-ended functional-normative classification

It is tempting to think of moral distress as 'a phenomenon' (for example: Epstein & Hamric 2009, Peter & Liaschenko 2013, Morley et al. 2019), but I think it is more helpful to think of 'moral distress' as a classification. To put it slightly differently: the expression 'moral distress' is used to depict a wide range of different types of situation as 'the same kind of thing'.

Any noun or noun phrase is used to refer to a group of objects, qualities, activities or abilities that are, in some sense, 'similar' or (colloquially) 'the same'. However, there are many different types of similarity. Physical similarity ('pebble'), taxonomic similarity ('tiger'), chemical similarity ('oxygen'), functional similarity ('furniture'), similarity based on forms of measurement ('pay increase'), relational similarity ('parent'), organisational similarity ('amateur dramatic society'), causal similarity ('narcotic'), similarity of location ('rock pool'), normative similarity ('generous gesture'), time structure similarity ('holiday') and many more.[3]

An important difference between these classifying terms concerns generalisations from one member (or one example) of the class to another. In particular, it concerns the extent to which such generalisations are secure or precarious. For instance, a generalisation from one sample of oxygen to another will, in the majority of cases, be secure. Both samples will behave in approximately the same way, given X, Y and Z conditions. Similarly for members of the class 'tiger', or 'pebble', or 'narcotic'. But generalisations about parents, items of furniture, holidays and generous gestures will be less secure. Parents do not all react in the same way to similar situations; you can sit on a chair, but not on a bookcase; one holiday may involve strenuous physical activity, another lying on a beach; one generous gesture means giving up your seat, another means giving up a large amount of money. Some generalisations about functional and normative classifications are, of course, possible; but they tend to be limited and not overly informative. Parents all have children; items of furniture can be found in homes; holidays involve time off work; and generous gestures mean doing something for someone. Like the 'composite nutshell' definition of moral distress, generalisations like these cover everything... but, in doing so, become information-depleted.

'Moral distress' is an open-ended functional-normative classification (open-ended in that new examples are still being added). Generalisation from one case to another is highly problematic. To illustrate this, consider some of the 'constraint' situations that have been proposed (I am setting aside non-constraint situations because the point can be made without them):

- Structural and economic constraints, such as understaffing
- Hospital policy and protocols
- Legal requirements
- Power of the medical profession
- Wishes of the patient's family
- Threats of physical violence or abuse, including those from patients
- Conflict of interests between patients, doctors, nurses, families
- Lack of supervisory support
- Personal failings, such as lack of resolve or an error in judgment

There are two ways of looking at this list. One is to say: 'They are all obstacles which make it difficult, or perhaps impossible, for the nurse to act in accordance with her moral judgment'. The other is to say: It is not clear why the reactions to such varied circumstances count as a single phenomenon. It is like suggesting that going for a walk, going on holiday, and popping out to the shops all count as examples of 'leaving the house', and that psychological reactions to these situations can be studied as examples of the same thing. I am not arguing that the first is wrong and the second is right. I am arguing that they are both legitimate ways of construing the same list.

To see why the second is legitimate, consider some of the generalisations that cannot be made from one category to another. The methods you adopt to correct lack of supervisory support will not help if you want to do something about understaffing; and the methods you adopt to improve staffing levels will not prevent conflicts with families who want 'everything done' for their loved ones, irrespective of whether (on the nurse's evaluation) this is in the patient's best interests. Finding ways to decrease the likelihood of errors in judgment will not lead to changes in the legislation or changes in the power gradient between nursing and medicine; nor will adopting measures to reduce the hegemony and/or indifference of doctors do anything to reduce the risk of abuse and violence from patients.

In a similar way, generalisations about the consequences of moral distress are unlikely to be replicable across different situations. For example, participating in unnecessary and aggressive treatment in critical care contexts may well lead to nurses leaving the job, or thinking about leaving (46%, according to one survey reported by Hamric and Blackhall 2007). However, it would be risky to assume that a comparable proportion of nurses in care homes would react in the same way to 'going along with relatives' wishes, even if I can tell that the client is not all that happy about this' (De Veer et al. 2013: 104). So generalisations such as the following one are incautious: 'An additional and dominant workplace consequence of moral distress is the issue of retention and staff shortages. Nurses not only think about leaving their current position but also consider leaving the nursing profession altogether' (Burston & Tuckett 2013: 319).

In this respect, one might suggest an analogy between moral distress and rashes. 'Rash' is not, in itself, a diagnosis. It is a symptom of many different conditions, including chronic dermatological problems, allergies, irritations caused by contact with various substances, infections – bacterial, viral, parasitic – and so on. Again, generalisations from one rash-inducing condition to another will tend to be insecure. The measures taken to treat a fungal infection will not be effective against eczema, for example. The implication of this (partial) analogy is that a response to moral distress should usually be focused more on the underlying pathology than on the distress itself. This is something which authors such as Austin (2012), Pauly et al. (2012), Varcoe et al. (2012) and Peter and Liaschenko (2013) fully appreciate.

It is the restricted ability to make causal generalisations from one case of moral distress to another – in contrast to generalisations from one sample of oxygen to another, or from one narcotic to another – that should make us wary of assuming that this is a single 'phenomenon' that can be 'defined'. Instead, we can think of 'moral distress' as a classification which, for reasons I will explore in a moment, groups together situations that resemble each other in one respect (situations giving rise to 'a negative feeling state'), but which are very different in other respects. In this sense, McCarthy and Deady (2008) are right to describe moral distress as an 'umbrella concept', though they did not comment on what underlies this metaphor: the precariousness of generalisations from one type of case to another.

12.5 Narrative transposition

I have referred to 'moral distress' as an open-ended functional-normative classification. In this section, I'll explain why. I should start by saying that, to some extent, all classifications are normative. Bowker and Star (1999) refer to 'the practical politics of classifying', and suggest that 'classification systems simultaneously represent the world "out there", the organizational context of their application ... and the political and social roots of that context' (Chapter 2). Schiappa (2003: 69) says: 'When are definitions political? Always'. Still, some classifications are more normative than others. 'Furniture', for example, is a functional-locational classification. It groups together items which are 'similar' in the sense that they are found in homes and offices, and have a particular kind of use. But it would be a bit of a stretch to say that the classification is 'normative' in any usual sense. In contrast, I will suggest that 'moral distress' is a functional and normative classification, with a specific (small-p) political twist in the tail.

What, then, is the function of the expression 'moral distress'? I suggest that it is discourse reframing or, putting it a somewhat different way, narrative transposition. It transposes a story about the problems of understaffing into a story about a virtuous moral agent being thwarted and, as a result, suffering. It transposes a story about the patient's family insisting that 'everything is done' for their loved one into a story about a virtuous moral agent being thwarted and, as a result, suffering. It transposes a story about doctors pursuing inappropriately aggressive treatment into a story about a virtuous moral agent being thwarted and, as a result, suffering. Schematically:

Political/economic issues	→	Virtuous moral agent thwarted, suffers
Clash of legitimate perspectives	→	Virtuous moral agent thwarted, suffers
Behaviour in organisations	→	Virtuous moral agent thwarted, suffers
Hospital policy and protocol	→	Virtuous moral agent thwarted, suffers

A series of very different narratives are transposed into a single type of narrative. Political discourse, economic discourse, organisational-behaviour discourse, personal failings discourse… all become a sort of Kryptonite discourse: the moral hero constrained, weakened, blocked and experiencing anguish.

The significance of the word 'transpose' in this discussion is the implied analogy with music. A piece of music can be transposed from one key to another. It's the same melody, but it is shifted from the key of C, say, to the key of G. Narrative transposition is a similar idea. The sequence of events remains more or less the same, but the recounting of the events is shifted from one narrative standpoint to another. For example, imagine a retelling of Hamlet from the viewpoint of Rosencrantz and Guildenstern (Stoppard 1973). Imagine a retelling of *Cinderella* from the viewpoint of Anna, one of the 'ugly sisters' (Campbell 2013), or *Snow White* told from the point of view of the Queen (Campbell 2014). The 'moral distress' transposition involves a retelling of stories about severely understaffed hospitals, insistent but possibly misguided families, and medical dominance in inter-professional relationships, from the standpoint of virtuous-but-defeated nurses.

The effect of this transposition is to elicit a different kind of response from the reader. Depending on the exact configuration of plot and character, a protagonist may elicit admiration, disapproval or sympathy (Paley & Eva 2005, Paley 2009). Stories in which the hero's virtue is rewarded invite admiration. Stories in which a central character suffers undeservedly invite sympathy. Stories which have an obvious villain invite disapproval or distaste. The 'moral distress' transposition converts a narrative about (for example) aggressive treatment of critical care patients into a narrative about suffering nurses. In doing so, it invites sympathy (for the nurse) rather than anger (on behalf of the patient). The emotional cadence (Velleman 2003) changes with the shift in narrative standpoint.

Let me illustrate this kind of transposition with an example from health care, but not nursing. Here is an extract from a newspaper article about the UK's 'hostile environment' policy, targeted at migrants, and its effects in schools, hospitals and homes. The article focuses on the way in which the NHS has become part of the 'hostile environment' front line, given that it is legally required to bill migrants, share data with the Home Office, and impose strict document checks in GP surgeries and hospitals (Usborne 2018).

Irial Eno, 28, a junior doctor in the West Midlands and part of *Docs Not Cops*, a group campaigning against the 'border in the NHS', says the hostile environment policies are 'a complete contradiction of everything we signed up to do'.

On most understandings of the expression, this is a clear example of 'moral distress': a conflict between the values of health care – 'everything we signed up to do' – and the institutional constraints imposed by UK law since 2014, compromising the professional integrity of health care staff (at least in Eno's view).

But imagine how the article would read if, instead, it told a moral distress story:

> Irial Eno, 28, a junior doctor in the West Midlands, says the hostile environment policies have led to doctors experiencing moral distress.

I cannot speak for anyone else, but my own reaction is something like this. The transposition changes my sense of the invited response to the story. Instead of anger and/or disgust at the NHS being co-opted into the government's 'hostile environment' policy, the narrative invites sympathy for doctors. Instead of migrants being represented as the targets of government policy, health care staff are represented as its victims. Instead of being about 'enforced NHS hostility to migrants', it's about 'suffering doctors'. If there were then to be a debate about how best to alleviate the doctors' distress, this would grotesquely miss the point, and trivialise an important political question. Dr Eno's membership of a campaigning group, *Docs Not Cops*, crystallises what is an intrinsically political issue. In contrast, the 'moral distress' version transposes the narrative in such a way that it is now 'all about the doctors', and in a way which, personally, I find a little distasteful. Some readers, of course, will have an entirely different reaction; but this is not a matter that is capable of proof or disproof. It is a question of using an object of comparison (in Wittgenstein's terms) to look at something from a slightly different angle.

12.6 Mandate and licence

The moral distress literature sometimes presents us with a choice. 'When we see moral distress as just an "individual's problem" we pathologize the individual ... This deflection away from organizational and systemic factors can camouflage the unethical features of organizational life' (Varcoe et al. 2012: 57). 'It is not the case that all nurses feel or perceive themselves to be powerless to act. Whether they do or not is very much a matter of personal character and aptitude, not "other" constraints' (Johnstone & Hutchinson 2015: 9). So Varcoe et al. focus on organisational/systemic factors; Johnstone and Hutchinson focus on an individual's character. Both agree that the concept of moral distress directs the attention to individual nurses, portraying them as moral agents, but constrained, powerless and suffering. However, Varcoe et al. argue that this deflects away from organisational structures, while Johnstone and Hutchinson argue that it deflects away from personal character and the capacity for self-assertion.

I think this dichotomy misses something potentially important. So in this section, I want to place 'moral distress' in the context of a tension between nursing's mandate and its licence (Dingwall & Allen 2001).

The narrative transposition represented by 'moral distress' reflects a wider discourse in which nursing's professional identity is constructed. In this respect, the 'moral distress' narrative can be read like this:

- It implicitly claims the moral high ground for nursing...
- ... portraying nurses as ethically sensitive agents...
- ... who are prevented from acting according to nursing values...
- ... with the consequence that they suffer moral and psychological harm...
- ... and so, to that extent, are victims...
- ... who should be listened to because, like patients, their stories of suffering need to be heard.

The possibility that moral distress discourse inclines towards a 'nurses as victims' perspective has been noted before (McCarthy & Deady 2008, Johnstone & Hutchinson 2015). Here, however, I want to focus on the idea of nurses as ethically aware agents intending to act on the basis of nursing values, and relate this idea to the concept of a mandate.

The distinction between mandate and licence is taken from the sociologist, Everett Hughes (1984). The *mandate* is the profession's chosen identity: the principles, culture and ideals which are promulgated, not only to the public and other professionals, but also to the profession's own members. In effect, it is a set of beguiling assertions which the profession makes about its contribution to society. The *licence*, on the other hand, represents the 'terms and conditions' on which members of the profession actually practise. It is an implied social contract which specifies what these practitioners are required to do in exchange for social and financial rewards. Importantly, mandate and licence do not always coincide. Indeed, the licence will almost invariably require practitioners – on some occasions – to undertake activities which threaten their occupational identity, creating a tension between the professional culture and institutional constraints. To some degree, this is endemic to any profession (Abbott 1988); but, as Allen (2004) notes, professional identities can sometimes be so divorced from reality that they might be termed pathological.

Dingwall and Allen (2001) claim that this is the situation in nursing, where the mismatch between licence and mandate has become a chronic source of dissatisfaction. The mandate still emphasises 'emotionally intimate therapeutic relationships with patients' (Allen 2004), an identity inherited from nurse theorists of the 1980s. However, this identity does not fit the role of nurses in modern health care structures. As a consequence, it creates 'exaggerated expectations' among its recruits, and 'fails to provide nurses with a knowledge base and a language with which to articulate what it is they do *in practice*' (Allen 2004: 279). So the mandate, and the theories which legitimate it, become 'a source of low morale and dissatisfaction'.

The discourse of moral distress – with its emphasis on nursing values, moral agency, psychological and moral harm, suffering nurses and compromised moral integrity as a result of institutional constraints – can be seen as a symptom of the tension between mandate and licence. It is like a flag, planted at some of the sensitive points where the mismatch is evident. This is a version of the idea that moral distress is an 'ethical canary' (Austin 2012, Varcoe et al. 2012). But whereas these authors see the discrepancy between mandate and licence as evidence that the licence is the problem, I'm arguing that we can see it as evidence that there may be something wrong with the mandate. Austin thinks that the *experience* of moral distress is an indication that 'the healthcare environment has become toxic'. I'm suggesting that the *discourse* of moral distress is an indication that, in some respects, nursing's mandate is (in Allen's terms) pathological, and a 'source of low morale and dissatisfaction'. On the first account, nurses-in-anguish show that the institution needs fixing. On the second, the discourse of moral distress shows that nursing's ideology might itself be part of the problem.

Let me illustrate this briefly. Allen suggests that the modern 'job description' of nursing includes '*inter alia* the requirement to reconcile the needs of individuals with the needs of the many; to balance the need for quality with the need for cost-effectiveness and efficiency; to mediate between standardisation and individualisation'. In 'moral distress' terms, however, standardisation, 'the needs of the many' and 'the need for cost-effectiveness and efficiency' would be classed as 'institutional constraints': structures and protocols which prevent nurses from doing 'the right thing' (that is, acting on nursing values). But if Allen is right, these 'constraints' are part of the weft and warp of contemporary nursing. They are not 'external' to 'what nurses do' (and so, potentially, obstacles to practice). They are an intrinsic feature of nursing work, one of the vectors by which practice is defined.

It may be objected, of course, that not all the suggested 'precipitating circumstances' fit Allen's account of the modern licence. True enough. But what motivates this objection is the 'craving for generality', the assumption that any observation, analogy or object of comparison must fit all cases. In making my own observations, I am drawing attention to what Wittgenstein (1963) called 'aspects'. Any one observation fits some cases, but not necessarily all. This does not prevent it from illuminating the cases it does apply to. In this context it doesn't prevent it from illuminating one aspect of 'moral distress' discourse. This is why I said earlier that the discourse of moral distress is an indication that, *in some respects*, nursing's mandate is a 'source of low morale and dissatisfaction'. It is also why I emphasised, in Section 12.4, that generalisations about moral distress are likely to be insecure. For the same reason, I acknowledge that, when we make the link to the mandate/ licence distinction, the 'rash' analogy breaks down. However, all analogies break down at some point. They throw light only on *some* aspects of the expression's use.

12.7 A compassion deficit?

So one final illustrative example. The Francis Report on the scandal at Mid Staffordshire Hospital in the UK (Francis 2013) is very clear that severe understaffing – 120 WTE nurses short of what was required, nearly 13% of the total nursing establishment – was a cause of the 'appalling care' at Mid Staffs. While many of the nurses at the hospital may have suffered distress, the focus of attention in the subsequent debate was on those whose response to the 'deplorable working conditions' was to develop a detached and dehumanising attitude towards patients. Received wisdom now has it that there was a 'compassion deficit' (Paley 2014) at Mid Staffs, and that the way to prevent something like this happening again is to 'embed compassionate care in both practice and pre-registration education' (MacArthur et al. 2017: 130).

However, if we interpret the Mid Staffs affair bearing in mind the mandate/licence distinction, we can suggest that there might be something a touch 'pathological' about an ideology that demands constant compassion from nurses who are run ragged by 13% understaffing, and who cope (in some cases) by switching off. Instead of examining the mandate for possible flaws, the standard academic response to the Mid Staffs affair was a retrenchment, accompanied by vitriol directed at the nurses whose reaction to the 'toxic' clinical environment did not (in compassion terms) measure up, and whose suffering did not take the officially approved form.

Notes

1 In fact, the expression 'moral distress' has been around much longer. One can find it in the early 19th century, according to *Google Books (Standard): American English*, an enormous corpus (155 billion words) hosted at Brigham Young University. Its original sense, however, was akin to 'moral depravity', although it could also refer to the various states occasioned by 'sin'. Later, it was used to designate the distress experienced by those whose attention was drawn to the dreadful conditions of other people. All this changed with Jameton's book. It would probably be impossible now to use the expression in its 19th- and early 20th-century senses, and still be understood.

2 See Section 7.4 on definitions, particularly Wittgenstein's remark: 'When I give the description "The ground was quite covered with plants" – do you want to say I don't know what I am talking about until I can give a definition of a plant?' (1963: §69). Similarly, if I distinguish between apples and oranges, do you want to say that I don't know what I'm talking about until I can give a definition of both?

3 For an interesting account of different types of similarity and classification, see Wierzbicka (1984).

References

Abbott, A. (1988). *The System of Professions: An Essay on the Division of Expert Labor*. Chicago, IL: University of Chicago Press.

Allen, D. (2004). Re-reading nursing and re-writing practice: Towards an empirically based reformulation of the nursing mandate. *Nursing Inquiry*, *11*(4), 271–283.

Austin, W. (2012). Moral distress and the contemporary plight of health professionals. *HEC Forum*, *24*(1), 27–38.

Bowker, G. C., & Star, S. L. (1999). *Sorting Things Out: Classification and Its Consequences*. Cambridge, MA: MIT Press.

Burston, A. S., & Tuckett, A. G. (2013). Moral distress in nursing: Contributing factors, outcomes and interventions. *Nursing Ethics, 20*, 312–324.

Campbell, J. (2013). *Cinderella Is Evil*. Kindle: Amazon Media.

Campbell, J. (2014). *Killing Snow White*. Kindle: Amazon Media.

Campbell, S. M., Ulrich, C. M., & Grady, C. (2016). A broader understanding of moral distress. *The American Journal of Bioethics, 16*(12), 2–9.

Corley, M. C. (1995). Moral distress of critical care nurses. *American Journal of Critical Care, 4*, 280–285.

Corley, M. C. (2002). Nurse moral distress: a proposed theory and research agenda. *Nursing Ethics, 9*(6), 636–650.

Corley, M. C., Elswick, R. K., Gorman, M., & Clor, T. (2001). Development and evaluation of a moral distress scale. *Journal of Advanced Nursing, 33*, 250–256.

Corley, M. C., Minick, P., Elswick, R. K., & Jacobs, M. (2005). Nurse moral distress and ethical work environment. *Nursing Ethics, 12*, 381–390.

De Veer, A. J., Francke, A. L., Struijs, A., & Willems, D. L. (2013). Determinants of moral distress in daily nursing practice: A cross sectional correlational questionnaire survey. *International Journal of Nursing Studies, 50*(1), 100–108.

Dingwall, R., & Allen, D. (2001). The implications of healthcare reforms for the profession of nursing. *Nursing Inquiry, 8*(2), 64–74.

Epstein, E. G., & Hamric, A. B. (2009). Moral distress, moral residue, and the crescendo effect. *Journal of Clinical Ethics, 20*(4), 330–342.

Fourie, C. (2015). Moral distress and moral conflict in clinical ethics. *Bioethics, 29*, 91–97.

Francis, R. (2013). *Report of the Mid Staffordshire NHS Foundation Trust Public Inquiry*. London: The Stationery Office.

Hamric, A. B. (2014). A case study of moral distress. *Journal of Hospice and Palliative Nursing, 16*(8), 457–463.

Hamric, A. B., & Blackhall, L. J. (2007). Nurse-physician perspectives on the care of dying patients in intensive care units: Collaboration, moral distress, and ethical climate. *Critical Care Medicine, 35*(2), 422–429.

Hanna, D. R. (2004). Moral distress: The state of the science. *Research and Theory for Nursing Practice: An International Journal, 18*, 73–93.

Hughes, E. C. (1984). *The Sociological Eye*. New Brunswick: Transaction Books.

Jameton, A. (1984). *Nursing Practice: The Ethical Issues*. Upper Saddle River, NJ: Prentice Hall.

Jameton, A. (2013). A reflection on moral distress in nursing together with a current application of the concept. *Bioethical Inquiry, 10*, 297–308.

Johnstone, M.-J., & Hutchinson, A. (2015). "Moral distress": Time to abandon a flawed nursing construct? *Nursing Ethics, 22*(1), 5–14.

Kälvemark, S., Höglund, A. T., Hansson, M. G., Westerholm, P., & Arnetz, B. (2004). Living with conflicts – ethical dilemmas and moral distress in the health care system. *Social Science and Medicine, 58*, 1075–1084.

Kopala, B., & Burkhart, L. (2005). Ethical dilemma and moral distress: Proposed new NANDA diagnoses. *International Journal of Nursing Terminologies and Classifications, 16*, 3–13.

Liaschenko, J. (1995). Artificial personhood: Nursing ethics in a medical world. *Nursing Ethics, 2*(3), 185–196.

Lützén, K., Cronqvist, A., Magnusson, A., & Andersson, L. (2003). Moral stress: synthesis of a concept. *Nursing Ethics, 10*(3), 312–322.

MacArthur, J., Wilkinson, H., Gray, M. A., & Matthews-Smith, G. (2017). Embedding compassionate care in local NHS practice: Developing a conceptual model through realistic evaluation. *Journal of Research in Nursing, 22*(1–2), 130–147.

McCarthy, J., & Deady, R. (2008). Moral distress reconsidered. *Nursing Ethics, 15*(2), 254–262.

McCarthy, J., & Gastmans, C. (2015). Moral distress: A review of the argument-based nursing ethics literature. *Nursing Ethics, 22*(1), 131–152.

Morley, G., Ives, J., Bradbury-Jones, C., & Irvine, F. (2019). What is 'moral distress'? A narrative synthesis of the literature. *Nursing Ethics, 26*(3), 646–662.

Nathaniel, A. (2006). Moral reckoning in nursing. *Western Journal of Nursing Research, 28*, 419–438.

Paley, J. (2009). Narrative machinery. In Y. Gunaratnam & D. Oliviere (Eds.), *Narrative and Stories in Health Care: Illness, Dying, and Bereavement* (pp. 17–32). Oxford: Oxford University Press.

Paley, J. (2014). Cognition and the compassion deciffit: The social psychology of helping behaviour in nursing. *Nursing Philosophy, 15*(4), 274–287.

Paley, J., & Eva, G. (2005). Narrative vigilance: the analysis of stories in health care. *Nursing Philosophy, 6*(2), 83–97.

Pauly, B. M., Varcoe, C., & Storch, J. (2012). Framing the issues: moral distress in health care. *HEC Forum, 24*(1), 1–11.

Peter, E., & Liaschenko, J. (2004). Perils of proximity: a spatiotemporal analysis of moral distress and moral ambiguity. *Nursing Inquiry, 11*(4), 219–225.

Peter, E., & Liaschenko, J. (2013). Moral distress reexamined: a feminist interpretation of nurses' identities, relationships, and responsibilities. *Bioethical Inquiry, 10*, 337–345.

Schiappa, E. (2003). *Defining Reality: Definitions and the Politics of Meaning.* 3rd ed. Carbondale, IL: Southern Illinois University Press.

Stoppard, T. (1973). *Rosencrantz and Guildenstern Are Dead.* London: Faber & Faber.

Usborne, S. (2018). How the hostile environment crept into UK schools, hospitals and homes. *The Guardian,* 1st August 2018. https://www.theguardian.com/uk-news/2018/aug/2001/hostile-environment-immigrants-crept-into-schools-hospitals-homes-border-guards.

Varcoe, C., Pauly, B., Webster, G. C., & Storch, J. (2012). Moral distress: tensions as springboards for action. *HEC Forum, 24*(1), 51–52.

Velleman, J. D. (2003). Narrative explanation. *The Philosophical Review, 112*(1), 1–25.

Webster, G. C., & Bayliss, F. (2000). Moral residue. In S. B. Rubin & L. Zoloth (Eds.), *Margin of Error: The Ethics of Mistakes in the Practice of Medicine* (pp. 217–230). Hagerstown, MD: University Publishing.

Wierzbicka, A. (1984). "Apples" are not a "kind of fruit": The semantics of human categorization. *American Ethnologist, 11*(2), 313–328.

Wilkinson, J. M. (1987). Moral distress in nursing practice: experience and effect. *Nursing Forum, 23*, 16–29.

Wittgenstein, L. (1963). *Philosophical Investigations.* Oxford: Basil Blackwell.

Index

Printed in the United States
By Bookmasters